PCEP

Perinatal Continuing Education Program

Maternal and Fetal Care

BOOK II

American Academy of Pediatrics

DEDICATED TO THE HEALTH OF ALL CHILDREN™

The original version of these self-instructional books was developed in 1978 at the University of Virginia under contract (#N09-HR-2926) from the National Heart, Lung, and Blood Institute. Subsequent versions have been developed independently by the authors and, for the current edition, an editorial board.

PCEP Original Authors
John Kattwinkel, MD
Lynn J. Cook, RNC, MPH
Hallam Hurt, MD
George A. Nowacek, PhD
Jerry G. Short, PhD

Primary authors for the original obstetrical content
Warren M. Crosby, MD
Lynn J. Cook, RNC, MPH

Several different approaches to specific perinatal problems may be acceptable. The PCEP books have been written to present specific recommendations rather than to include all currently acceptable options. The recommendations in these books should not be considered the only accepted standard of care. We encourage development of local standards in consultation with your regional perinatal center staff.

Library of Congress Control Number: 2012937490

ISBN: 978-1-58110-658-9

The PCEP books are one part of a larger perinatal program. Information about the books, and the educational program, may be obtained by visiting the PCEP Web site at www.pcep.org and by obtaining the *PCEP Implementation Manual* CD, available through www.aap.org/bookstore. Information about obtaining CME and CEU credit (up to 54 hours) for book study may be obtained by visiting www.cmevillage.com.

Brand names are furnished for identification purposes only. No endorsement of the manufacturers or products mentioned is implied.

Every effort has been made to ensure that the drug selection and dosage set forth in this text are in accordance with the current recommendations and practice at the time of publication. It is the responsibility of the health care provider to check the package insert of each drug for any change in indications and dosage and for added warnings and precautions.

The publishers have made every effort to trace the copyright holders for borrowed material. If they have inadvertently overlooked any, they will be pleased to make the necessary arrangements at the first opportunity.

Printed in the United States of America

PC0010
5-263/0512

1 2 3 4 5 6 7 8 9 10

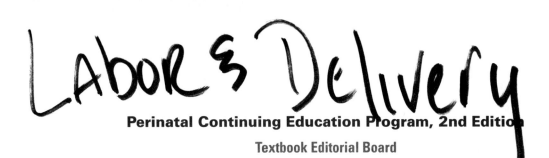

Labor & Delivery

Perinatal Continuing Education Program, 2nd Edition

Textbook Editorial Board

Editor

John Kattwinkel, MD, FAAP
Charles Fuller Professor of Neonatology
Department of Pediatrics
University of Virginia
Charlottesville, VA

Associate Editor, Obstetrics

Christian A. Chisholm, MD
Associate Professor of Obstetrics and Gynecology
University of Virginia School of Medicine
Charlottesville, VA

PCEP Textbook Editorial Board Members

Robert J. Boyle, MD, FAAP
Professor of Pediatrics
University of Virginia School of Medicine
Charlottesville, VA

Susan B. Clarke, MS, RNC-NIC, CPN
Clinical Nurse Specialist, Continuing Education
  and Outreach
Professional Development Department
Children's Hospital Colorado
Aurora, CO

Brenda P. Daugherty, MSN, NNP-BC
NNP Manager
West Virginia University Department
  of Pediatrics
Morgantown, WV

Victoria Flanagan RN, MS
Perinatal Outreach Educator
Regional Program for Women's and Children's
  Health
Dartmouth-Hitchcock Medical Center
Lebanon, NH

Martha D. Mullett, MD, MPH
Professor of Pediatrics
West Virginia University
Morgantown, WV

Susan Niermeyer, MD, MPH, FAAP
Professor of Pediatrics
University of Colorado School of Medicine
Section of Neonatology
Aurora, CO

Barbara O'Brien, RN, MS
Program Director
Office of Perinatal Quality Improvement
The University of Oklahoma Health
  Sciences Center
Department of OB/GYN
Oklahoma City, OK

E. Rebecca Pschirrer, MD, MPH
Department of Obstetrics & Gynecology
Dartmouth-Hitchcock Medical Center
Lebanon, NH

Roger E. Sheldon, MD, MPH, FAAP
Emeritus Professor of Pediatrics
College of Medicine
University of Oklahoma
Oklahoma City, OK

Gautham K. Suresh, MD, FAAP
Neonatology
Dartmouth-Hitchcock Medical Center
Lebanon, NH

Sarah M. Wilson, RN, BSN
Neonatal Intensive Care Unit
University of Virginia
Charlottesville, VA

PCEP Implementation Manual CD

Lynn J. Cook, RNC, MPH, Editor
Landenberg, PA

George A. Nowacek, PhD, Layout and Evaluation
Charlottesville, VA

Continuing Education Credit

Continuing education credit is available for every perinatal health care provider who studies the Perinatal Continuing Education Program (PCEP) books. The American Medical Association's *AMA PRA Category 1 Credit(s)™* or contact hours/continuing education units (CEUs) are available to physicians, nurses, nurse practitioners, nurse midwives, respiratory therapists, and any other professional who provides care to pregnant women or newborn babies.

Accreditation and Designation Statements

The University of Virginia School of Medicine is accredited by the Accreditation Council for Continuing Medical Education (ACCME) to provide continuing education for physicians.

The University of Virginia School of Medicine designates this enduring material for a maximum of 54 *AMA PRA Category 1 Credit(s)™*. Physicians should claim only the credit commensurate with the extent of their participation in the activity.

The University of Virginia School of Medicine awards 0.1 CEU per contact hour to each nonphysician participant who successfully completes this educational activity. The CEU is a nationally recognized unit of measure for continuing education and training activities that meet specific educational planning requirements. The University of Virginia School of Medicine maintains a permanent record of participants who have been awarded CEUs.

Disclosure of Financial Relationships

All the authors and editorial board members listed on the previous pages have disclosed that they have no relevant financial relationships with any commercial interest.

AMA PRA Category 1 Credit(s)™ or Contact Hour Credit

Credit is given only for complete books, not individual educational units. Possible hours: Book I, 14.5; Book II, 15.5; Book III, 16.5; Book IV, 7.5.

To register for education credits, visit www.cmevillage.com.

BOOK II

Maternal and Fetal Care

For more information, see the other books in the PCEP series.

Book I: Maternal and Fetal Evaluation and Immediate Newborn Care

Book III: Neonatal Care

Book IV: Specialized Newborn Care

Unit 1: Hypertension in Pregnancy

Objectives

In this unit you will learn

A. What risks hypertension poses to the pregnant woman and to the fetus

B. How to identify chronic hypertension and pregnancy-related hypertension and how to define the various types of hypertension during pregnancy

C. How to manage chronic hypertension during pregnancy and which fetal surveillance measures to use

D. How to manage pregnancy-related hypertension and which fetal surveillance measures to use

E. When to seek help with the care of a woman with hypertension

F. How to stabilize a woman who has worsening preeclampsia or eclampsia

G. Which anticonvulsant and antihypertensive drugs to use and how to administer them, and which antihypertensive drugs to avoid

H. How to manage chronic hypertension during labor and delivery, and what to anticipate for the care of the baby

I. How to manage the various forms of pregnancy-related hypertension during labor and delivery, and what to anticipate for the care of the baby

J. How to manage hypertension during the postpartum period

Unit 1 Pretest

Before reading the unit, please answer the following questions. Select the *one* **best** answer to each question (unless otherwise instructed). Record your answers on the test and check them against the answers at the end of the book.

1. A woman with chronic hypertension is at increased risk during pregnancy for all the following, *except*
   A. Post-term pregnancy
   B. Growth-restricted baby
   C. Compromised renal function
   D. Preeclampsia

2. **True** **False** A blood pressure of 160/110 mm Hg in a pregnant woman with proteinuria and persistent headache represents severe preeclampsia.

3. **True** **False** Magnesium sulfate is used for the acute reduction of blood pressure in women with severe preeclampsia.

4. **True** **False** If gestational hypertension occurred in one pregnancy, there is an increased risk of it occurring in subsequent pregnancies.

5. **True** **False** Slowing of fetal growth rate may occur before preeclampsia is evident.

6. **True** **False** In cases of severe preeclampsia, early delivery for the health of the pregnant woman and/or the baby may be necessary.

7. **True** **False** Women with hypertension during pregnancy are at increased risk for placenta previa.

8. **True** **False** When thrombocytopenia is present, epidural anesthesia is the preferred method of pain relief during labor.

9. All of the following are possible maternal complications of hypertension during pregnancy, *except*
   A. Intracranial hemorrhage
   B. Renal failure
   C. Pulmonary edema
   D. Diabetes mellitus

10. Which of the following should be done *first* if a woman with preeclampsia has a seizure?
   A. Give an intravenous bolus of magnesium sulfate.
   B. Give intravenous glucose.
   C. Page anesthesia personnel so a cesarean section can start immediately.
   D. Give intravenous diazepam.

11. Which of the following is *most* likely to be present at birth in a newborn whose mother received large amounts of magnesium sulfate?
   A. Low blood sodium
   B. High blood pressure
   C. Poor urine output
   D. Poor respiratory effort

3

12. Which of the following is *least* likely to be present in a woman with HELLP syndrome?
A. Elevated liver transaminases
B. Elevated serum bilirubin
C. Hydramnios
D. Thrombocytopenia (low platelet count)

13. In women with severe preeclampsia, lowering blood pressure below 140/90 mm Hg should be avoided because blood pressure below that level is likely to result in
A. Increased maternal cardiac output
B. Decreased placental perfusion
C. Venous stasis and thrombosis formation
D. Inadequate blood flow to the lungs

14. Which of the following should a woman with hypertension report immediately to her health care provider?

Yes	No	
____	____	Urine positive for protein
____	____	Weight gain of 1 lb/week
____	____	Persistent headache
____	____	Right upper abdominal pain
____	____	Blurred vision
____	____	Uterine contractions

15. Which of the following are appropriate measures for a woman with *un*complicated chronic hypertension?

Yes	No	
____	____	Use serial ultrasound examinations to assess fetal growth.
____	____	Check liver transaminases monthly, starting at 28 weeks' gestation.
____	____	Check creatinine clearance and blood urea nitrogen monthly, starting at 28 weeks' gestation.
____	____	Use narcotic analgesia liberally during labor.
____	____	Consult with maternal-fetal medicine specialist if preeclampsia develops.
____	____	Plan for cesarean delivery.

16. Which of the following are appropriate postpartum care measures for a woman who had severe preeclampsia?

Yes	No	
____	____	Provide invasive cardiac output monitoring for 1 to 2 days.
____	____	Continue magnesium sulfate infusion for 12 to 48 hours.
____	____	Arrange for home blood pressure monitoring for 1 to 2 weeks.
____	____	Continue hospitalization and bed rest for 1 to 2 weeks.

1. What Are the Risks of Peripartum Hypertension?

High blood pressure during pregnancy may be due to

- Chronic hypertension that was present before pregnancy
- A rise in blood pressure that occurs only with pregnancy (pregnancy-related hypertension)
- A combination of both conditions

Regardless of the cause, hypertension during pregnancy poses a potentially serious threat to the health of a pregnant woman and her fetus. In the United States and worldwide, hypertension is a major cause of maternal mortality and morbidity, and adversely affects fetal and neonatal health too.

High blood pressure increases the risk for each of the following complications:

A. Maternal Risks
   - Intracranial hemorrhage
   - Stroke
   - Seizures
   - Congestive heart failure
   - Pulmonary edema
   - Renal failure
   - Liver failure
   - Abruptio placentae
   - Death

B. Fetal/Neonatal Risks
   - Impaired placental blood flow and function
   - Intrauterine growth restriction
   - Oligohydramnios
   - Non-reassuring antepartum tests of fetal well-being
   - Preterm birth induced due to declining maternal and/or fetal health
   - Perinatal death

2. What Are the Types of Peripartum Hypertension?

Much of prenatal care is devoted to identifying hypertension and treating it before it threatens the health of a woman or fetus. It is important to distinguish pregnancy-related hypertension from other causes of hypertension because treatment is different.

A. Chronic Hypertension
   Women with chronic hypertension may be identified in 2 ways.

   1. History of chronic hypertension before pregnancy, whether or not the hypertension was treated

   2. Persistent elevation of blood pressure to 140/90 mm Hg or higher *before* 20 weeks' gestation or *after* 12 weeks' postpartum

      Chronic hypertension may occur by itself or may be a complication of another disease, such as renal dysfunction, cardiac disease, or thyroid disorders. Women with chronic hypertension, regardless of the cause, are at increased risk for developing superimposed preeclampsia.

B. Pregnancy-Related Hypertension
   The cause of pregnancy-related hypertension is unknown. It occurs *only* during pregnancy, with the onset of blood pressure elevation first noted *after* 20 weeks' gestation.

5

Several types of hypertension can develop during pregnancy, with escalating severity and risk to the woman and the fetus. These types include gestational hypertension; preeclampsia; severe preeclampsia; eclampsia; and hemolysis, elevated liver enzymes, and low platelets (HELLP) syndrome. Progression through these conditions is usually slow and may not go beyond mild preeclampsia. Occasionally, a woman's condition may worsen, however, within days or even hours to severe preeclampsia or eclampsia.

Pregnancy-related hypertension generally resolves within a few days after delivery, but may take as long as 12 weeks for complete resolution. Infrequently, symptoms worsen after delivery. In rare cases, pregnancy-related hypertension may not become evident until as late as 10 days postpartum. Table 1.1 summarizes the clinical and laboratory characteristics.

 Prompt detection and unrelenting surveillance of pregnancy-related hypertension is important to reducing perinatal mortality and morbidity from this disease.

1. *Gestational Hypertension* is defined as
   - Blood pressure of 140/90 mm Hg, after 20 weeks' gestation in a woman who had normal blood pressure before 20 weeks' gestation
   - No proteinuria

   The term is used only during pregnancy. After delivery and the postpartum period, a specific diagnosis can be made.
   - Additional signs and symptoms may develop during pregnancy, identifying the condition as preeclampsia, eclampsia, or HELLP syndrome.

   OR
   - Preeclampsia does not develop, and blood pressure returns to normal by 12 weeks' postpartum, allowing identification of the condition as *transient* gestational hypertension.

   OR
   - Blood pressure remains elevated postpartum and the diagnosis of chronic hypertension is confirmed.

2. *Mild Preeclampsia* is defined as
   - Blood pressure of 140 to 159 mm Hg systolic and/or 90 to 109 mm Hg diastolic

   PLUS
   - Proteinuria 1+ or greater (≥0.3 g protein in a 24-hour urine specimen)

3. *Severe Preeclampsia* includes the changes that define preeclampsia, plus one or more of the following:
   - Blood pressure of 160/110 mm Hg on 2 occasions at least 6 hours apart with the woman at bed rest
   - Proteinuria 2+ or 3+ on 2 random urine samples collected at least 4 hours apart (≥5 g protein in a 24-hour urine specimen)
   - Cerebral disturbances (persistent headache in particular)
   - Visual disturbances (blurred vision, scotomata ["spots before the eyes"—*not* what is commonly called "floaters" but rather dark spots and/or color changes in a woman's visual field])
   - Epigastric or right upper quadrant pain
   - Thrombocytopenia
   - Pulmonary edema or cyanosis (rare)

Table 1.1. Hypertension in Pregnancy: Types and Characteristic Findings*					
Signs and Symptoms	**Gestational Hypertension**	**Mild Preeclampsia**	**Severe Preeclampsia**	**Eclampsia**	**HELLP Syndrome**
			Findings of pre-eclampsia, plus one or more of the following:		
Maternal Factors					
Blood pressure	**140/90 mm Hg**† (in woman normotensive before 20 weeks)	**140-159 mm Hg systolic and/or 90-109 mm Hg diastolic**†	160/110 mm Hg (or higher)	Usually elevated, but may not be	Usually elevated, but often not
Proteinuria occurring first in pregnancy and regressing postpartum	**None**† (<0.3 g/24 hours)	**1+ or greater**† (≥0.3 g/24 hours)	2+ (≥5 g/24 hours)	**3+ or greater**	Usually present
Neurologic changes	None	None	Cerebral disturbances (especially headache), visual disturbances (especially blurred vision, scotomata), clonus, and/or hyperreflexia	**Seizure(s) and/or coma**†‡	May be present
Urine output	Normal	Normal	May be decreased	Usually decreased	Usually decreased
			(decreased = <500 mL/24 hours)		
Creatinine clearance	Normal	Normal	Decreased	Decreased	Variable
			(decreased = serum creatinine >1.2 mg/dL)		
Serum uric acid	Normal	Increased	Increased	Increased	Variable
Epigastric or right upper quadrant abdominal pain	None	None	May be present	May be present	Persistent pain
Liver function	Normal	Normal	AST and ALT may be elevated	AST and ALT elevated	AST, ALT, and bilirubin elevated
Pulmonary edema or cyanosis	None	None	May be present	May be present	May be present
Platelets	Normal	Normal	<variable	<variable	<100,000/mm³
Fetal Factors					
Fetal growth	May be restricted	May be restricted	May be restricted	May be restricted	May be restricted

*AST, aspartate aminotransferase; ALT, alanine aminotransferase.
†Defining characteristics of condition shown in bold.
‡The occurrence of a seizure or the onset of coma differentiates eclampsia from preeclampsia.

- Oliguria: urine output less than 500 mL in 24 hours
- Serum creatinine greater than 1.2 mg/dL
- Elevated liver enzymes
- Fetal growth restriction

Note: Only *one* of these findings needs to be present for the diagnosis of severe pre-eclampsia to be made.

4. *Eclampsia* is defined by the occurrence of a grand mal seizure and/or onset of coma, with no other known cause, in a woman with preeclampsia.

5. *HELLP Syndrome* is a form of severe preeclampsia that can be difficult to identify. While it most commonly occurs in the setting of other symptoms of severe preeclampsia, the woman may not develop hypertension or proteinuria until after she has other symptoms. Initial signs and symptoms of HELLP syndrome can mimic those of gastroenteritis or gall bladder disease and typically include

- Nausea
- Vomiting
- Abdominal pain

Mild jaundice is often detectable. Examine the woman carefully and obtain liver function tests if nausea, vomiting, abdominal pain, and/or jaundice are found.

Abnormalities of liver function usually include mildly elevated

- Aspartate aminotransferase (AST) and alanine aminotransferase (ALT) (liver transaminases)
- Serum bilirubin

Blood studies typically reveal

- Platelet count below 100,000/mm^3
- Hemolysis (elevated lactate dehydrogenase and haptoglobin; abnormal blood smear)

C. ,Preeclampsia Superimposed on Chronic Hypertension

The onset of preeclampsia in a woman with chronic hypertension dramatically increases the risk of serious complications for the woman and her fetus.

The condition is diagnosed by

- New-onset proteinuria ($\geq$0.3 g in 24-hour urine specimen) in a woman with hypertension present before 20 weeks' gestation and no prior evidence of proteinuria
- Sudden increase in proteinuria if it is already present
- Sudden increase in hypertension in a woman whose hypertension has been well-controlled
- Thrombocytopenia (platelets <100,000/mm^3)
- Increase in ALT or AST to abnormal levels

Development of persistent headache, scotomata, or epigastric pain also may indicate superimposed preeclampsia in a woman with chronic hypertension.

Self-test

Now answer these questions to test yourself on the information in the last section.

A1. What blood pressure changes define gestational hypertension?
_____

A2. What is the difference between gestational hypertension and preeclampsia?
_____

A3. What is the difference between preeclampsia and eclampsia?
_____

A4. Which of the following are typical findings in HELLP syndrome?

Yes	No	
____	____	Nausea and vomiting
____	____	Jaundice
____	____	Elevated blood glucose
____	____	Elevated platelet count
____	____	Elevated liver transaminases

A5. **True** **False** The diagnosis of preeclampsia is made when a pregnant woman develops a blood pressure of 140/90 mm Hg or higher and proteinuria.

A6. **True** **False** Initially, blood pressure is markedly elevated in women who develop HELLP syndrome.

A7. **True** **False** During pregnancy, a woman with hypertension, whether preexisting chronic hypertension or pregnancy-related hypertension, is at higher risk for complications than a woman with normal blood pressure.

A8. Which of the following risks are increased when maternal hypertension is present?

Yes	No	
____	____	Preterm birth
____	____	Abruptio placentae
____	____	Maternal congestive heart failure
____	____	Placenta previa
____	____	Intrauterine growth restriction
____	____	Non-reassuring tests of fetal well-being
____	____	Congenital anomalies
____	____	Maternal seizures
____	____	Maternal stroke

Check your answers with the list that follows the Recommended Routines. Correct any incorrect answers and review the appropriate section in the unit.

3. How Is Chronic Hypertension Managed During Pregnancy?

Women with *un*complicated hypertension generally tolerate pregnancy well. Preconception control of blood pressure is important to optimal outcome.

Due to the decrease in vascular resistance that normally occurs in pregnancy, many women with chronic hypertension have a fall in blood pressure during the second trimester. This may influence whether antihypertensive medication is needed. Occasionally, however, women with uncomplicated chronic hypertension develop hypertensive crisis, which may seriously jeopardize maternal and/or fetal health.

Management largely depends on whether complications of chronic hypertension, such as impaired renal function, and/or other medical diseases are present. If complications are present, or develop during pregnancy, the threat to maternal and/or fetal health is significantly increased. Management can be extremely complicated.

A. Initial Evaluation
 1. *At First Prenatal Visit, Look for Factors That May Be Associated With or Further Complicate Chronic Hypertension*
   - Previous pregnancy with perinatal loss
   - Elevation in blood pressure above the woman's usual (nonpregnant) level
   - Other illnesses that have vascular components (lupus erythematosus, diabetes mellitus, chronic renal disease, etc)
   - Assess maternal renal function
     - Creatinine clearance
     - Total protein excretion
     - Urinalysis
     - Blood urea nitrogen (BUN)
   - Perform physical examination, including
     - Retinoscopy (assess for hypertensive changes)
     - Echocardiogram or electrocardiogram (rule out cardiomyopathy)

 2. *Serious Complications and/or Superimposed Preeclampsia* are more likely to develop if any of the following are found:
   - Unstable blood pressure that cannot be controlled to stay below 150 to 160 mm Hg systolic or 100 to 110 mm Hg diastolic
   - Presence of other vascular diseases (diabetes mellitus, lupus erythematosus, renal disease, etc)
   - Creatinine clearance below 100 mL/minute
   - Persistent proteinuria
   - Abnormal urinalysis (in particular, casts and renal cells)
   - Elevated BUN
   - Retinopathy
   - Cardiomyopathy

    Women with complicated hypertension can become seriously, sometimes suddenly, ill during pregnancy. If complications are present or if superimposed preeclampsia develops, referral of the patient to maternal-fetal medicine specialists for prenatal care and delivery is strongly recommended.

B. Prenatal Management
For women with uncomplicated chronic hypertension, assess maternal and fetal health frequently. If complications develop, it is essential to detect them early.

 1. *Instruct the Woman*
   - On how to obtain home blood pressure measurements
   - To record blood pressure frequently, preferably at least once per day
   - To report any change in blood pressure

2. *Provide Antihypertensive Medication, as Needed:* As long as blood pressure remains below 150/100 mm Hg, antihypertensive medication likely provides no added benefit.

   a. *Women NOT being treated with antihypertensive medication before pregnancy*
- Blood pressure may decline to normal levels and stay there throughout pregnancy.
- Even for these women, the risk of developing preeclampsia and/or fetal growth restriction is increased.

   b. *Women being treated with antihypertensive medication before pregnancy*
- Because of the normal fall in blood pressure, antihypertensive medication may not be needed during pregnancy.
- If blood pressure reaches and persists at 150 to 160/100 to 110 mm Hg, or if end-organ disease is present, administration of antihypertensive medication is recommended. Some common antihypertensive drugs should be *avoided* during pregnancy. (See Table 1.2.)
- Diuretic therapy is generally avoided in pregnant women. Diuretics can potentiate the antihypertensive effects of other medications, but the associated plasma volume reduction may have seriously adverse effects on the fetus, especially when placental perfusion is already reduced, as it may be in maternal hypertension. Consultation with regional center specialists is strongly recommended.

3. *Schedule Frequent Prenatal Visits,* every 2 weeks until approximately 28 weeks, then every week until delivery.

4. *Periodically Reassess Maternal Urine Protein Excretion* at least monthly.

5. *Assess Fetal Growth and Well-being*
- Ultrasound measurements of fetal growth at 18 to 20 weeks and 28 to 32 weeks. Additional ultrasounds may be performed at monthly intervals until delivery, as clinically indicated by fundal height measurements, maternal blood pressure trends, and prior sonographic assessment of fetal growth.
- Daily fetal activity determinations, from approximately 28 weeks until delivery.
- Test of fetal well-being (eg, nonstress test [NST] and/or biophysical profile [BPP]) beginning at a gestational age and at a testing interval determined by baseline maternal health status, blood pressure trend during pregnancy, and evidence or lack thereof of fetal growth restriction or oligohydramnios.

6. *Allow the Onset of Spontaneous Labor, unless* decline in maternal and/or fetal health dictates earlier intervention.

7. *Consider Induction* if spontaneous onset of labor has not occurred before 41 weeks' gestation.

 If a woman with chronic hypertension develops increased blood pressure and proteinuria, and/or declining creatinine clearance, hospitalization may be necessary. Consult with regional center maternal-fetal medicine specialists.

Table 1.2. Antihypertensive Medication During Pregnancy		
A. Drugs for Ongoing Control of *Chronic* Hypertension During Pregnancy		
Medication	**Administration**	**Comments and Cautions**
Methyldopa	*Total daily dose:* 750-2,000 mg *Given:* 250-500 mg *Schedule:* 2-4 times/day *Route:* oral	Often considered a first-line medication for the management of chronic hypertension during pregnancy.
Labetalol HCl	*Total daily dose:* 200-2,400 mg/day *Dose:* starting: 100 mg usual: 200-400 mg *Schedule:* 2-3 times/day *Route:* oral	May have misleading effect on fetal heart rate (may cause mild bradycardia and/or fetus may not be able to mount a tachycardic response to stress). May be associated with fetal growth restriction.
B. Antihypertensive Drugs That Should Be *Avoided* During Pregnancy		
Medication	**Comments and Cautions**	
Angiotensin-converting enzyme inhibitors (captopril, etc) and angiotensin receptor blockers (losartan, etc)	1. Associated with birth defects and impaired fetal renal function. 2. Not recommended for use, even short-term use, during pregnancy.	
Nitroprusside (used only for hypertensive emergency)	1. May cause fetal toxicity as drug metabolizes into cyanide. 2. Maternal hypotension and poor placental perfusion are likely because drug effects are rapid and pronounced. 3. If used during pregnancy for hypertensive crisis, administration for <24 hours is recommended.	
Atenolol	1. Associated with fetal growth restriction. 2. Avoid use in early pregnancy; use with caution in late pregnancy.	

C. Intrapartum Management
1. *Provide Pain Control* by means of
   - Narcotic analgesia
   - Epidural anesthesia (except when thrombocytopenia is present)
2. *During Labor, Further Elevation in Blood Pressure May Occur* due to normal hemodynamic changes, maternal fear, pain, and/or superimposed preeclampsia. Because it may not be possible to determine the cause of an increase in blood pressure, all women who develop blood pressure elevation and proteinuria during labor should be treated as if they have superimposed preeclampsia.
3. *Placental Function May Be Impaired.* Anticipate possible need for emergency cesarean delivery and/or neonatal resuscitation.
4. *Be Aware That the Risk of Abruptio Placentae Is Increased.*

D. Postdelivery Management

1. *Maternal*
   - Methylergonovine has a tendency to cause vasospasm and increase blood pressure. Therefore, administration of this drug for the management of postpartum hemorrhage is *contraindicated* in women with symptomatic heart disease or hypertension.
   - Women with chronic hypertension can develop encephalopathy, pulmonary edema, and heart and/or renal failure postpartum, depending on the complications that were experienced during pregnancy. Close blood pressure and laboratory monitoring should continue until the findings are stable.

2. *Neonatal*
   - If resuscitation is needed, monitor for possible post-resuscitation complications. (See Book I: Maternal and Fetal Evaluation and Immediate Newborn Care, Unit 5, Resuscitating the Newborn.)
   - Screen for hypoglycemia. (See Book I: Maternal and Fetal Evaluation and Immediate Newborn Care, Unit 8, Hypoglycemia.)
   - Blood tests, as indicated.
     – Hydrochlorothiazide given to the mother may cause a transient decrease in platelets in the newborn as well as fetal hemoconcentration.
     – Women with hypertension that develops during pregnancy, particularly those with HELLP syndrome, frequently have babies with thrombocytopenia and neutropenia.

Self-test

Now answer these questions to test yourself on the information in the last section.

B1. True   False   Angiotensin-converting enzyme inhibitor antihypertensive medications are the drugs of choice for treatment of chronic hypertension during pregnancy.

B2. True   False   Women with uncomplicated chronic hypertension usually tolerate pregnancy well.

B3. True   False   In women with chronic hypertension, blood pressure rarely declines during pregnancy.

B4. True   False   Women requiring antihypertensive medication before pregnancy will always need such medication during pregnancy.

B5. Which of the following factors increase the risk associated with chronic hypertension during pregnancy?

Yes	No	
____	____	Walking 2 miles a day
____	____	Multiple sclerosis
____	____	Creatinine clearance below 100 mL/minute
____	____	Diabetes mellitus
____	____	Development of gestational hypertension
____	____	Lupus erythematosus

B6. Which of the following are appropriate measures for a pregnant woman with *un*complicated chronic hypertension?

Yes	No	
____	____	Allow spontaneous onset of labor if it occurs before 41 weeks.
____	____	Use narcotic analgesia liberally during labor.
____	____	Treat for preeclampsia if blood pressure increases and proteinuria develops.
____	____	Plan for cesarean delivery.

Check your answers with the list that follows the Recommended Routines. Correct any incorrect answers and review the appropriate section in the unit.

4. Are Some Women at Increased Risk for Development of Hypertension During Pregnancy?

Yes. Women with any of the following factors are more likely to develop hypertension during pregnancy:

- Pregnancy-related hypertension in a previous pregnancy
- Multifetal gestation
- Chronic hypertension
- Renal disease or medical illnesses that affect vascular and connective tissue, such as diabetes mellitus, lupus erythematosus, etc
- Obesity
- Antiphospholipid antibody syndrome
- Age 35 years or older
- Primigravida
- African American heritage
- Family history of preeclampsia
- Hydatidiform mole and fetal hydrops are associated with hypertension onset before 20 weeks

While some women are at increased risk for pregnancy-related hypertension, the illness can occur in any woman. All women should be monitored for possible onset of hypertension.

5. What Are the Management Guidelines for Gestational Hypertension?

Gestational hypertension (hypertension of 140/90 mm Hg, without proteinuria) by itself does not require treatment. Close monitoring is needed, however, because there is an increased risk that a woman with gestational hypertension will develop preeclampsia.

  A. Home Care

    Carefully review the implications of the following care measures, determine if each can realistically be carried out in the home (eg, does the woman have a scale to weigh herself?), modify the regimen, and/or make arrangements for care to be provided as needed.

- Frequent blood pressure measurement
- Daily dipstick testing of urine for protein
- Daily weight
- Daily fetal activity determinations
- Instructions for the woman to report promptly *any* of the following:
  - Increase in blood pressure
  - Protein in her urine
  - Persistent headache
  - Abdominal pain
  - Blurred vision, "spots before the eyes," etc
  - Weight gain of more than 2 lbs in 1 day
  - Decrease in fetal movement
  - Uterine contractions

B. Prenatal Care

The goal is to detect preeclampsia, if it develops, as early as possible.

- Provide prenatal visits once to twice a week (office, clinic, or patient's home), in addition to the monitoring measures being done daily in the home.
- Obtain baseline laboratory tests at the time of diagnosis of gestational hypertension, including hematocrit, hemoglobin, platelet count, and serum creatinine. Comparison to test results obtained later will help establish an early diagnosis of preeclampsia, if it develops.
- Develop a plan for antenatal testing for fetal well-being.
- Use serial ultrasound examinations to evaluate fetal growth. While assessment of fetal growth is important in itself, it also may allow early detection of maternal illness. Slowing of the normal rate of fetal growth sometimes occurs several weeks before preeclampsia becomes clinically evident.
- Plan for spontaneous onset of labor. If gestation goes beyond 40 weeks, however, consider induction of labor.
- If preeclampsia develops, hospitalize the patient. Consultation with regional center maternal-fetal medicine specialists is strongly recommended.

C. Intrapartum Care

Provide routine labor care. Women with gestational hypertension often develop preeclampsia during labor. Monitor closely for

- Rise in blood pressure
- Onset of proteinuria
- Decrease in urine output

6. What Are the Prenatal Management Guidelines for Preeclampsia and Eclampsia?

A. Mild Preeclampsia (blood pressure of 140 to 159 mm Hg systolic and/or 90 to 109 mm Hg diastolic with proteinuria)

When hypertension is present, the onset of proteinuria often precedes a sudden worsening of the disease. The earlier in pregnancy preeclampsia occurs, the less likely any treatment will be successful. As soon as evidence of preeclampsia is detected, evaluation *in a hospital* is needed for adequate assessment of maternal condition.

 Preeclampsia is a serious illness that requires hospitalization and treatment. Multiple organ systems may be affected.

Rise in blood pressure is not the only important finding. Some women will be seriously ill but have minimal blood pressure elevation.

1. *Institute Bed Rest and Evaluate/Monitor Condition for 4 to 8 Hours*
   a. *Check blood pressure at least every hour* to be sure it is not increasing rapidly
   b. *Physical examination* every 4 to 8 hours, including
      - Reflexes. (Check patellar or antecubital reflexes; if hyperreflexia [exaggerated reflexes] is present, check for clonus.)
      - Central nervous system involvement, including headache, visual disturbances, and/or disorientation.
      - Epigastric pain and right upper quadrant tenderness.

c. *Retinoscopy.* (Look for spasm of retinal vessels and blurring of disc margins.)

d. *Blood tests.*
- Complete blood count with platelet count
- Serum uric acid
- AST and ALT
- Serum creatinine

e. *Urine tests.*
- Urinalysis/urine culture (to rule out proteinuria due to urinary tract infection)
- Dipstick at least once every 4 hours
- Consider 12- to 24-hour urine collection for total protein and creatinine clearance
- Measure output

f. *Evaluate fetal well-being, growth, and amniotic fluid volume* when preeclampsia is first diagnosed. If results are normal, obtain NST and BPP twice weekly, and assess fetal size and amniotic fluid volume every 3 weeks.

2. *Respond to Patient Condition*: After several hours of hospitalized bed rest, with the woman lying on her side, her condition will either be

a. Improved: Fetal assessment is reassuring, and maternal blood pressure is stable or decreased.
- If fetus is mature and cervix is ripe, consider induction of labor.
- If fetus is immature or cervix is not ripe, consider return to outpatient management with close surveillance of maternal and fetal condition.

b. Unchanged: Consider outpatient management if the woman can be followed closely, or continue hospitalization if needed for adequate surveillance of patient condition. If the fetus is near term and has evidence of pulmonary maturity, consider delivery. If the fetus is small and/or immature, consult with maternal-fetal medicine specialists regarding further management.

 BEWARE: Mild preeclampsia can sometimes progress to eclampsia within a few hours.

c. *Worsened:* Blood pressure and proteinuria increase, or symptoms of severe preeclampsia develop. In many cases, the fetus will need to be delivered, regardless of fetal size or length of gestation. Even if symptoms decline, the underlying disease will not improve until after delivery. As the disease continues, the lives of the woman and her fetus are in jeopardy. Generally, it is advisable to proceed with delivery as soon as the woman's condition is stable.

B. Severe Preeclampsia (preeclampsia, plus one or more of the findings listed in Section 2 and in Table 1.1)

The risk of eclampsia, abruptio placentae, maternal intracranial hemorrhage, and fetal death is significantly increased with the onset of severe preeclampsia. Hospitalize the patient and stabilize her condition (see protocol below). Transfer of the woman to a regional center should be considered.

 Severe preeclampsia may necessitate delivery, regardless of fetal age, size, or maturity. Delivery may be necessary to preserve the health of the woman, the baby, or both.

C. Eclampsia (preeclampsia plus seizure[s] or development of coma)

If convulsions or coma develop, the risk of maternal and/or fetal death increases dramatically.

 Regardless of blood pressure or proteinuria, any woman pregnant beyond 20 weeks who has a seizure or becomes comatose should be assumed to have eclampsia and treated accordingly.

Self-test

Now answer these questions to test yourself on the information in the last section.

C1. List at least 3 signs and symptoms a woman with gestational hypertension should be taught to report promptly to her health care provider.

_____

_____

_____

C2. Which of the following conditions increase the likelihood a woman will develop pregnancy-related hypertension?

Yes	No	
____	____	Age 35 or older
____	____	Twins
____	____	Renal disease
____	____	Short stature
____	____	Obesity
____	____	First pregnancy
____	____	Chronic hypertension

C3. **True** **False** Women with preeclampsia should be evaluated in a hospital.

C4. **True** **False** Any pregnant woman can develop hypertension during pregnancy.

C5. **True** **False** If severe preeclampsia develops, maternal condition will not improve until the baby is delivered.

C6. **True** **False** Delivery may be necessary for a woman who develops severe preeclampsia or eclampsia, regardless of fetal gestational age.

Check your answers with the list that follows the Recommended Routines. Correct any incorrect answers and review the appropriate section in the unit.

7. How Do You

- **Manage the Labor of a Woman With Preeclampsia?**
- **Stabilize a Woman With Worsening Preeclampsia or Eclampsia?**

Although the situations outlined below are quite different, the treatment is almost identical.

- Woman *in labor* with apparently *stable preeclampsia*
- Woman *not in labor* but with *deteriorating condition*

For women with preeclampsia, even those in stable condition, labor is often associated with a worsening of their condition. For these women, therapy is generally instituted as soon as labor begins to prevent seizures.

Women with worsening preeclampsia or eclampsia need to be treated aggressively to prevent further deterioration of their condition, whether or not they are in labor.

A. Prevent Seizures From Occurring and/or From Recurring

1. *Give Magnesium Sulfate:* Patients with worsening preeclampsia often develop neurological irritability. However, hyperreflexia is not currently considered in the diagnosis of preeclampsia or as a marker for impending eclampsia.

   Magnesium sulfate is used to prevent and treat convulsions due to preeclampsia or eclampsia, but has little direct effect on blood pressure.

   Use an intravenous (IV) infusion of magnesium sulfate for women

   - In labor with stable preeclampsia
   - With worsening preeclampsia or eclampsia whether or not they are in labor
   - With preeclampsia who develop hyperreflexia or clonus

   Give loading dose of 4 to 6 g, given over 20 minutes, followed by continuous infusion of 1 to 3 g/hour (usually 2 g/hour is used). *Continue* administration of magnesium sulfate throughout labor and for 12 to 48 hours, or longer if necessary, following delivery.

   Note: *Myasthenia gravis, heart block, and recent myocardial infarction are absolute contraindications for the use of magnesium sulfate. Magnesium sulfate is especially hazardous for women with renal failure. The usual loading dose may be given, but maintenance doses should be reduced and may not be needed at all. Therapy should be guided by magnesium blood levels checked regularly.*

2. *Monitor Magnesium Levels:* Check serum magnesium levels 4 to 6 hours after therapy is started, and periodically thereafter depending on the woman's clinical status. Adjust dosage as necessary to maintain serum level between 4 and 8 mg/dL.

   Check vital signs and deep tendon reflexes (DTRs) every hour.

   - If DTRs diminish or disappear, stop the magnesium sulfate infusion and check serum magnesium levels.
   - In the rare event that respirations become depressed as a result of magnesium toxicity, stop the magnesium infusion, perform endotracheal intubation, and ventilate the woman. Then give calcium gluconate (1 g) by *slow* IV push.

   Monitor oxygen saturation. Repeat calcium gluconate as necessary until spontaneous respirations return.

   Signs of magnesium sulfate toxicity include loss of DTRs, depressed respiration, cardiac arrest, and visual symptoms. (Blurred vision, however, is more likely to be a symptom of worsening preeclampsia.)

Magnesium level in blood
- 10 mEq/L = 12 mg/dL: Associated with loss of DTRs
- 12 to 14 mEq/L = 14 to 18 mg/dL: Associated with respiratory depression
- Greater than 18 mEq/L = greater than 15 mg/dL: Associated with cardiac arrest

3. *If Magnesium Sulfate Fails:* Very rarely, a woman may continue with seizures in spite of a magnesium level in the therapeutic range (4 to 8 mg/dL). Under such circumstances, give diazepam (Valium), 5 to 10 mg, intravenously over 5 to 10 minutes. This anticonvulsant stops eclamptic seizures quickly, but IV administration may cause respiratory arrest. Be prepared with personnel and equipment (endotracheal tubes, laryngoscope, ventilation bag, etc) to intubate and provide assisted ventilation. Diazepam readily crosses the placenta and can depress the fetus, too, necessitating resuscitation and prolonged ventilatory support for some newborns.

4. *If Magnesium Sulfate and Diazepam Both Fail:* Sodium amytal or sodium thiopental may be given intravenously. It is advisable that this be done by practitioners skilled in the use of these drugs, such as an anesthesiologist or anesthetist.
Patients who fail anticonvulsant therapy may have intracranial bleeding as the *cause* of their seizures. Consultation with a regional center specialist(s) and/or a local neurologist is recommended.

B. Control Hypertension
Hypertension needs to be controlled in both of these situations to
- Prevent dangerous blood pressure elevation during labor in women with preeclampsia.
- Provide acute blood pressure reduction in women with worsening preeclampsia or eclampsia.

In either case, a blood pressure above 160/105 mm Hg needs to be lowered promptly, to the range of 140 to 150/90 to 100 mm Hg. This lower blood pressure reduces the risk of intracranial hemorrhage and stroke, but does not cure the preeclampsia/eclampsia. Pressure lowered too far, however, may compromise placental blood flow.

 Blood pressure should be lowered quickly, but not too far. Avoid bringing it below 140/90 mm Hg because, below this pressure, placental perfusion may decrease, leading to fetal distress.

Guidelines for the administration of medications (Table 1.3) for the acute reduction of blood pressure are

1. Check maternal blood pressure every 5 to 10 minutes (maximal effect usually occurs within 5 minutes of injection for both of the drugs listed).

2. Repeat dose every 10 to 30 minutes, until desired blood pressure (with woman resting on her side) is achieved.

3. Goal is stable blood pressure 140 to 150/90 to 100 mm Hg.

4. Assess woman for postural hypotension because it may occur with tachycardia, headaches, nausea, and/or difficulty sitting or standing.

Table 1.3. Antihypertensive Medication for *Acute Reduction* in Blood Pressure During Pregnancy*
During Labor for Women With Preeclampsia and/or to Stabilize Women With Worsening Preeclampsia or Eclampsia
Hydralazine HCl • 5-10 mg, given IV bolus over 2-5 minutes. • Repeat dose every 20-30 minutes until desired effect is achieved, then repeat as necessary. **Labetalol HCl** • Initially, 10 mg, given IV bolus over 2-5 minutes and repeated after 10-20 minutes if insufficient improvement in blood pressure. • If BP is not reduced appropriately in 10-20 minutes, increase does to 20 mg; may repeat as above. • If BP is not reduced appropriately in another 10-20 minutes, increase dose to 40 mg; may repeat as above. • If BP is not reduced appropriately in another 10-20 minutes, give the maximum single dose of 80 mg; may repeat as above. • Maximum recommended total dose is 300 mg/day. • Avoid use in women with asthma or congestive heart failure.

Note: See Table 1.2 for drugs that should be avoided.
*IV, intravenous; BP, blood pressure.

   C. Monitor Fetal Well-being and Maternal Health

      1. *Be Sure to Evaluate All Aspects of Maternal and Fetal Health* as you stabilize maternal condition in preparation for delivery. Other complications, related or unrelated to hypertension, can occur too (eg, maternal infection, cord prolapse, abruptio placentae, etc). While appropriate treatment of hypertension is critical to maternal and fetal health, be careful not to focus exclusively on it.

      2. *Record Fluid Intake and Output*, beginning at the time of hospital admission and continuing through 24 hours after delivery. Fluid balance is often altered with preeclampsia, particularly during labor and if oxytocin is administered. Fluid overload with pulmonary edema may occur. If evidence of pulmonary edema or oliguria (urine output of less than 20 mL/hour) develops, consultation with regional center staff is recommended.

Self-test

Now answer these questions to test yourself on the information in the last section.

D1. When eclampsia is present, _____ is generally used to prevent recurrence of maternal seizures.

D2. Signs of magnesium sulfate toxicity include

Yes	No	
___	___	Exaggerated reflexes
___	___	High serum sodium
___	___	Slow respiratory rate
___	___	Loss of deep tendon reflexes
___	___	Deceased urine output

D3. **True** **False** When maternal blood pressure is 160/105 mm Hg or higher, it should be lowered as quickly and as much as possible.

D4. **True** **False** Diazepam (Valium) may be used if magnesium sulfate fails to control seizures in a woman with eclampsia.

D5. **True** **False** For women with severe preeclampsia, the goal for antihypertensive treatment is to achieve a blood pressure of 90/60 mm Hg.

D6. **True** **False** If magnesium sulfate is given during labor, it should be stopped as soon as the baby is delivered.

D7. What can happen if maternal blood pressure is lowered too far?

_____

_____

D8. If magnesium sulfate fails to stops seizures in a woman with eclampsia, what should be done?

Yes	No	
___	___	Consult a neurologist and/or regional center specialists.
___	___	Give diazepam (Valium) intravenously.
___	___	Be prepared to provide assisted ventilation to the woman.
___	___	Perform a cesarean section immediately.
___	___	Consider that intracranial hemorrhage may have occurred.
___	___	Be prepared to assist the baby's respirations.

Check your answers with the list that follows the Recommended Routines. Correct any incorrect answers and review the appropriate section in the unit.

8. What Should You Do When a Seizure Occurs?

A seizure is a dramatic event. You need to react immediately, but *calmly*. Stay focused on what needs to be done to help the woman, not on the seizure itself. A team response should be as practiced and as planned as it is for cardiopulmonary resuscitation.

A. Initial Response

1. *Protect the Woman From Skeletal and Soft tissue Injury.* Wait for the seizure to subside.

2. *Give Oxygen by Mask.* Be sure the mask fits tightly and use a flow rate of 6 to 10 L/min, to keep oxygen saturation above 90%.

3. *Apply Pulse Oximeter* to allow continuous monitoring of oxygen saturation.

4. *Consider Providing an Oral Airway or Endotracheal Intubation* if the woman cannot maintain adequate oxygenation.

5. *Take Maternal Blood Pressure.* If higher than 160/105 mm Hg, give hydralazine, 5 mg, by IV bolus or labetalol 10 mg by IV bolus over 2 to 5 minutes. Recheck blood pressure every 5 to 10 minutes and follow stabilization protocol in Section 7.

6. *Give Magnesium Sulfate.*
   - Use loading dose of 4 to 6 g, given intravenously over 20 minutes, of a magnesium sulfate solution containing 40 g of magnesium per 1,000 mL sterile water; follow with continuous infusion of 2 g/hour. (See stabilization protocol in Section 7.)
   - If infusion of magnesium sulfate is already running, DTRs are present (check knee jerk), and the patient is breathing spontaneously, give another dose of magnesium sulfate, 4 g, intravenously over 20 minutes.

7. *Check and Monitor Fetal Heart Rate.* Fetal bradycardia often occurs soon after a maternal seizure. The woman may be cyanotic, with slow and deep respirations. The woman will recover spontaneously, given an open airway (in rare cases, assisted ventilation may be needed), oxygen, and time. As the woman recovers her oxygenation, fetal heart rate and condition will also recover.

This is the time a woman is in the most danger from overzealous drug therapy, anesthesia, and surgery. The first actions you should take are to stabilize the woman's condition. Once stabilized, delivery should be carried out promptly.

Cesarean delivery before stabilization is dangerous. Even if fetal bradycardia is present, the woman's condition should be stabilized before delivery is undertaken.

B. Post-seizure Care

Follow the stabilization protocol, given in Section 7. Consult with maternal-fetal medicine specialists. Arrange for patient transfer and delivery, as appropriate.

9. How Do You Know When a Woman With Eclampsia or Worsening Preeclampsia Has Been Stabilized?

A. **Woman Is Awake and Aware:** A stable patient knows where she is, can answer questions appropriately, can carry on a conversation, and can cooperate with her care.

B. **Blood Pressure Is Stable:** Blood pressure remains at the same level for 4 to 6 hours.

C. **No Findings That Indicate Worsening Conditions:** A woman whose condition is stable will have *none* of the following:
   - Oliguria (urine output <20 mL/hour)
   - Headache
   - Blurred vision, "spots before the eyes"
   - Epigastric/abdominal pain
   - Shortness of breath, cyanosis, or pulmonary edema
   - Clonus

10. What Should Be Done After Maternal Condition Has Been Stabilized?

A. Consult With Regional Center Experts

Complex assessment and management of maternal and fetal condition is required for optimal outcome for women with severe preeclampsia, eclampsia, or HELLP syndrome. Even if stabilized initially, maternal or fetal condition may become unstable and

22

deteriorate further, requiring rapid reassessment and intervention. Decisions regarding location, timing, and route of delivery require careful weighing of fetal condition, maternal condition, and fetal gestational age.

Consultation with maternal-fetal medicine and neonatal intensive care specialists is recommended, whether or not you plan to transfer the woman to a regional center.

B. Transfer the Woman to a Regional Perinatal Center

Women with severe preeclampsia, eclampsia, or HELLP syndrome can be extremely sick. Central hemodynamic monitoring, while uncommonly used in pregnancy, may be necessary during labor. Intensive care of the baby may be needed after delivery. Transfer of the pregnant woman to a regional center may be indicated, even for a term pregnancy. Transport generally should not be undertaken until a woman's condition is stabilized but, once stabilized, should be accomplished without delay, *unless* she is in labor.

C. Prepare for Delivery

If the woman is in active labor, or transfer to a regional perinatal center is not advisable for other reasons, proceed with plans for delivery. Consult pediatric specialists to prepare for the delivery room and neonatal care of the baby.

1. *Consider Administration of Corticosteroids:* If the pregnancy is 24 to 34 weeks' gestation, administration of corticosteroids is generally recommended to promote fetal lung maturity, even if delivery is expected to occur in less than 24 hours. See Unit 7, Preterm Labor, in this book and/or consult with regional center maternal-fetal medicine specialists.

2. *Induce Labor*
   - In general, it is recommended that women with eclampsia or worsening preeclampsia be delivered within 24 hours of their condition being stabilized.
   - General anesthesia carries particularly high risks for these women, making vaginal delivery safer than cesarean section.
   - Provide routine care and pain management, with use of narcotics.
   - Cervical ripening agents may be appropriate to use.
   - Induction of labor may be successful even if the cervix is not ripe and the pregnancy is far from term.
   - If placental function is diminished due to hypertension, the fetus is more likely to have a Category II or III fetal heart rate tracing during labor. Anticipate possible need for emergency cesarean delivery and/or neonatal resuscitation.

3. *Cesarean Delivery:* If induction of labor failed, cesarean delivery may be appropriate. Timing and location of delivery should be based on maternal and fetal condition. If cesarean delivery becomes necessary, anesthesia considerations are complex, and consultation with regional center experts is recommended.

4. *Prepare for Care of the Baby*
   - Be prepared for a hypotonic baby with poor respiratory effort if the mother received prolonged administration of magnesium sulfate.
   - Feed early and screen for hypoglycemia. (See Book I: Maternal and Fetal Evaluation and Immediate Newborn Care, Unit 8, Hypoglycemia).
   - If resuscitation is needed, monitor for possible post-resuscitation complications. (See Book I: Maternal and Fetal Evaluation and Immediate Newborn Care, Unit 5, Resuscitating the Newborn.)

11. How Should Women With HELLP Syndrome Be Managed?

Women with HELLP syndrome are at increased risk for serious maternal complications, including disseminated intravascular coagulation, hepatic hematoma and/or necrosis, and death. The risk for fetal complications, including intrauterine death, is also increased. Once the diagnosis of HELLP syndrome is made, delivery is a short-term goal and transfer to a regional perinatal center is strongly recommended. Consultation with maternal-fetal medicine specialists regarding therapy and pre-transport stabilization is also recommended.

In the event that a woman is in labor when HELLP syndrome is diagnosed, and labor is too far advanced and/or the woman's condition too unstable for safe transfer, provide management as outlined previously for severe preeclampsia and eclampsia.

12. Are the Risks From Hypertension Eliminated After Delivery?

No. Intensive monitoring of a woman's condition is usually needed for 1 to 2 days postpartum. If started before delivery, magnesium sulfate is generally continued postpartum for 12 to 48 hours or longer. The duration of magnesium therapy after delivery is determined by the severity of maternal illness and evidence of resolution of preeclampsia.

While gestational hypertension will resolve completely after delivery, it does not do so immediately. Occasionally, the condition of women with pregnancy-related hypertension worsens during the postpartum period, before it starts to resolve. Women may become seriously ill with severe preeclampsia or eclampsia. The highest risk period for development of eclampsia is the first 24 hours postpartum. Worsening hypertension and seizures develop most commonly within 1 or 2 days after delivery but, in rare cases, may not occur until 10 days' postpartum.

Chronic hypertension also may be unstable following delivery. Continued use and/or readjustment of antihypertensive medication may be needed during this time. A few patients may continue to be hypertensive. For these women, labetalol or nifedipine therapy is often used.

A woman's blood pressure should be normal, or have declined to safer levels, before hospital discharge, and she should have evidence of sustained diuresis.

Home monitoring for 1 to 2 weeks' postpartum is appropriate for women whose pregnancies were complicated by chronic hypertension, preeclampsia, or eclampsia. Assessment includes

- Frequent blood pressure measurement
- Daily dipstick testing of urine for protein
- Prompt reporting of any of the following:
  - Increase in blood pressure
  - Protein in urine
  - Persistent headache
  - Epigastric/abdominal pain
  - Blurred vision or other visual disturbances

Signs and symptoms of pregnancy-related hypertension can be expected to resolve by the time of the 6-week postpartum examination. If they have not, the woman should be reexamined at 12 weeks' postpartum.

Self-test

Now answer these questions to test yourself on the information in the last section.

E1. **True** **False** In general, women who have severe preeclampsia, eclampsia, or HELLP syndrome should be stabilized and then transferred for delivery at a regional perinatal center.

E2. **True** **False** Cesarean delivery is usually safer than vaginal delivery for a woman with hypertension.

E3. **True** **False** Hypertension can worsen postpartum, causing serious illness in the mother.

E4. **True** **False** If fetal bradycardia is present in a woman experiencing an eclamptic seizure, an emergency cesarean delivery should be done immediately, regardless of maternal condition.

E5. Which of the following is appropriate post-discharge postpartum care for a woman who had severe preeclampsia?

Yes	No	
____	____	Continue blood pressure monitoring at home for 1 to 2 weeks
____	____	Complete bed rest
____	____	Daily dipstick check of urine for protein
____	____	Low-salt diet

E6. You see a woman with preeclampsia begin to have a seizure. What would you do?

Immediately	Within Several Minutes	Not Indicated	
____	____	____	Take blood pressure.
____	____	____	Check serum potassium.
____	____	____	Apply pulse oximeter.
____	____	____	Protect the woman from soft-tissue and skeletal injury.
____	____	____	Give magnesium sulfate.
____	____	____	Prepare for cesarean delivery within 30 minutes.
____	____	____	Give oxygen by mask.

Check your answers with the list that follows the Recommended Routines. Correct any incorrect answers and review the appropriate section in the unit.

Hypertension in Pregnancy

Recommended Routines

All the routines listed below are based on the principles of perinatal care presented in the unit you have just finished. They are recommended as part of routine perinatal care.

Read each routine carefully and decide whether it is standard operating procedure in your hospital. Check the appropriate blank next to each routine.

**Procedure Standard
in My Hospital**

**Needs Discussion
by Our Staff**

_____ _____ 1. Establish guidelines for the consistent classification, and reclassification if condition changes during pregnancy, of pregnant women with hypertension as having
  • Chronic hypertension
  • Chronic hypertension with superimposed preeclampsia
  • Pregnancy-related hypertension, including
    – Gestational hypertension
    – Preeclampsia
    – Severe preeclampsia
    – Eclampsia
    – HELLP syndrome

_____ _____ 2. Establish written instructions for the home care of women who develop hypertension during pregnancy, including a list of findings to report to their health care provider.

_____ _____ 3. Establish guidelines for the assessment of women admitted to the hospital for evaluation of preeclampsia.

_____ _____ 4. Establish guidelines for the immediate stabilization of a woman who has rapidly worsening preeclampsia or eclampsia.

_____ _____ 5. Establish a protocol for response to maternal seizure(s) due to eclampsia.

_____ _____ 6. Establish guidelines for intravenous infusion of
  • Magnesium sulfate
  • Antihypertensive medication

_____ _____ 7. Establish guidelines for the postpartum assessment for every woman whose pregnancy was complicated by hypertension.

Self-test Answers

These are the answers to the self-test questions. Please check them with the answers you gave and review the information in the unit wherever necessary.

A1. Rise in blood pressure to 140/90 mm Hg after 20 weeks' gestation

A2. Proteinuria is present with preeclampsia but not with gestational hypertension.

A3. Preeclampsia becomes eclampsia when a pregnant woman has a grand mal seizure or becomes comatose and no other cause is known.

A4.

Yes	No	
X		Nausea and vomiting
X		Jaundice
	X	Elevated blood glucose
	X	Elevated platelet count
X		Elevated liver transaminases

A5. True

A6. False. Initially, blood pressure *may not* be elevated in women with the hemolysis, elevated liver enzymes, low platelets (HELLP) syndrome. In this form of severe preeclampsia, other symptoms, which may, at first, suggest gastroenteritis or gall bladder disease, are sometimes present before hypertension and proteinuria develop.

A7. True

A8.

Yes	No	
X		Preterm birth
X		Abruptio placentae
X		Maternal congestive heart failure
	X	Placenta previa
X		Intrauterine growth restriction
X		Non-reassuring tests of fetal well-being
	X	Congenital anomalies
X		Maternal seizures
X		Maternal stroke

B1. False. Angiotensin-containing enzyme inhibitors, such as Captopril, can cause fetal deformity or renal failure, as well as severely reduce placental perfusion. These drugs should not be used during pregnancy.

B2. True

B3. False. In women with chronic hypertension, blood pressure often declines during pregnancy, due to the decrease in vascular resistance that normally occurs in all women when they are pregnant.

B4. False. Women with chronic hypertension who needed antihypertensive medication prepregnancy may not need it during pregnancy. (See question B3.)

B5.

Yes	No	
	X	Walking 2 miles a day
	X	Multiple sclerosis
X		Creatinine clearance below 100 mL/minute
X		Diabetes mellitus
X		Development of gestational hypertension
X		Lupus erythematosus

B6.

Yes	No	
X		Allow spontaneous onset of labor if it occurs before 41 weeks.
X		Use narcotic analgesia liberally during labor.
X		Treat for preeclampsia if blood pressure increases and proteinuria develops.
	X	Plan for cesarean delivery.

C1. Any 3 of the following: persistent headache, visual disturbance, epigastric pain, weight gain of more than 2 pounds in 1 day, protein in her urine, blood pressure increase, fetal movement decrease, uterine contractions

C2. Yes   No

Yes	No	
X	____	Age 35 or older
X	____	Twins
X	____	Renal disease
____	X	Short stature
X	____	Obesity
X	____	First pregnancy
X	____	Chronic hypertension

C3. True

C4. True

C5. True

C6. True

D1. Magnesium sulfate

D2. Yes   No

Yes	No	
____	X	Exaggerated reflexes
____	X	High serum sodium
X	____	Slow respiratory rate
X	____	Loss of deep tendon reflexes
____	X	Deceased urine output

D3. False. When maternal blood pressure is 160/105 mm Hg or higher, it should be lowered as quickly as possible; but care should be taken to avoid dropping the blood pressure below 140/90 mm Hg because, below that pressure, placental perfusion may be reduced, resulting in fetal distress.

D4. True

D5. False. Treatment goal is to keep the blood pressure no lower than 140/90 mm Hg and no higher than 160/105 mm Hg.

D6. False. If magnesium sulfate is given during labor, the infusion is continued for 12 to 48 hours, or longer, after delivery.

D7. Placental perfusion may decrease, which can, in turn, lead to fetal distress.

D8. Yes   No

Yes	No	
X	____	Consult a neurologist and/or regional center specialists.
X	____	Give diazepam (Valium) intravenously.
X	____	Be prepared to provide assisted ventilation to the woman.
____	X	Perform a cesarean section immediately.
X	____	Consider that intracranial hemorrhage may have occurred.
X	____	Be prepared to assist the baby's respirations.

E1. True

E2. False. Anesthesia and surgery nearly always carry more risks than a vaginal delivery.

E3. True

E4. False. If the condition of a woman who has had an eclamptic seizure is *un*stable, a cesarean delivery should *not* be done, even if the fetus appears to be in distress. The risk of maternal death from surgery and anesthesia is very high. Surgery should not be undertaken until the woman's condition has been stabilized. The fetus, however, usually recovers from the stress brought on by the mother's convulsion.

E5.

Yes	No	
X	___	Continue blood pressure monitoring at home for 1 to 2 weeks
___	X	Complete bed rest
X	___	Daily dipstick check of urine for protein
___	X	Low-salt diet

E6.

Immediately	Within Several Minutes	Not Indicated	
___	X	___	Take blood pressure.
___	___	X	Check serum potassium.
___	X	___	Apply pulse oximeter.
X	___	___	Protect the woman from soft-tissue and skeletal injury.
___	X	___	Give magnesium sulfate.
___	___	X	Prepare for cesarean delivery within 30 minutes.
___	X	___	Give oxygen by mask.

Note: If an intravenous line is in place, magnesium sulfate also can be started immediately. All of the "within several minutes" responses should be done as soon as the seizure stops.

Unit 1 Posttest

If you are applying for continuing education credits, a posttest for this unit is available online. Completion of unit posttests and the book evaluation form are required to achieve continuing education credit. For more details, visit www.cmevillage.com.

Unit 2: Obstetric Hemorrhage

Objectives

In this unit you will learn

A. What risks obstetric hemorrhage carries for a woman and a fetus

B. How to respond to life-threatening obstetric hemorrhage when the cause is unknown

C. How to identify and treat the causes of early pregnancy bleeding

D. How to identify and treat the causes of late pregnancy bleeding

E. How to determine the difference between placenta previa and abruptio placentae

F. How to recognize and provide emergency treatment for disseminated intravascular coagulation (DIC)

G. What care to anticipate for a baby born to a woman with obstetric hemorrhage

H. Which women should receive Rh immune globulin and when it should be administered

I. What routine measures are needed to prevent or reduce postpartum hemorrhage

J. How to recognize postpartum hemorrhage and identify its causes

K. How to treat postpartum hemorrhage

L. What every hospital needs to respond to obstetric hemorrhage

Unit 2 Pretest

Before reading the unit, please answer the following questions. Select the *one best* answer to each question (unless otherwise instructed). Record your answers on the test and check them against the answers at the end of the book.

1. **True   False**   In a woman being treated for obstetric hemorrhage, declining urine output suggests blood is being lost from her vascular system.

2. **True   False**   Cesarean section is the recommended route of delivery when a total placenta previa is present, even if no bleeding has occurred.

3. **True   False**   A woman who had an abruptio placentae with one pregnancy has an increased risk for having another abruptio placentae with a subsequent pregnancy.

4. **True   False**   Even with fetal death, in severe cases of abruptio placentae, cesarean delivery of the dead fetus may be necessary for maternal health.

5. **True   False**   Placenta accreta is more common with placenta previa.

6. **True   False**   The most common cause of postpartum hemorrhage is disseminated intravascular coagulation.

7. **True   False**   Abruptio placentae usually can be prevented.

8. **True   False**   Steady, slow, persistent bleeding postpartum suggests uterine atony.

9. Abruptio placentae
   A. Is usually caused by a perinatal infection
   B. May be associated with disseminated intravascular coagulation
   C. Most often occurs in women who are heroin users
   D. Is always accompanied by visible bleeding

10. When late-pregnancy placental bleeding occurs,
    A. The fetus will almost always go into severe shock.
    B. The degree of fetal blood loss correlates closely with the degree of maternal bleeding.
    C. Maternal blood, but not fetal blood, is lost.
    D. Fetal health may be compromised by decreased placental perfusion.

11. Which of the following would be especially important to check in a baby whose mother had a bleeding placenta previa?

Yes	No	
____	____	Hematocrit
____	____	Serum creatinine
____	____	Bilirubin
____	____	Blood pressure
____	____	Blood culture

12. **True   False**   Maternal tachycardia and declining blood pressure are usually the first signs of abruptio placentae.

13. **True   False**   With certain types of obstetric hemorrhage, most blood loss occurs internally and is not visible externally.

14. **True   False**   Any bleeding during pregnancy requires investigation.

15. **True** **False** Disseminated intravascular coagulation can develop with either abruptio placentae or hemolysis, elevated liver enzymes, and low platelets (HELLP) syndrome.

16. **True** **False** An Rh-negative unsensitized woman had an episode of significant bleeding at 10 weeks' gestation and received Rh immune globulin at that time. At 25 weeks' gestation, she has another episode of bleeding and should receive Rh immune globulin again, within 72 hours of the bleeding.

17. Which of the following is *most* likely to be associated with postpartum hemorrhage?
   A. Primigravida
   B. Preterm delivery
   C. Post-term delivery
   D. High parity

18. All of the following statements about ectopic pregnancy are accurate, *except:*
   A. Surgical removal or chemotherapy may be used to destroy the pregnancy.
   B. Significant maternal internal bleeding may occur.
   C. The implantation site is most often in a fallopian tube.
   D. Symptoms rarely occur before 12 to 14 weeks' gestation.

19. All of the following are generally an indication of abruptio placentae, *except:*
   A. Sudden increase in fundal height
   B. Bright red, painless bleeding
   C. Uterus that is tender when palpated
   D. Increased uterine tone

20. Which of the following should you do *first* when postpartum hemorrhage is detected?
   A. Prepare for immediate surgery.
   B. Check clotting studies.
   C. Palpate the uterus.
   D. Give an intravenous bolus of 40 units oxytocin.

21. All of the following increase the risk for placenta previa, *except:*
   A. Maternal hypertension
   B. Multifetal gestation
   C. High parity
   D. Previous cesarean section

1. What Is Obstetric Hemorrhage?

A. Definition

Obstetric hemorrhage is bleeding from the vagina, cervix, placenta, or uterus during pregnancy. Obstetric hemorrhage is also excessive postpartum uterine bleeding.

B. Maternal Versus Fetal Blood Loss

When the source of the bleeding is the placenta, blood lost is primarily maternal blood, but may be fetal blood too. Because of the relatively small blood volume of the fetus, even a small amount of fetal blood loss can be life-threatening.

Fetal health may be severely compromised due to loss of fetal blood and/or to decreased placental perfusion from maternal blood loss.

C. Necessity for Prompt Evaluation

In the past, obstetric hemorrhage caused more deaths in pregnant and postpartum women than all other causes of maternal mortality combined. Even today, obstetric hemorrhage can be fatal for a woman and/or her fetus. Regardless of the source of the bleeding, maternal blood loss may be minor or may rapidly progress to severe hemorrhage. When bleeding first starts, it is impossible to know how severe it may become.

 Any bleeding during pregnancy should be evaluated in a hospital, without delay.

D. Estimation of Blood Loss

Most young, pregnant women have expanded blood volume and efficient autonomic vascular reflexes, so that even heavy blood loss may not be accompanied initially by the usual signs of shock. This can be misleading. Visible blood loss also may be misleading. With certain types of obstetric hemorrhage, profuse bleeding can occur behind the placenta or into the woman's abdomen. The amount of blood that can be seen after it flows out of the body through the vagina may be only a small portion of the total volume of blood lost from a woman's vascular system.

Monitor urine output each hour. Renal blood flow is particularly sensitive to changes in blood volume. Diminishing urine output suggests renal perfusion is diminished because, somewhere, blood is being lost from the circulatory system. Crystalloid and/or colloid solutions should be given intravenously to keep urine output of 30 mL/hour or more.

Furthermore, visual estimation of blood loss is notoriously inaccurate. Blood loss is usually underestimated by as much as 50%. Bloody items, such as pads, towels, and sheets, should be weighed and their weight should be compared with the standard dry weight of identical items. The difference in weight, in grams, is approximately equal to the volume of blood in milliliters.

2. What Does Your Hospital Need to Manage Obstetric Hemorrhage?

Although certain conditions increase the risk for obstetric hemorrhage, profuse bleeding also can occur suddenly and without warning in any woman. Every hospital with a delivery service needs to be fully capable of managing obstetric hemorrhage.

Three resources are needed.

1. A clear plan of action that is familiar to and understood by all staff members
2. Access to adequate blood supplies and technician support (within ≤30 minutes) 24 hours/day, 7 days/week
3. Capability for emergency cesarean section (within 30 minutes) and hysterectomy 24 hours/day, 7 days/week

3. What Emergency Care Should You Give a Woman Who Presents With Life-Threatening Hemorrhage From an Unknown Cause?

Occasionally, a woman will come into a hospital with sudden onset of profuse vaginal bleeding with no history of placenta previa or other easily identified reason for the bleeding. Your first actions should be to stabilize the woman's condition, and then to determine the source of the hemorrhage.

Your intervention on behalf of a woman with obstetric hemorrhage needs to be prompt and aggressive.

Your intervention on behalf of a fetus, even if fetal condition is worrisome, should wait until maternal condition has been stabilized. Until the woman's condition is stabilized, the life of the woman and the fetus may be in serious jeopardy.

A. Get Help

Many actions need to be taken with extreme speed and skill. Often, 2 physicians and several experienced nurses are needed to provide the care that a hemorrhaging pregnant woman needs. Emergency surgery may be needed, so all surgical support and blood bank services also need to be mobilized immediately. Pediatric practitioners should be notified of a woman's status so that preparations for delivery room and nursery care of the baby can be made.

B. Give Volume Expansion and Stabilize the Woman's Condition

It is much better to prevent shock than it is to treat it.

Whenever possible, replacement therapy for obstetric hemorrhage should begin BEFORE the woman develops signs of shock.

If the visible volume of blood lost constitutes a life-threatening amount, you suspect a large amount of internal bleeding, and/or the woman shows signs of shock, institute general life support measures *immediately,* without taking time for invasive diagnostic examinations. These measures include the following:

- *Insertion of large-bore intravenous (IV) lines* (18 gauge or larger): Massive hemorrhage can deplete blood volume so quickly that several IV lines may be needed to pump replacement fluids into a woman with sufficient speed.
- *Rapid infusion of saline solutions.*
- *Infusion of blood products as soon as possible:* Under the circumstance of massive hemorrhage, the use of type-specific (rather than crossmatched) packed red blood cells may be appropriate.

Severe anemia can dramatically worsen the effects of blood loss. If hemorrhage occurs in a woman with hemoglobin below 6 g/dL, it is more likely to be fatal. When a woman is severely anemic, enough red blood cells may be lost, even with relatively light bleeding, that oxygen supply to body tissues can be seriously compromised. Death may result from inadequate oxygen perfusion of vital organs.

C. Evaluate Fetal Well-being and Gestational Age

Fetal status may influence the timing and type of intervention taken. Determine if the fetus is alive. This can be done simply by finding a fetal heartbeat with a Doppler monitor or fetoscope.

If the fetus is alive, then estimation of fetal gestational age may be important. This can be done by asking the woman, checking her records (if available), or with a clinical or ultrasound examination. In the most critical cases, however, surgical intervention may be needed to save the woman's life, regardless of fetal gestational age.

Measures such as turning the woman onto her side and giving her oxygen by mask may be appropriate, and may benefit fetal health, as long as they do not interfere with the resuscitation or life support measures needed for the woman.

D. Obtain Maternal Blood Tests

1. *Send Blood Samples*
   - Type and crossmatch (at least 4 units of packed red cells)
   - Complete blood count (CBC)
   - Prothrombin time (PT) and partial thromboplastin time (PTT)
   - Platelet count
   - Fibrinogen level

2. *Collect a 5-mL Clot Tube of Blood and Tape It to the Patient's Bed:* The tube should be free of anticoagulant. If a clot does not form within 10 to 15 minutes, DIC is probably present.

E. Deliver the Baby Promptly

If the *bleeding does **not** stop,* the uterus must be emptied as soon as the woman is stable enough to tolerate surgery. If the woman shows signs of labor, examine her under a double setup to determine whether a vaginal delivery can be carried out promptly and safely.

F. Determine the Cause of the Bleeding

If the *bleeding stops,* the woman's condition is stable, and fetal heart rate monitoring is reassuring, proceed with testing to identify the source of the bleeding (described in the sections that follow).

Self-test

Now answer these questions to test yourself on the information in the last section.

A1. What are the 3 things every hospital should have to manage obstetric hemorrhage?

_____

_____

_____

A2. Obstetric hemorrhage is bleeding from the _____ during pregnancy or postpartum.

A3. Blood loss with obstetric hemorrhage may be visible, or it may be _____.

A4. With obstetric hemorrhage, significant blood loss may occur before signs of _____ appear in the woman.

A5. **True** **False** When the source of the bleeding is the placenta (placenta previa, abruptio placentae), the blood lost may come from the woman and from the fetus.

A6. Which actions should you take as soon as a woman is admitted with late pregnancy obstetric hemorrhage from an unknown source?

Yes	No	
____	____	Get help immediately.
____	____	Take blood pressure.
____	____	Insert large-bore intravenous lines.
____	____	Begin infusion of saline solutions.
____	____	Type and crossmatch blood.
____	____	Obtain tube of blood; tape it to the patient's bed.
____	____	Give oxygen by mask to the pregnant woman.

A7. What amount of bleeding during pregnancy requires investigation?

_____

Check your answers with the list that follows the Recommended Routines. Correct any incorrect answers and review the appropriate section in the unit.

4. What Are the Causes of Bleeding in Early Pregnancy?

When any woman in the reproductive years (approximately 12 to 48 years of age) misses a menstrual period and then has vaginal bleeding and/or lower abdominal pain, a spontaneous abortion or ectopic pregnancy should be suspected.

Obtain a serum beta human chorionic gonadotropin (β-hCG) titer to help differentiate normal intrauterine pregnancy from spontaneous abortion, ectopic pregnancy, and non-obstetric causes of vaginal bleeding and/or lower abdominal pain. Interpret the results as follows:

- **Negative** serum β-hCG: Woman is not pregnant, but may have a gynecological problem.

- **Positive** serum β-hCG: If it is 5 to 6 weeks or longer since a woman's last menstrual period, or the β-hCG value is greater than 1,500 to 2,000 mIU/mL, an intrauterine pregnancy should be identifiable within the uterus by ultrasound (particularly if a vaginal, rather than an abdominal, probe is used).

    1. If the *uterus contains an intact pregnancy* (gestational sac, fetal "pole," and/or fetal heart can be identified), the bleeding indicates that a spontaneous abortion is threatened, or is in the process of occurring.

2. If the *uterus appears empty,*
- The pregnancy is elsewhere (ectopic), usually in a fallopian tube.

or
- The pregnancy dates are incorrect with the gestational sac too small to be visualized by ultrasound.

or
- Complete spontaneous abortion has occurred.

3. If a *pregnancy cannot be detected either in the uterus or a fallopian tube* by ultrasound, and the woman is stable, wait 48 hours and repeat the serum β-hCG.
- If pain and bleeding continue, and the β-hCG titer is falling, this indicates a failed pregnancy, which most likely is within a fallopian tube (ectopic pregnancy).
- If the bleeding stops and/or the serum β-hCG titer continues to rise, the pregnancy may be normal and is probably within the uterus. If a gestational sac still cannot be seen, repeat the serum β-hCG again. When the serum β-hCG reaches 1,500 mIU/mL, a gestational sac is almost always large enough to be seen. When the serum β-hCG level is 1,500 mIU/mL or higher, obtain another transvaginal ultrasound examination to determine whether the pregnancy is within the uterus.

A. Spontaneous Abortion

Of all recognized pregnancies, approximately 10% to 15% are lost through spontaneous abortion, sometimes called miscarriage. More than 60% of spontaneous abortions are caused by abnormal development of either the fetus or the placenta, and usually occur within the first 5 to 10 weeks of pregnancy.

When a threatened abortion occurs, subsequent ultrasound examination may reveal an intact gestational sac and a fetal heartbeat. Many such pregnancies stop bleeding and continue to term with no additional problems.

A threatened abortion may progress to increased vaginal bleeding, uterine cramps, and passage of tissue. If tissue is passed, the pregnancy will not continue. Approximately 10% to 20% of spontaneous abortions are complete, but it may be difficult to determine that from clinical findings. In many cases, vaginal probe ultrasound examination, together with physical examination, can be used to distinguish between incomplete and complete abortion.

Surgical scraping of the uterus (dilation and curettage) or suction curettage (dilation and evacuation) may be needed to be sure that all fetal and placental tissues are removed so the bleeding will stop and the uterus can heal.

B. Ectopic Pregnancy

An ectopic pregnancy is one that has implanted somewhere other than inside the uterus. The abnormal site of implantation is usually in a fallopian tube but may, less commonly, be elsewhere in the abdomen. Women with prior tubal surgery, a prior ectopic pregnancy, an intrauterine device in place, or history of pelvic inflammatory disease are at higher risk, but an ectopic pregnancy can occur in any woman.

Initially, an embryo may grow, but usually dies after a few weeks because the tissues on which the placenta is implanted cannot provide adequate support for continued growth. Serious internal bleeding may occur due to placental separation from the implantation site or from rupture of the fallopian tube by the growing embryo.

Bleeding from the vagina often occurs, along with abdominal pain, but may represent only a small portion of the total volume of blood lost; the remainder may be hidden within the abdomen. Vaginal bleeding is from the uterus as the lining established in response to a pregnancy is sloughed when the pregnancy dies. Internal bleeding, if it occurs, is from the ectopic pregnancy itself because the growing placenta has invaded blood vessels in the tissue on which it is implanted, and caused those vessels to bleed. Depending on the woman's condition, immediate intervention may be needed to stop internal bleeding. Surgery is often used to locate and remove an ectopic pregnancy.

If the woman is stable, consultation with specialists skilled in the management of ectopic pregnancy is recommended. Referral to a regional center for therapy may be indicated, especially if preservation of future fertility is desired by the woman. Laparoscopic removal of the ectopic pregnancy with preservation of the fallopian tube or chemotherapy with methotrexate to end the pregnancy may be used.

5. What Are the Causes of Bleeding in Late Pregnancy?

A. Bloody Show

Vaginal discharge of a mixture of blood and mucus is a normal occurrence in early labor. There is almost always less bleeding with bloody show than with menstrual flow, and will not result in significant blood loss.

Other causes of obstetric bleeding, however, often progress to serious hemorrhage. In general, *any* bleeding should be considered abnormal and investigated in a hospital.

B. Placental Bleeding

1. *Placenta Previa* (placenta is implanted low in the uterus, partially or completely covering the cervical os, as shown in Figure 2.1)

Sometimes, an ultrasound examination obtained early in pregnancy shows what appears to be a placenta previa. A placenta that appears to cover the internal cervical os in early pregnancy very often, however, does not cover it at term. In most cases, the development of the lower uterine segment in late pregnancy will "move" the placenta away from the internal os.

Women with the appearance of a placenta previa by ultrasound *before* 20 weeks' gestation usually do *not* require special management, unless bleeding ensues.

True placenta previa is a common cause of vaginal bleeding during late pregnancy and should be suspected with any bleeding, particularly bright red, painless bleeding, occurring after 24 weeks' gestation. Significant bleeding can occur with any type of placenta previa, whether marginal, partial, or complete.

Placenta previa is more likely to occur

- With multifetal gestation
- In women who have had a previous cesarean section
- In women with high parity
- With large and/or numerous fibroids
- If it occurred in a previous pregnancy

It also is associated with abnormal fetal presentation (fetal position may be influenced by the location of a low-lying placenta).

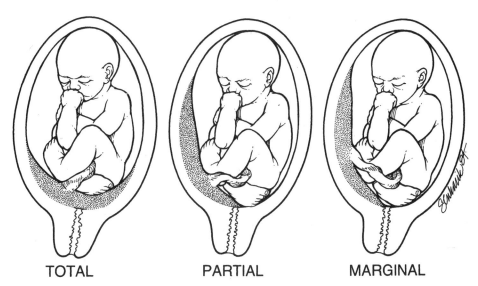

Figure 2.1. Types of Placenta Previa
Reproduced with permission from Gabbe SG, Niebyl JR, Simpson JL. Obstetric hemorrhage. In: Gabbe SG, Niebyl JR, Simpson JL, eds, *Obstetrics: Normal and Problem Pregnancies*. 3rd ed. New York, NY: Churchill Livingstone; 1996:511.

Bleeding from a placenta previa will always be visible externally. Initial bleeding may not be heavy and may instead be characterized by intermittent but persistent spotting. Alternatively, significant blood loss may occur with the first episode of bleeding. Sometimes, a placenta previa is not recognized until labor, when cervical changes cause the previa to bleed for the first time. Cervical dilatation, uterine contractions, or digital examination may cause the bleeding to worsen dramatically.

2. *Abruptio Placentae* (premature separation of a normally implanted placenta from the uterine wall; part or all of the placenta may separate)

Placental separation is unpredictable and can occur at any time during pregnancy. Most late pregnancy abruptions begin before the onset of labor. Signs of abruption include increasing uterine resting tone and sudden vaginal bleeding. Bleeding is usually accompanied by uterine cramps and/or a uterus that is tender and firm to palpation. The blood lost may be bright red, but is more commonly dark red with clots. Bleeding may be visible vaginally, but also may be completely concealed behind the placenta. Sometimes, the center of a placenta separates but the edges remain adhered, trapping all blood lost between the placenta and the uterine wall. Even if completely concealed, the volume of blood lost can still be very large.

Although most abruptions occur spontaneously with no known cause, the risk is increased with
- History of an *abruption in a previous pregnancy* (risk of recurrence is approximately 10%)
- *Acute abdominal trauma* (traffic accident, domestic violence, maternal fall, etc)
- *Hypertension* (either chronic or pregnancy-specific)
- *Smoking* (vasoconstrictive effects of smoking are known to limit placental perfusion and may foster premature separation of the placenta)

- *Sudden uterine decompression* (particularly if the uterus was over-distended)
  - Multifetal gestation (abruption of Twin B placenta may occur after Twin A is delivered)
  - Rupture of membranes (especially if hydramnios was present)
  - Following amniocentesis (this is rare)
- *High parity* (several previous births)
- *Uterine tumors* (fibroids) or *malformations* (thought to create an inadequate site for placental growth and adherence of the anchoring villi)
- *Short umbilical cord* (may pull placenta off the uterine wall as the fetus descends during the second stage of labor)
- *Cocaine use* (substance users sometimes use cocaine to induce labor and/or to relieve labor pains, but the vascular effects of acute cocaine use can result in placental abruption)
- *Premature rupture of membranes* (abruptio placentae affects approximately 10% of women with premature rupture of membranes)

In addition to the risks posed by hemorrhage, a woman with placental abruption is also at risk for the development of DIC, which is a life-threatening complication.

C. Cervical Bleeding

Significant bleeding from the cervix itself (not from the placenta or uterus above it) is unusual. The most common cause is chronic cervicitis. Other causes include cervical polyps and, rarely, cervical carcinoma. In some cases, women mistake bleeding hemorrhoids or hemorrhagic cystitis as blood coming from the vagina.

An even more unusual, but possible, cause of cervical bleeding is cervical pregnancy. Signs and symptoms, as well as evaluation, of this are similar to those for ectopic pregnancy, but the hemorrhage is likely to be much greater and occur later in pregnancy (usually the second trimester).

D. Obstetric Bleeding of Unknown Cause

It is not always possible to determine the cause of bleeding. For approximately one-third of all cases of significant late pregnancy bleeding, the cause is never identified. Even if a cause cannot be identified, late pregnancy bleeding makes it more likely the pregnancy will experience additional problems.

Self-test

Now answer these questions to test yourself on the information in the last section.

B1. **True** **False** The initial signs and symptoms of ectopic pregnancy and threatened abortion are similar.

B2. **True** **False** More than half the time, the cause of late pregnancy bleeding cannot be identified.

B3. **True** **False** Women with placenta previa are at high risk for disseminated intravascular coagulation.

B4. **True** **False** Much of the bleeding that accompanies ectopic pregnancy may be internal, into the woman's abdominal cavity.

B5. **True** **False** Women with placenta previa may present with sudden onset of profuse bleeding or with persistent, intermittent spotting.

B6. **True** **False** Undetected cancer of the cervix is the most common cause of cervical bleeding during pregnancy.

B7. **True** **False** Bloody show is a mixture of blood and mucus that is normally passed vaginally during early labor.

B8. List at least 3 causes of abnormal late-pregnancy bleeding.

_____

_____

_____

B9. Identify whether the following factors are associated with placenta previa, abruptio placentae, both, or neither.

	Placenta Previa	Abruptio Placentae	Neither
Multifetal gestation	_____	_____	_____
Acute abdominal trauma	_____	_____	_____
Maternal cocaine use	_____	_____	_____
Maternal diabetes mellitus	_____	_____	_____
Uterine fibroids	_____	_____	_____
Multiparous woman	_____	_____	_____
Occurred in a previous pregnancy	_____	_____	_____
Previous cesarean delivery	_____	_____	_____
Maternal hypertension	_____	_____	_____
Abnormal fetal presentation	_____	_____	_____
First pregnancy	_____	_____	_____
Short umbilical cord	_____	_____	_____
Maternal smoking	_____	_____	_____
Hydramnios	_____	_____	_____

Check your answers with the list that follows the Recommended Routines. Correct any incorrect answers and review the appropriate section in the unit.

6. How Do You Determine the Cause of Late-Pregnancy Bleeding?

Emergency management of severe obstetric hemorrhage, prior to identification of the bleeding source, was described earlier in this unit. Most women with late-pregnancy bleeding, however, will *not* have life-threatening hemorrhage on admission to the hospital. Take the following steps to identify the source of the bleeding:

A. Obtain History

1. *Estimate Blood Loss* by asking the woman about her bleeding.
   - How does this compare to your normal menstrual flow?
   - When did the bleeding start?
   - What color has the blood been?
   - How many pads did you use?
   - Have there been cramps, contractions, and/or abdominal pain?

2. *Review Prenatal Care:* If the prenatal record is not available, obtain full history from the patient.

B. Examine the Woman

1. *Physical Examination*
   a. *Check vital signs*
   b. *Measure fundal height:* Mark fundal height with ink on the woman's abdomen for comparison with subsequent measurements. Remeasure every hour. A sudden increase in fundal height suggests abruptio placentae with ongoing bleeding concealed behind the placenta.
   c. *Assess uterine tenderness, contractions, and baseline tonus:* With abruptio placentae (usually not with placenta previa), the uterus will be tender with increased tonus. Generally, an external monitor cannot detect these changes as well as the palpating hand of an experienced perinatal care provider.
   d. *Vaginal examination:* **A digital vaginal examination should *not* be done in patients who have bleeding during late pregnancy, unless you are *certain* a placenta previa is *not* present.**

2. *Laboratory Tests*
   a. *For all women with late-pregnancy bleeding, obtain*
      - Type and crossmatch, so blood will be immediately available if the need for it arises (request at least 4 units of packed red blood cells)
      - CBC
   b. *If abruptio placentae is suspected, investigate the possibility of DIC and obtain*
      - PT and PTT
      - Platelet count
      - Fibrinogen level
      - Fibrin Degradation Products, Fibrin Split Products, or D-Dimer

3. *Ultrasound Examination*
   a. *Ultrasound can be used to determine whether a placenta previa is present.* Scan first with an abdominal transducer. If a placenta previa is present, a vaginal probe may stimulate further bleeding. Once a placenta previa has been ruled out, a vaginal probe may be used. Check when the woman's bladder is empty because false-positive results may occur when the bladder is full.

b. *Abruptio placentae cannot be reliably ruled in or out by ultrasound scan.*
Even results that appear to show a partial abruption can be misleading. Sometimes, what is thought to be a retroplacental clot turns out not to be one at all.

Placenta previa can be identified with ultrasound examination.

Abruptio placentae cannot reliably be identified with ultrasound examination, and ultrasound results may be misleading.

4. *Double Setup Vaginal Examination*: This is a pelvic examination done in an operating room, with the woman on the operating table and all preparations and personnel for an immediate cesarean delivery in place.

a. *When should you do a double setup examination?*
In nearly all situations, ultrasound examination will confirm the presence or absence of placenta previa. If the diagnosis is not certain, the fetus is mature, and the woman is in labor, a double setup examination should be done. If the placenta is felt on digital examination, a cesarean section should be undertaken. If the placenta is not felt, vaginal delivery may be possible. A marginal placenta previa, not detectable on double setup digital examination, may begin to bleed as the cervix dilates further during labor, and cesarean delivery may become necessary.

If placenta previa is present and the examination causes further separation of the placenta from the uterine wall, profuse, life-threatening bleeding can ensue, necessitating *immediate* cesarean delivery. The double setup ensures that a cesarean delivery can be carried out without delay.

If placenta previa is not present, vaginal or cervical causes of bleeding can be investigated with gentle, careful speculum examination.

b. *When should you NOT do a double setup or any digital examination?*
Any examination where the examining finger(s) enters the uterus above the cervix can precipitate bleeding if a placenta previa is present. Massive bleeding can put the woman and the fetus in immediate danger.

When the amount of blood being lost is *not* life-threatening and the fetus is preterm, the bleeding usually will slow or stop by itself. If a double setup examination stimulates uncontrollable hemorrhage, an immediate cesarean delivery would be necessary. Maternal health would be threatened by the hemorrhage; fetal health would be threatened by the hemorrhage and by being delivered preterm.

When vaginal bleeding is present, do not undertake a double setup examination or any digital examination unless you are

• *Willing and prepared to proceed with an immediate cesarean delivery OR*
• *Certain a placenta previa is not present*

47

5. *Assess the Fetus*

    a. *Estimate or reconfirm fetal age:* If gestational age was not previously established, use ultrasound to measure biparietal diameter, abdominal circumference, femur length, etc, to estimate it.

    b. *Evaluate fetal well-being:* Obtain a biophysical profile and/or monitor fetal heart rate.

    c. *Provide external fetal heart rate monitoring:* Do *not* attempt to insert an internal fetal scalp electrode or uterine pressure transducer.

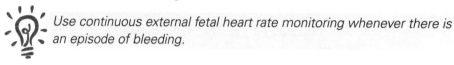 *Use continuous external fetal heart rate monitoring whenever there is an episode of bleeding.*

7. What Are the Typical Differences Between Placenta Previa and Abruptio Placentae?

While Table 2.1 shows the classic characteristics of placenta previa and abruptio placentae, the signs and symptoms may vary for an individual woman. Some women may have findings suggestive of one cause of bleeding when, in fact, the bleeding is due to a different cause. *Presentation can be confusing. Thorough assessment of each woman is essential.* Distinguishing between placenta previa and placental abruption is vital to optimal management.

Table 2.1. Usual Characteristics of Placenta Previa Versus Abruptio Placentae		
Finding	**Placenta Previa**	**Abruptio Placentae**
Maternal		
Blood color	Bright red	Dark red, clots
Pain	Painless (unless in labor)	Painful (constant, uterine pain)
Uterine tenderness	Absent	Usually present
Uterine tone	Normal	Increased, may feel tense, hard, and/or rigid to palpation
Shock	Uncommon	Frequent, especially with severe grades
Disseminated intravascular coagulation	Very rare	Frequent, especially with severe grades
Ultrasound	Almost always determines location of placenta	Appearance of clots behind placenta rarely are actual clots; may not be possible to identify true clots; useful to rule out placenta previa
Fetal		
Fetal non-reassuring status	Rare, unless maternal shock and/ or significant fetal blood loss	Frequent, especially with severe grades

Self-test

Now answer these questions to test yourself on the information in the last section.

C1. List the classic characteristics of placenta previa and abruptio placentae.

Finding	Placenta Previa	Abruptio Placentae
Blood color	_____	_____
Pain	_____	_____
Uterine tenderness	_____	_____
Uterine tone	_____	_____
Shock	_____	_____
Disseminated intravascular coagulation	_____	_____

C2. What is the reason a digital vaginal examination should not be done when third-trimester bleeding from an unknown source is present? _____

C3. When late pregnancy bleeding from an unknown source is present, what is the likely explanation for a sudden increase in fundal height? _____

C4. **True** **False** When late-pregnancy bleeding occurs, ultrasound is used to locate the placenta.

C5. **True** **False** Continuous external fetal monitoring should be used during any episode of bleeding.

C6. **True** **False** Whenever a woman is admitted with late-pregnancy bleeding, her blood should be typed and crossmatched, with at least 4 units of packed red blood cells readied for possible transfusion.

C7. **True** **False** Uterine tenderness is usually present with placenta previa but rarely with abruptio placentae.

C8. Which of the following blood tests should be obtained when abruptio placentae is suspected?

Yes	No	
____	____	Prothrombin time and partial thromboplastin time
____	____	Complete blood count
____	____	Serum electrolytes
____	____	Platelet count
____	____	Blood urea nitrogen and creatinine
____	____	Fibrinogen level

C9. When placenta previa is present or suspected, a double setup examination should *not* be done unless _____.

Check your answers with the list that follows the Recommended Routines. Correct any incorrect answers and review the appropriate section in the unit.

8. How Do You Manage Placenta Previa and Abruptio Placentae?

A. Placenta Previa

1. *Confirm Presence of Placenta Previa*

Repeat an ultrasound examination at 26 to 28 weeks to confirm the continued presence of a placenta that completely or partially covered the cervical os earlier in pregnancy. If a placenta previa is present, repeat the ultrasound again at 34 to 36 weeks.

2. *Manage According to Maternal Condition and Fetal Gestational Age*

 When a placenta previa is known to be present, hospitalization is required during any episode of bleeding.

a. *Preterm*

For some women, strict bed rest at home may be possible during stable periods, when there is *no* bleeding. It may be appropriate to follow patients who have minimal, intermittent bleeding to term with periodic blood replacement to keep maternal hematocrit above 30% to 35%. Instruct the woman that *any* episode of vaginal bleeding should be reported promptly and treated as an emergency.

What may begin as slight bleeding can suddenly become heavy bleeding. The pattern of bleeding or spotting with placenta previa can vary widely. Some women will have intermittent bleeding with relatively little blood loss. Other women may have one minor episode of bleeding, followed by no spotting or bleeding until later in pregnancy or when labor begins. Massive hemorrhage may then occur, without warning.

For many women, hospitalization is required until the pregnancy reaches term, severe bleeding occurs, or labor begins. Hospitalization at a regional center equipped to care for preterm and/or sick babies is advisable because life-threatening hemorrhage can occur at any time and without any warning. Transfer of the woman, however, should not be undertaken until she is stable and all bleeding has stopped.

Assess fetal well-being frequently with nonstress test and/or biophysical profile. Use external fetal heart rate monitoring during any episode of bleeding.

Determine fetal gestational age. Unless uncontrollable bleeding dictates emergency intervention, plan for a cesarean delivery when the fetus's lungs are mature and the woman's condition is stable. Consider amniocentesis to assess fetal pulmonary maturity.

b. *Term*

If the presence of a placenta previa has been confirmed but there is no bleeding, plan for a cesarean delivery at term. This is not an emergency situation but could become one because heavy bleeding could start at any time.

c. *Preterm or term*

Inform the patient that placenta previa carries serious risks. If bleeding starts, the woman and/or the fetus can lose a significant proportion of their blood volume very quickly. Profuse bleeding can occur even after delivery. Because a placenta previa is implanted in an area of the uterus that may not contract well, postpartum hemorrhage is more common and can be difficult to control.

Discuss with the pregnant woman the possibility of placenta accreta (when placental tissue invades the uterine muscle, making separation of the placenta difficult or impossible) and the resulting need for a hysterectomy as the only means to control bleeding. Placenta accreta is more common with placenta previa, especially in women who have had a previous cesarean delivery.

B. Abruptio Placentae

1. *Clinical Findings*

   Placental separation may be partial or complete. In general, the condition of the woman and the fetus depends on the amount of placental surface separated from the uterine wall.

   Study Table 2.2 to learn the risks and characteristic findings for the different grades of abruptio placentae.

2. *Management*

   Management corresponds to the degree of placental separation (grade of abruption) and depends on the presence or absence of fetal non-reassuring status, maternal shock, and/or maternal DIC.

    Regardless of the degree of abruption, blood products need to be available at all times in case they are required. An abruption can worsen suddenly and dramatically at any time.

Grade I:	Vaginal delivery is often possible for these less serious abruptions. If labor progress is good, maternal status is stable, and there is no evidence of fetal non-reassuring status, then normal vaginal delivery can be expected.
Grade II:	Emergency cesarean delivery is performed if there is *any* evidence of fetal non-reassuring status. If fetal distress occurs in this situation, it is likely that the placental separation is worsening. Therefore, prompt intervention should be undertaken when non-reassuring findings of fetal condition first occur.
Grade III:	With complete abruption and fetal death, vaginal delivery is indicated if maternal status is stable and labor progresses well. In most cases, vaginal delivery is safer for the woman, especially if her fibrinogen and platelet levels have not declined to critical levels (platelets = 50,000/mm³ or fibrinogen = 100 mg/dL). When a woman is already in active labor, it may be appropriate to allow labor to continue. Give volume replacement and provide blood components to correct clotting defects (see Section 9), as necessary. Because of high risk for maternal DIC, cesarean delivery of a dead fetus may become necessary.

   Consultation with regional center staff is recommended.

   When complete (Grade III) abruption occurs, do the following:

   1. Insert intrauterine pressure transducer.
   2. Begin oxytocin infusion. (See Unit 8, Inducing and Augmenting Labor, in this book.)
   3. Obtain platelet count and fibrinogen level frequently.

Women who had Grades II or III placental abruption should continue to be monitored during the postpartum period for the development of DIC. If DIC develops, it can be life-threatening.

Table 2.2. Abruptio Placentae: Grades of Placental Separation			
Finding	**Grade I**	**Grade II**	**Grade III**
General			
Amount of placenta separated from uterine wall	10%-25%	25%-50%	>50%
Diagnostic criteria	Vaginal bleeding and maternal signs clearly indicate an abruption	Fetal compromise is present (see Book I: Maternal and Fetal Evaluation and Immediate Newborn Care, Unit 3, Fetal Well-being)	Fetal death
Maternal Signs			
Maternal bleeding (may be concealed)	Present, usually visible externally; rarely progresses	Present, high risk that abruption will progress (worsen)	Present and continues, often concealed
Need for blood transfusion	Usually not	May be needed	Usually needed
Shock	No	May develop	Present
Disseminated intravascular coagulation (DIC)	No	May develop	Likely to develop
Uterus	Tender, may be tense	Tender, firm	Tender, hard
Life-threatening	No	Rarely	Yes
Labor	Usually normal	Fetal death unless delivered promptly	Uterus may be contracting strongly but progress often poor
Delivery	Usually vaginally	Emergency cesarean section usually required for fetal health	If DIC present, cesarean section may be needed to stop the process
Fetal Signs			
Non-reassuring status	If does not develop within 2 hours, unlikely it will later	Present	By definition of Grade III, the fetus is dead

Self-test

Now answer these questions to test yourself on the information in the last section.

D1. **True**   **False**   Placental abruption may be complete or partial.

D2. **True**   **False**   Regardless of the degree of abruption, cesarean delivery is always required.

D3. **True**   **False**   A placenta found by ultrasound examination to cover the internal cervical os at 12 to 16 weeks will almost always cover (completely or partially) the os at term.

D4. **True**   **False**   A rising platelet count and fibrinogen level signal the onset of disseminated intravascular coagulation in a woman with a Grade II abruptio placentae.

D5. **True**   **False**   When placental abruption occurs, disseminated intravascular coagulation may not be present before delivery but may develop after delivery.

D6. Which of the following risks apply to a woman with placenta previa diagnosed at 34 weeks' gestation?

	Yes	No	
	____	____	Preterm delivery may be necessary.
	____	____	Placenta accreta may be present and necessitate a hysterectomy after delivery.
	____	____	Acute preeclampsia is likely to occur.
	____	____	If bleeding occurs, the woman and the fetus can lose large amounts of blood.
	____	____	Postpartum hemorrhage is more likely to occur.
	____	____	Disseminated intravascular coagulation is likely to develop.

D7. A total placenta previa (completely covers the internal cervical os) is diagnosed at 32 weeks' gestation. Bleeding has stopped, maternal vital signs and laboratory values are stable, and tests of fetal well-being are reassuring. What should you do?

   A. Begin administration of steroids to the woman and deliver the baby by cesarean section 24 hours later.

   B. Hospitalize the woman, at bed rest, and continue observation until fetal maturity is achieved, unless bleeding or labor ensue and necessitate cesarean delivery.

   C. Perform cesarean delivery within the next several hours, before the placenta begins to bleed again.

   D. Give the woman a blood transfusion and deliver the baby by cesarean section within the next 24 hours.

Check your answers with the list that follows the Recommended Routines. Correct any incorrect answers and review the appropriate section in the unit.

9. How Do You Recognize and Treat Disseminated Intravascular Coagulation?

A. What Is Disseminated Intravascular Coagulation?

Disseminated intravascular coagulation occurs when some event triggers the release of a surplus amount of thromboplastins into the bloodstream. Thromboplastic substances normally cause or accelerate clot formation, but the overstimulation of the clotting system results in clots being formed more rapidly than the thromboplastins can be replaced. Rather than one large clot forming, however, numerous microscopic clots appear throughout the vascular system. Because these tiny clots are so numerous, they consume the factors required for clotting. Because the microscopic clots have "tied up" all the clotting factors, the remaining blood cannot clot. If bleeding is present for any reason, it will worsen significantly because of the lack of available clotting factors. Overwhelming hemorrhage can result.

Whenever possible, women with DIC should be treated in a regional medical center, but do not transfer a woman who is in unstable condition.

B. Who Is at Risk for DIC?

A variety of conditions can lead to DIC. In severe infections, thromboplastins produced by bacteria (in particular, *Escherichia coli*) can cause septic shock and DIC. When a fetus dies but is not delivered for several weeks (termed retained dead fetus syndrome), DIC may develop slowly, over a period of 4 to 8 weeks. With either abruptio placentae or amniotic fluid embolism, DIC can develop within hours. Pregnant women at risk for DIC include those with

- Abruptio placentae (most common cause of DIC in pregnant women).
- Amniotic fluid embolism.
- Fetal death with the dead fetus retained for 4 weeks or longer.
- HELLP syndrome (a severe form of pregnancy-specific hypertension. (See Unit 1, Hypertension in Pregnancy, in this book.)

In addition, women with profuse bleeding who are transfused with a massive amount of blood to replace the blood lost may develop clotting problems. Because the blood lost contained clotting factors, but banked blood is treated with anticoagulants, transfusion of large volumes of either whole blood or packed red blood cells dilute the natural clotting proteins and may significantly reduce the capability of the blood to coagulate.

C. Which Blood Tests Are Important?

For some tests, it can take several hours to obtain results. While the tests should be checked, it may not be prudent to wait for the results before beginning therapy. For this reason, also collect 5 mL of the patient's blood in an anticoagulant-free tube. Tape the tube to her bedside. Check it every few minutes. If a clot does not form within 10 to 15 minutes, DIC is probably present.

 If DIC is strongly suspected, do not delay therapy while awaiting laboratory test results. Proceed with treatment, according to the woman's clinical condition.

Obtain the following tests. If checked earlier, consider rechecking every hour.
- PT and PTT. (If these are prolonged but the tests listed below are all normal, it suggests the patient does not have DIC but may have another problem.)
- Low platelet count (<50,000/mm³).
- Low fibrinogen level (<150 mg/dL) indicates DIC.

D. How Is DIC Treated?

Overall treatment of a pregnant woman with DIC has 3 goals.
- Give blood components to provide clotting factors.
- Stabilize the woman.
- Deliver the baby.

This sounds simple, but is not. A woman with placental abruption and DIC may be critically ill, with a fetus that is dead or in serious jeopardy, and require complex management and multiple critical care resources and personnel. Treatment will depend, in part, on whether the woman is bleeding heavily.

The management plans that follow are designed as a guide for emergency therapy when the patient is too unstable for safe transport to a regional center.

 Consultation with maternal-fetal medicine specialists at a regional center is recommended as soon as DIC is suspected.

1. *Blood Components That Are Used When Clotting Factors Are Needed*
   Fresh frozen plasma (FFP) and cryoprecipitate provide clotting factors, but in different volumes of fluid. All the blood components listed may be used to provide clotting factors, but none should be used to provide blood volume. If large amounts of clotting factors are needed, such as in the treatment of DIC, the blood component that contains these factors in the smallest volume is preferred. For this reason, cryoprecipitate is preferred over FFP in the management of DIC.

   In certain cases with extremely low platelet count, transfusion of platelets also may be indicated.
   a. *Cryoprecipitate*
      - Each bag (40 to 50 mL) contains approximately the same amount of fibrinogen as a unit of FFP plus some other clotting factors, including factor VIII.
      - Usual starting dose is 1 bag of cryoprecipitate.
   b. *FFP*
      - FFP is available in 2 forms.
        – Regular 200- to 250-mL bags
        – 400- to 600-mL bags prepared by plasmapheresis
      - Each unit contains fibrinogen, plus all other clotting factors, including a higher level of factor VIII than in cryoprecipitate.
      - Usual starting dose is 2 bags of regular FFP or 1 bag of plasmapheresis-prepared FFP.
   c. *Platelets:* Platelets (5 to 10 units) may be needed, although rarely.

 If these blood components are not kept in your hospital, know where and how to obtain them quickly, 24 hours/day, 7 days/week.

2. *Management of Women* Without *Severe Hemorrhage*
   a. *Provide continuous monitoring* of fetal heart rate and the woman's blood pressure and other vital signs.
   b. *Give clotting factors* by IV infusion. Use cryoprecipitate or FFP to bring the fibrinogen level above 100 mg/dL.
   c. *Recheck.*
      - Serum fibrinogen level every hour
      - Platelet count every hour
      - CBC every 8 to 12 hours

    d. *Consider giving platelets.* Transfusion may occasionally be indicated depending on the platelet level and the route of delivery.
- Vaginal delivery: Consider platelet transfusion if count is less than 20,000/mm^3 and there is evidence of poor clot formation in spite of adequate fibrinogen level (>100 mg/dL).
- Cesarean delivery: Consider platelet transfusion if count is less than 50,000/mm^3; if possible, delay surgery until level reaches 50,000/mm^3.

    e. *Assess progress of labor.* If vaginal delivery seems possible, it is safer for the woman than cesarean delivery. If labor is not expected to progress, however, delivery by cesarean section should be undertaken as soon as the serum fibrinogen level is above 100 mg/dL and the platelet count is above 50,000/mm^3.

3. *Management of Women* With *Severe Hemorrhage*

Management of a woman with DIC and bleeding crisis should be carried out in an area equipped for intensive care. Multiple, large-bore IV lines are needed (fluids may need to be pumped into the woman, rather than passively infused). Monitor the patient's blood pressure and other vital signs continuously. Provide life-support measures, as needed.

 A patient in shock with DIC is better treated in the original hospital than transported in unstable condition.

    a. *Give blood components and fluid volume*
- Packed red blood cells through one IV line
- Cryoprecipitate or FFP through a second IV line
- Platelets or saline through a third IV line

    b. *Recheck serum fibrinogen level and platelet count* every 30 to 60 minutes.

    c. *Perform emergency cesarean delivery* as soon as the fibrinogen level exceeds 100 mg/dL and the platelet count is greater than 50,000/mm^3, whether or not the fetus is alive.

10. What Care Should You Anticipate for the Newborn?

Obstetric hemorrhage may have little effect on the fetus, or it can result in significant fetal blood loss, fetal compromise, fetal death, and/or a sick newborn. At delivery, you should be prepared with personnel and equipment for resuscitation of the newborn (Book I: Maternal and Fetal Evaluation and Immediate Newborn Care, Unit 5, Resuscitating the Newborn). You should be able to assess the baby for signs of acute blood loss, check blood pressure, and give blood volume replacement, if necessary, in the delivery room.

A central (not heelstick) hematocrit should be measured soon after delivery, and other therapy provided as indicated by clinical and laboratory findings. (See Book III: Neonatal Care, Unit 4, Low Blood Pressure, for neonatal hypovolemia [low blood volume] and hypotension [low blood pressure] management.)

11. What Additional Care Do You Need to Provide to Rh-Negative Women?

Women who are Rh-negative and unsensitized (negative Rh antibody screening test) may become sensitized during an episode of bleeding at any point during pregnancy. When bleeding occurs, fetal blood may enter the maternal circulation. If the fetus is Rh-positive, an Rh-negative woman may develop antibodies in response. This rarely affects the current pregnancy but may cause Rh disease in subsequent pregnancies. For this reason, sensitization needs to be prevented. This is done with the administration of Rh immune globulin (RhIG).

Regardless of the cause of bleeding, RhIG should be given with the first episode and needs to be administered within 72 hours of the onset of bleeding. Protection lasts for approximately 12 weeks. Depending on the course of the pregnancy, subsequent doses may be needed.

A. Early Pregnancy Bleeding

Feto-maternal (from the fetus to the mother) transfusion may or may not occur with early pregnancy bleeding. The safe assumption is that some bleeding may have occurred. When the fetus is small, the amount of bleeding is also small. Therefore, less RhIG needs to be given. Within the first trimester, 50 micrograms (µg) is recommended. If a repeat episode(s) of bleeding occurs within the first 12 weeks, there is no need to repeat RhIG administration.

B. Late-Pregnancy Bleeding

During late-pregnancy bleeding, the volume of feto-maternal hemorrhage is likely to be greater than during early pregnancy bleeding. For this reason, a minimum dose of 300 µg RhIG is recommended.

When there has been significant maternal bleeding, such as may occur with placenta previa, abruptio placentae, etc, a Kleihauer-Betke test is used to estimate the amount of fetal blood that may have entered the maternal circulation. The volume of fetal red cells estimated by the Kleihauer-Betke test is divided by 15. This then gives the number of doses of 300 µg of RhIG that are needed (each 300 µg of RhIG is adequate for each 15 mL of fetal cells that entered the maternal circulation).

Administration of RhIG should be repeated if bleeding episodes are separated by 12 weeks or more.

C. During Pregnancy for All Rh-Negative Women

Even in pregnancies with no evidence of obstetric bleeding, feto-maternal transfusion may still occur. Nearly all Rh-negative women who deliver an Rh-positive baby will be protected from sensitization by the dose of RhIG given after delivery. However, it is recommended that all unsensitized Rh-negative women receive RhIG at 28 weeks' gestation to protect the small number of women who may have unrecognized feto-maternal bleeding during pregnancy. Because term delivery would be 12 weeks after this dose of RhIG, all women who received RhIG during pregnancy should also receive a dose postpartum.

D. Following Delivery

Feto-maternal transfusion also can occur during delivery of a healthy baby from an uncomplicated pregnancy. The recommended dose following delivery of an Rh-positive baby to an unsensitized Rh-negative woman is 300 µg of RhIG. Every unsensitized Rh-negative woman who has an Rh-positive baby should receive a dose of RhIG postpartum. This postpartum dose should be given whether or not a dose was given earlier in pregnancy.

Self-test

Now answer these questions to test yourself on the information in the last section.

E1. **True** **False** Disseminated intravascular coagulation is a complicated, life-threatening condition that, whenever possible, should be treated at a regional medical center.

E2. **True** **False** When a woman has disseminated intravascular coagulation, whether her condition is stable or unstable, rapid transfer to a regional medical center is advisable.

E3. **True** **False** If a tube of blood drawn from a woman with abruptio placentae fails to clot within 15 minutes, disseminated intravascular coagulation is probably present.

E4. **True** **False** The need for resuscitation of the newborn cannot be predicted by the amount of blood the woman has lost.

E5. What are the 3 main goals for treatment of a woman with disseminated intravascular coagulation?

_____
_____
_____

E6. Name 3 fluids that are used to provide clotting factors.

_____
_____
_____

E7. A woman has a Grade III placental abruption with vaginal bleeding and disseminated intravascular coagulation. Cryoprecipitate, packed red blood cells, and saline solutions are being infused rapidly to provide clotting factors and blood volume expansion. Maternal blood pressure is stable, but heavy vaginal bleeding continues. The fetus is dead. An oxytocin infusion has been started, membranes were ruptured, but labor does not progress well. What should you do?
  A. Perform cesarean delivery as soon as the platelet count is above 50,000/mm³ and fibrinogen level is above 100 mg/dL.
  B. Continue to give clotting factors and increase the oxytocin infusion until vaginal delivery occurs.
  C. Perform immediate cesarean delivery.
  D. Transfer the woman immediately to a regional medical center.

E8. When a woman has obstetric hemorrhage, what should you do for the baby at delivery?

_____
_____
_____

Check your answers with the list that follows the Recommended Routines. Correct any incorrect answers and review the appropriate section in the unit.

12. What Is Postpartum Hemorrhage?

Estimated blood loss of more than 500 mL following delivery of the placenta after a vaginal delivery has traditionally been classified as postpartum hemorrhage. Because the blood volume of an average woman at term is increased more than 1,000 mL above her non-pregnant blood volume, most patients with postpartum hemorrhage are not ill and do not require treatment beyond the routine prophylaxis that should be given to all women to minimize postpartum bleeding.

Despite that most women, even those with heavy bleeding, do well with little or no treatment, postpartum hemorrhage remains a major cause of maternal mortality.

NOTE: Immediate postpartum bleeding after the placenta has been delivered may be caused by cervical laceration. The cervix should be examined carefully if the uterus seems to be firmly contracted.

13. What Are the Causes of Postpartum Hemorrhage?

Blood supply to the uterus increases as gestation advances. At term, at least 500 mL of blood flows through the uterus each minute. After delivery of the placenta, bleeding from the placental site is normally controlled by uterine contractions that dramatically reduce the volume of blood flowing through the arteries and veins of the uterus. Life-threatening hemorrhage can occur in any of the following situations:

A. Uterine Atony

Uterine contractions are not strong enough or frequent enough to stop bleeding from the placental site. This is called atony. Atony accounts for 60% to 70% of the cases of postpartum hemorrhage, and is more likely to occur

- In women who have had several previous births
- In women with hypertension
- With a previously overdistended uterus (hydramnios, multifetal gestation)
- When fibroid tumors are present
- After prolonged labor (lasting ≥20 hours)
- After precipitate labor (lasting ≤3 hours)
- In women with chorioamnionitis
- In women with a history of previous postpartum hemorrhage

B. Retained Placental Fragments

When the placenta is torn and part of it remains in the uterus, the arteries and veins of the placental site are left open. Often the uterus cannot contract strongly enough to control the bleeding. Significant hemorrhage can result, even if the retained fragment is small. Retained placental fragments account for about 25% of the cases of postpartum hemorrhage.

C. Lacerations

Lacerations include tears in blood vessels, at any point from the cervix to the perineum, that cannot be controlled by uterine contractions. Such lacerations account for 5% to 10% of the cases of postpartum hemorrhage and are more likely to occur

- With precipitate labor
- When the fetus is very large
- Following forceps or vacuum extraction delivery

D. Uterine Rupture

Although rare (<1% of cases of postpartum hemorrhage), this occurs most often

- Following precipitate labor in multiparous women
- In patients who had previous uterine surgery (cesarean section, hysterotomy, etc)
- Following difficult forceps or vacuum extraction delivery

E. Abnormal Blood Clotting

Also rare (<1% of the cases of postpartum hemorrhage), coagulopathy most often accompanies a disease known to be associated with DIC, such as abruptio placentae, septic shock, retained dead fetus syndrome, or amniotic fluid embolism.

Other extremely rare inherited bleeding disorders may interfere with blood clotting in affected women. Such conditions almost always will be known before pregnancy, and maternal-fetal medicine specialists and/or hematology experts should be involved in the woman's care throughout pregnancy.

F. Uterine Inversion

This is an extremely rare but potentially devastating complication. It occurs when the uterus turns inside out, with the inverted fundus coming through the cervix into the vagina, and sometimes beyond. Complete prolapse of the uterus can occur. Uterine inversion may be caused by vigorous pulling on a cord that is attached to a placenta implanted at the very top of the fundus. Pulling on the cord may pull the placenta, with the fundus still attached, into the lower uterus, through the cervix, and into the vagina, rather than separate the placenta from the uterine wall. The placenta may separate and be delivered just before the diagnosis of inversion is made, or (especially in cases of inversion with placenta accreta) may remain attached to the inverted fundus.

There may be other, unexplained causes for uterine inversion. Whatever the cause, blood loss can be extremely heavy and shock may ensue. With rapid diagnosis and treatment, hypovolemic shock usually can be avoided.

14. What Should You Do *Routinely* to Prevent or Reduce Postpartum Hemorrhage?

A. Administer Uterotonic Medication

Oxytocin or methylergonovine are used routinely to cause uterine contractions immediately *following* delivery of the placenta, to prevent or reduce postpartum hemorrhage from uterine atony. One of these drugs should be given as soon as the placenta is delivered, but *not before* placental delivery.

If given before delivery of the placenta, increased postpartum hemorrhage may result. This is because the contracting uterus may trap the separated placenta. The bulk of the trapped placenta then prevents the uterus from contracting well enough to close off the bleeding arteries and veins.

1. *Oxytocin*
   a. Give intravenously for patients with an IV line in place.

 Do not give an IV bolus of undiluted oxytocin because hypotension and cardiac arrhythmia can result.

   • Use a dilute solution: 10 to 40 units/1,000 mL of normal saline or lactated Ringer's solution.
   • Infuse at a rate of approximately 100 to 200 mL/hour.
   b. Give intramuscularly for patients without an IV line: 10 to 15 units of oxytocin.

2. *Methylergonovine* (Methergine)
   a. Because of the possible side effects of this drug, it is the second choice to oxytocin.
   • Give intramuscularly: 0.2 mg, 1 dose
   OR
   • Give orally: 0.2 mg, every 4 hours for 24 hours (6 doses)
   b. Methylergonovine is a smooth muscle stimulant and may cause serious adverse effects.

   Venospasm: Blood return to the heart and cardiac output are reduced, and severe hypotension and cardiac arrhythmias can result, which may be fatal for women with symptomatic heart disease.

   Arteriospasm: May cause acute blood pressure elevation, which may be fatal for women with either chronic or pregnancy-specific hypertension.

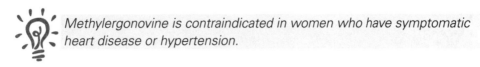
Methylergonovine is contraindicated in women who have symptomatic heart disease or hypertension.

B. Inspect the Placenta

Routinely inspect *every* placenta for missing segments (cotyledons). Do this by holding the placenta in your 2 cupped hands, with the uterine side facing you. If the placenta is torn, it suggests a fragment is retained in the uterus. Manually explore the uterus and retrieve any missing pieces of the placenta.

C. Inspection

After *every* delivery, visually inspect the cervix, vagina, and perineum for lacerations.

D. Provide Intensive Surveillance for First Postpartum Hour

The first hour following delivery, a period sometimes called the "fourth stage" of labor, is when most postpartum hemorrhage occurs. Bleeding may be minimal immediately after delivery, but become massive 20 or 30 minutes later. Intensive monitoring of maternal condition during this immediate postpartum period is recommended for *all* women.

15. How Do You Recognize Postpartum Hemorrhage?

Postpartum hemorrhage usually presents in 1 of 2 ways.

- Large gush of blood and clots (suspect uterine atony).

or

- Steady, slow, unrelenting flow of blood. While not a large amount of blood at one time, the flow is clearly more than usual postpartum bleeding, both in volume and in persistence (suspect retained placental fragments).

16. How Do You Treat Postpartum Hemorrhage?

Treatment requires prompt, coordinated actions of all health care team members to achieve optimal outcome. Precise documentation is also important. Postpartum hemorrhage can occur at any time, even in women with low-risk, uncomplicated pregnancies. Every hospital, including those with relatively few deliveries, needs to be able to respond appropriately and efficiently to this crisis situation.

Adequate response is facilitated when a

- Comprehensive but simple plan of action is established, and is familiar to all team members
- Clear, easily used documentation form is available, and is familiar to all team members

The plan outlined below starts with the most common cause of postpartum hemorrhage and proceeds to less common causes, which generally require more invasive intervention. Some actions will need to be taken simultaneously. Early detection of postpartum hemorrhage is an essential component of treating it. Typical signs of shock may develop so late in some women that death can occur despite emergency intervention and blood transfusion.

Simultaneously with beginning to determine the cause of the hemorrhage, you need to prevent the woman from becoming hypotensive. While beginning to investigate the cause of obstetric hemorrhage, the care team must simultaneously implement clinical resuscitation measures to prevent hypotension and hemorrhagic shock and their potential complications.

- Establish IV access.
- Give volume expansion, as needed. (See Section 3.)
- Send blood for crossmatch.

61

Postpartum hemorrhage is an emergency. Begin treatment at the first evidence of hemorrhage, BEFORE rapid heart rate, hypotension, or other signs of shock develop.

A. Palpate the Uterus

Uterine atony is the most common cause of postpartum hemorrhage and, therefore, should be investigated first.

1. *If the Fundus Is as Firm* and round as a baseball and located at or below the umbilicus, uterine atony is not the problem. Look for another cause, such as retained placental fragment(s) or birth canal laceration.

2. *If the Uterus Is "Boggy,"* with a soft fundus, easily indented by examining fingers and well above the umbilicus, uterine atony is most likely the cause of the bleeding. Fundal massage usually will result in contraction of the uterus.

   a. *First maneuver*
   - *Stabilize the position of the uterus:* Slide one hand over the symphysis pubis and press your fingers into the lower abdomen, below the fundus; keep your fingers firmly pressed in this position to stabilize the uterus and prevent it from being pushed into the pelvis during massage. (Massage is much less effective if the fundus is compressed in the pelvis.)
   - *Massage the top of the fundus:* Use your other hand to massage the fundus to cause it to contract.

   b. *Second maneuver:* If abdominal massage of the fundus does not result in firming and uterine contraction, with marked reduction in bleeding, manual compression of the uterus may be needed.

   - *Continue to massage the fundus:* Keep your hand that is above the umbilicus and massaging the fundus in place. (See first maneuver, above, and Figure 2.2.)
   - *Insert your other hand into the vagina:* Form a fist with that hand.
   - *Compress the uterus against the vaginal fist:* Continue to massage the fundus.

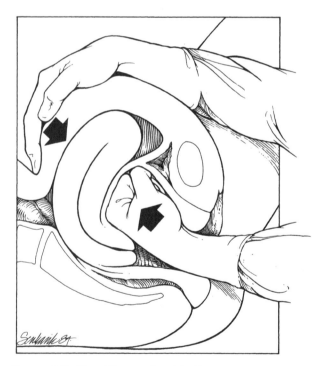

Figure 2.2. Manual Compression of the Uterus.
Reproduced with permission from Gabbe SG, Niebyl JR, Simpson JL. Obstetric hemorrhage. In: Gabbe SG, Niebyl JR, Simpson JL, eds. *Obstetrics: Normal and Problem Pregnancies*. 3rd ed. New York, NY: Churchill Livingstone; 1996:518.

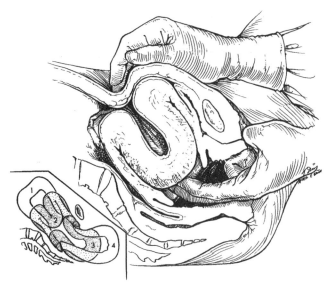

Figure 2.3. Uterine Inversion.
Reproduced with permission from Cunningham FG, MacDonald PC, Gant NF, et al.
Hemorrhage. In: Cunningham FG, MacDonald PC, Gant NF, et al. *Williams Obstetrics.*
20th ed. Stamford, CT: Appleton & Lange; 1997:768.

3. *If the Fundus Cannot Be Found,* consider that uterine inversion may have occurred. The diagnosis is certain if a large, round mass, covered by the shaggy decidual lining of the uterus, is found in the vagina.

Management of uterine inversion varies from the approach used for other forms of postpartum hemorrhage. Response to this uncommon emergency is presented separately, at the end of this section.

Figure 2.3 shows incomplete inversion, comparable to stage 2 in the inset. Round mass of inverted fundus can be felt in the vagina.

The inset shows progression as the uterus turns completely inside-out. In stage 4, the uterus has prolapsed outside the woman's body.

B. Administer Uterotonic Medication

Drugs that cause contraction of uterine muscle should be given. *The only exception is the very rare case of uterine inversion, when uterotonic medication should **not** be given until the uterus is restored to its normal position.*

1. *Begin Infusion of Dilute Oxytocin.*
   - If an oxytocin infusion is already in place for the prevention of postpartum hemorrhage, simply increase the rate of infusion.
   - If an oxytocin infusion is *not* in place, start an IV line. Give a dilute solution of oxytocin, even if the woman received an earlier intramuscular (IM) injection of oxytocin. Use a solution of 10 to 40 units/1,000 mL and infuse at a rate of approximately 100 to 200 mL/hour.

   AND/OR

2. Give misoprostol, 400 to 1,000 μg, sublingual, buccal, or rectal dosing. Vaginal dosing also may be used; however, significant bleeding usually makes this route less than optimal. Mistoprostol may be used in women with hypertension or asthma.

3. *Give Methylergonovine*, 0.2 mg, IM, every 2 to 4 hours.
   Methylergonovine, 0.2 mg, may be given IM. Do *not*, however, give this drug to a woman with hypertension (from any cause) or symptomatic heart disease. (See possible side effects and warnings in Section 14.)

   AND/OR

4. *Give Carboprost Tromethamine* (Hemabate), 250 μg IM or directly into uterine muscle (fundus). This dose may be repeated at 15-minute intervals up to 8 doses. If severe bleeding continues after 2 to 3 doses, however, a hysterectomy is usually necessary.

C. Perform Surgery
   If the actions above do not produce prompt firming of the fundus and decreased bleeding, prepare to go to the operating room to look for uterine rupture and/or birth canal tears.

1. *Prepare for Surgery*
   a. *Continue to hold the uterus out of the pelvis and to massage the fundus.*
   b. *Summon anesthesia staff and surgical personnel.*
   c. *Consider starting a second, or third, IV line* with pump tubing for rapid infusion of additional fluids if bleeding is profuse.
   d. *Send blood for crossmatch* (if not already done), request that at least 4 units of packed red cells be prepared.
   e. *Draw blood samples.*
      • CBC
      • Platelet count
      • PT and PTT
      • Fibrinogen level
      Tape an anticoagulant-free tube to the patient's bedside and check for clot formation every few minutes. (If a clot does not form within 10 to 15 minutes, see management of DIC in Section 9.)
   f. *Discuss the woman's status with her family* (as soon as time permits).

2. *Manual Exploration:* General anesthesia is usually required. In extreme cases, when the woman is moribund from shock, general anesthesia may not be needed. Anesthesia personnel should be continuously available, however, to provide intensive monitoring of vital signs and life-support measures, as needed.
   a. *Explore the vagina and cervix:* Repair lacerations as they are encountered.
   b. *Explore the uterus:* If lacerations were not found, or if found and repaired but bleeding continues from the uterus, examine the uterus.
      • *Search for retained placental fragments.* If found, remove them. If bleeding continues, recheck the uterus.
      • *Search for uterine rupture.* If found, a laparotomy will be necessary to repair it or to remove the uterus to stop the bleeding.

3. *Perform Laparotomy:* If the uterus and vagina have been explored and no lacerations found, or if lacerations were found and repaired but uterine hemorrhage continues, a laparotomy is necessary.
   a. Explore the pelvis for uterine rupture or upward extension of cervical lacerations. If lacerations are found, repair them. If vaginal bleeding persists, the source of the bleeding must be within the uterus. Under these circumstances, a prompt hysterectomy (total or subtotal) may be life-saving.

b. If there are compelling reasons to preserve fertility, however, an attempt can be made to interrupt the main arteries that supply blood to the uterus without removing the uterus itself. Uterine artery ligation is done with large figure-8 stitches taken through the broad ligament at the vesicouterine peritoneal fold and into the wall of the uterus. Care should be taken not to include the ureters in this stitch. If necessary, the utero-ovarian and infundibulopelvic ligaments also may be ligated without sacrificing either the ovaries or the uterus. Ligating these vessels may diminish uterine blood flow sufficiently to slow bleeding enough for clot formation to occur. The remaining uterine blood supply is generally sufficient to allow for future pregnancies.

c. In the past, bilateral ligation of the hypogastric arteries also was used for the purpose of diminishing uterine blood flow in the treatment of postpartum hemorrhage. Ligation of these arteries is more difficult, is more likely to result in complications including ureteral injury, and is not as effective as uterine artery ligation.

d. In the most severe cases, a woman may remain in shock after the vaginal bleeding has been stopped during the hysterectomy. In this situation, a subtotal hysterectomy may be quicker, with less blood loss, than a total hysterectomy. A subtotal hysterectomy involves removal of the fundus, above the point where the uterine arteries have been tied off, leaving the cervix in place.

e. Regardless of the surgical procedure used to control the hemorrhage, the fallopian tubes and ovaries rarely need to be removed.

17. How Do You Manage Uterine Inversion?

Although very rare, when uterine inversion occurs, it is an emergency that requires an immediate, knowledgeable response. Follow the steps described below.

 Do not give uterotonic medication (oxytocin, methylergonovine, misoprostol, or carboprost) until after the uterus is restored to its proper position.

A. Prepare for Surgery; Begin Blood Volume Expansion

Provide management, as outlined previously, for any type of postpartum hemorrhage. Surgery may not be needed but, if it is, it will be an emergency situation, so all preparations and personnel should be in place. If the placenta is still attached, do not remove it until blood volume expansion fluids are being given. Bleeding is likely to worsen as soon as the placenta is separated from the fundus, and continue profusely until the uterus is re-inverted.

B. As Soon as the Placenta Is Separated

Once the placenta is detached, try to re-invert the uterus by placing your fingers in the center of the inverted fundus and pushing inward, trying to push the leading point of the fundus back through the cervix and turning the uterus right-side-out again.

If the cervix and lower uterine segment have contracted to form a tight, unyielding ring so the fundus cannot be pushed back through it, give magnesium sulfate (4 to 6 g intravenously over 5 to 10 minutes) or terbutaline (0.25 mg, IV) for uterine relaxation.

C. If These Maneuvers Do Not Achieve Re-inversion

If attempts at uterine re-inversion fail, administer deep general anesthesia to obtain relaxation of the cervix. Halothane provides optimal uterine relaxation. Attempt again to re-invert the uterus by pushing it back through the cervix.

D. If the Cervix Remains Unyielding

If the cervix remains too tight to allow uterine re-inversion, cut it in the midline posteriorly. Keep traction on the cut edges with ring forceps. Re-invert the uterus and repair the cervical incision.

E. If the Uterus Still Cannot Be Re-inverted Vaginally

If all previous attempts, as outlined above, fail, continue the anesthesia and proceed promptly to surgical intervention with a laparotomy.

Place a figure-8 suture in the highest part of the fundus that can be seen abdominally. With one person pulling on the suture and a second person pushing on the fundus from the vagina, the uterus may return to its normal position.

F. As Soon as the Uterus Is Re-inverted

1. *Give Uterotonic Medications*
   - Begin infusion of dilute oxytocin solution.
   and
   - Give methylergonovine 0.2 mg IM or misoprostol 400 µg.
   Uterotonic medication may inhibit manipulation of the uterus and should not be given until after the uterus has been re-inverted.

2. *Hold the Fundus and Compress the Uterus* until it begins to contract. This will help prevent inversion from occurring again, as well as help control the bleeding until uterine tone is regained. The technique used is the same as shown earlier in the first maneuver for management of uterine atony. If this does not control the bleeding or keep the uterus from re-inverting, use the second maneuver. (See Section 16.)

3. *Repair the Cervical Incision* (if one was made). It may not be possible to do this abdominally. If that is the case, use a vaginal approach.

G. Check Vaginal and Abdominal Examinations

1. Continue examinations for 4 to 6 hours to be sure inversion does not recur.
2. Check at any time if an increase in postpartum bleeding develops.

Self-test

Now answer these questions to test yourself on the information in the last section.

F1.   **True**   **False**   Uterine atony is the most common cause of postpartum hemorrhage.

F2.   **True**   **False**   In an emergency, undiluted oxytocin may be given by intravenous push to stop massive postpartum hemorrhage.

F3.   **True**   **False**   After *every* delivery, the placenta should be inspected for missing segments.

F4.   **True**   **False**   Early detection of postpartum hemorrhage is one of the most important components of treating it.

F5.   **True**   **False**   If uterine inversion occurs with the placenta still attached, the placenta should be removed immediately.

F6.   **True**   **False**   An oxytocin infusion should be started as soon as uterine inversion is recognized.

F7.   What are 4 things that should be done routinely to help prevent postpartum hemorrhage?

_____

_____

_____

F8.   Methylergonovine should not be given to women who have _____ or

_____ .

F9.   Steady, slow, unrelenting flow of blood postpartum suggests _____ .

F10.   List at least 3 causes of postpartum hemorrhage.

_____

_____

_____

F11.   If uterine inversion occurs, uterotonic medication should be given _____ the uterus is restored to its normal position.

Check your answers with the list that follows the Recommended Routines. Correct any incorrect answers and review the appropriate section in the unit.

18. What Needs to Be Documented?

What needs to be documented is the same as the documentation needed for care given in any situation. This can, of course, be extremely difficult when multiple intensive care measures need to be provided simultaneously and rapidly.

As with any response to a life-threatening crisis, your actions and those of other team members in your hospital need to be practiced and rehearsed. Team members may have assigned tasks, so everything gets done and no effort is duplicated. For example, one person is responsible for managing IV lines and fluids, another for medications, another for monitoring vital signs, another for recording the woman's response to therapy and medications, etc.

A flow diagram format with columns of different headings that allow charting of several actions in the same time frame (horizontally across the page), as well as multiple actions over time (vertically down the page), may allow the clearest and most concise format for record keeping. For items that will be repeated, such as blood transfused or CBC results, preprinted headings with those labels allow simple recording of corresponding numbers indicating fluid volume or laboratory values, rather than writing out complete descriptions.

Flow diagrams should minimize the amount of writing needed by having standard columns and labels for common, frequently repeated items, yet do not confuse or obscure the "flow" of care and corresponding patient responses by providing a check-off box for every possible action that might be taken. There should be a column for comments that allow unique items to be noted as they occurred in the sequence of care provided.

Consider including the following:

1. *Delivery:* Time and date

2. *Condition of Patient When Problem Was First Identified*

3. *Therapy*
   - Medication(s): Drug name/dosage/route/time given/response
   - Fluid(s): *Crystalloid:* Type/amount/time given/response
     Blood/blood components: type/amount/time given/response
   - Laboratory: Test(s)/time sent/result(s)
   - Vital signs: Values/time/relation to therapy given

4. *Periodic Reassessment* of patient condition and/or cause of the bleeding

5. *Surgical Intervention*
   - Time decision made, anesthesia and other staff notified
   - Discussion with family
   - Time surgery started
   - Results of exploration: Vagina/cervix/uterus
   - Lacerations repaired, placental fragment(s) retrieved, other surgical repair

6. *Summary*
   - Estimation of total blood loss
   - Urine output
   - Total fluids given: Crystalloid/blood/blood components
   - Patient condition: Findings/therapy/response to therapy
   - Ongoing management plan

Obstetric Hemorrhage

Recommended Routines

All the routines listed below are based on the principles of perinatal care presented in the unit you have just finished. They are recommended as part of routine perinatal care.

Read each routine carefully and decide whether it is standard operating procedure in your hospital. Check the appropriate blank next to each routine.

Procedure Standard   **Needs Discussion**
in My Hospital   **by Our Staff**

_____ _____ 1. Develop a system whereby an emergency cesarean delivery can be started within 30 minutes from the time the decision to operate is made, at any time of the day or night, any day of the week.

_____ _____ 2. Develop a system whereby an emergency hysterectomy can be carried out urgently at any time of day or night, any day of the week.

_____ _____ 3. Establish guidelines for the emergency treatment and stabilization of women with
   • Obstetric hemorrhage of unknown origin
   • Bleeding placenta previa
   • Abruptio placentae
   • Disseminated intravascular coagulation
   • Postpartum hemorrhage

_____ _____ 4. Establish a routine to ensure the prevention and/or early detection of postpartum hemorrhage for _every_ woman, including
   • Administration of uterotonic medication following placental delivery
   • Visual inspection of the placenta
   • Visual inspection of the birth canal
   • Intensive monitoring during first postpartum hour

_____ _____ 5. Establish written instructions for obtaining blood components quickly, 24 hours/day, 7 days/week.

_____ _____ 6. Develop flow diagram(s) for quick and clear recording of events and actions during crisis management of
   • Severe antepartum obstetric hemorrhage
   • Disseminated intravascular coagulation
   • Severe postpartum hemorrhage

Self-test Answers

These are the answers to the self-test questions. Please check them with the answers you gave and review the information in the unit wherever necessary.

A1. • Clear plan of action with staff trained in implementing it
   • Access to adequate blood supplies and technical personnel 24 hours/day, 7 days/week
   • Capability for emergency cesarean delivery or hysterectomy within 30 minutes, 24 hours/day, 7 days/week

A2. Cervix, placenta, vagina, or uterus

A3. Hidden

A4. Shock

A5. True

A6. Yes   No

    X   ____   Get help immediately.
    X   ____   Take blood pressure.
    X   ____   Insert large-bore intravenous lines.
    X   ____   Begin infusion of saline solutions.
    X   ____   Type and crossmatch blood.
    X   ____   Obtain tube of blood; tape it to the patient's bed.
    X   ____   Give oxygen by mask to the pregnant woman.

A7. Any bleeding during pregnancy should be investigated in a hospital, without delay.

B1. True

B2. False. Approximately one-third of the cases of significant late pregnancy bleeding never have a cause identified.

B3. False. Women with abruptio placentae are at high risk for disseminated intravascular coagulation. Disseminated intravascular coagulation rarely occurs with placenta previa.

B4. True

B5. True

B6. False. Undetected cancer of the cervix is a rare but important cause of cervical bleeding.

B7. True

B8. *Placental bleeding:* Placenta previa and abruptio placentae; *cervical bleeding:* chronic cervicitis, cervical polyps or, rarely, cervical cancer, or more rarely, cervical pregnancy; *unknown causes*

B9.

	Placenta Previa	Abruptio Placentae	Neither
Multifetal gestation	X	X (with second twin)	
Acute abdominal trauma		X	
Maternal cocaine use		X	
Maternal diabetes mellitus			X
Uterine fibroids	X	X	
Multiparous woman	X	X	
Occurred in a previous pregnancy	X	X	
Previous cesarean delivery	X		
Maternal hypertension		X	
Abnormal fetal presentation	X		
First pregnancy			X
Short umbilical cord		X	
Maternal smoking		X	
Hydramnios		X (with sudden decompression when membranes rupture)	

C1.
Finding	Placenta Previa	Abruptio Placentae
Blood color	Bright red	Dark red—old clots
Pain	Painless	Painful
Uterine tenderness	Absent	Present
Uterine tone	Normal	Increased—firm, hard, rigid
Shock	Uncommon	Frequent
Disseminated intravascular coagulation	Very rare	Frequent

Note: The chart for C1 shows the classic characteristics of these placental abnormalities. Findings, however, may vary for an individual woman.

C2. If placenta previa is present, the examining finger may disrupt the placental attachment to the lower uterine segment, which may start or worsen bleeding, sometimes with a dramatic increase in the volume of blood lost. A digital examination should not be done until you are certain a previa is not present.

C3. Abruptio placentae is present, with active bleeding and accumulation of blood concealed behind the placenta.

C4. True

C5. True

C6. True

C7. False. Uterine tenderness is usually present with abruptio placentae, but rarely with placenta previa.

C8.
Yes	No	
X	___	Prothrombin time and partial thromboplastin time
X	___	Complete blood count
___	X	Serum electrolytes
X	___	Platelet count
___	X	Blood urea nitrogen and creatinine
X	___	Fibrinogen level

C9. You are willing and completely prepared to perform an immediate cesarean delivery.

D1. True

D2. False. Vaginal delivery is often possible with Grade I abruptions, and may be possible with Grade III.

D3. False. A placenta that covers the cervical os early in pregnancy usually does not cover the os at term.

D4. False. A *falling* platelet count and fibrinogen level are hallmarks of disseminated intravascular coagulation with placental abruption.

D5. True

D6.
Yes	No	
X	___	Preterm delivery may be necessary.
X	___	Placenta accreta may be present and necessitate a hysterectomy after delivery.
___	X	Acute preeclampsia is likely to occur.
X	___	If bleeding occurs, both the mother and the fetus can lose large amounts of blood.
X	___	Postpartum hemorrhage is more likely to occur.
___	X	Disseminated intravascular coagulation is likely to develop.

D7. B

E1. True

E2. False. Any pregnant woman, especially one with disseminated intravascular coagulation, should not be transferred in *unstable* condition.

E3. True

E4. True

E5. 1. Give blood components to provide clotting factors.
    2. Stabilize the woman's condition.
    3. Deliver the baby.

E6. Fresh frozen plasma, cryoprecipitate, and platelets

E7. A. Perform cesarean delivery as soon as platelet count is above 50,000/mm³ and fibrinogen level is above 100 mg/dL.

E8. • Provide neonatal resuscitation, as needed.
  • Assess the baby for signs of acute blood loss.
  • Check blood pressure.
  • Give blood volume replacement, if necessary.
  • Check central (not heelstick) hematocrit soon after delivery.

F1. True

F2. False. Intravenous injection of undiluted oxytocin can cause maternal cardiac arrhythmia and hypotension.

F3. True

F4. True

F5. False. Bleeding is likely to worsen dramatically as soon as the placenta is removed. It should not be removed until just before you begin to try to re-invert the uterus.

F6. False. Oxytocin (or any uterotonic medication) will make the uterus harder to manipulate and should not be given until the uterus has been re-inverted. As soon as the uterus is back in its normal position, begin uterotonic medications.

F7. 1. Give oxytocin and methylergonovine or give misoprostol after delivery of the placenta.
  2. Inspect the placenta for missing pieces.
  3. Inspect the birth canal for tears.
  4. Provide intensive monitoring during first hour after delivery.

F8. Hypertension (from any cause) or symptomatic heart disease

F9. There are retained placental fragments.

F10. Any 3 of the following: Uterine atony, retained pieces of the placenta, birth canal tears, uterine rupture, abnormal maternal blood clotting, or uterine inversion

F11. After

Unit 2 Posttest

If you are applying for continuing education credits, a posttest for this unit is available online. Completion of unit posttests and the book evaluation form are required to achieve continuing education credit. For more details, visit www.cmevillage.com.

Unit 3: Perinatal Infections

Objectives

In this unit you will learn

A. Which infections are particularly important during pregnancy and after delivery

B. What factors govern the effects of infection on a woman, her fetus, and newborn

C. What risks each of the perinatal infections pose to a woman, her fetus, and newborn

D. How each of the perinatal infections is transmitted

E. How each of the perinatal infections is treated

F. Antimicrobial therapy that should, and should not, be used during pregnancy

G. What should be done for the woman, and for the newborn after delivery, if infection is suspected or identified

Note: This unit is a bit different from other units in this book. Unlike the other units, which provide information important in the day-to-day care of women and newborns, many of the infections presented are uncommon, and some are rare.

Information concerning these infections is important, however, because perinatal infections are responsible for a large portion of maternal, fetal, and neonatal mortality and morbidity. Nevertheless, a specific infection may be encountered infrequently, or never, by an individual perinatal care provider.

For this reason, study the unit to learn the essential information, but do not try to memorize the material. Instead, use the unit as a reference.

Material in this unit is intended to be consistent with the *Guidelines for Perinatal Care*, 6th ed, American Academy of Pediatrics and American College of Obstetricians and Gynecologists, 2007; the *Red Book: 2009 Report of the Committee on Infectious Diseases*, 28th ed, American Academy of Pediatrics, 2009; and various statements issued by the Centers for Disease Control and Prevention, the American College of Obstetricians and Gynecologists, and the American Academy of Pediatrics. However, you are also encouraged to consult the most recent version of those documents for any specific infection.

Unit 3 Pretest

Before reading the unit, please answer the following questions. Select the *one* *best* answer to each question (unless otherwise instructed). Record your answers on the test and check them against the answers at the end of the book.

1. Which of the following babies should be isolated from other babies?

Yes	No	
____	____	Baby with congenital rubella infection
____	____	Baby with chlamydial conjunctivitis
____	____	Baby whose mother has untreated gonorrhea at the time of delivery
____	____	Baby with suspected herpes infection
____	____	Congenital cytomegalovirus infection

2. A 32-year-old primigravida has active genital herpes. Her membranes rupture at 38 weeks' gestation. Two hours later, she comes to the hospital, but she is not in labor. What should be done?

   A. Bed rest and antibiotic therapy

   B. Cesarean delivery as soon as possible

   C. Amniocentesis for fetal pulmonary maturity studies

   D. Biophysical profile

3. **True** **False** If a mother is a hepatitis B carrier, the only neonatal treatment available is to isolate the baby from the mother.

4. **True** **False** Positive urine cultures, whether a pregnant woman has symptoms or not, should be treated with appropriate antibiotics.

5. **True** **False** A woman with gonorrhea is at increased risk for premature rupture of the amniotic membranes.

6. **True** **False** Transplacental infection of the fetus always causes congenital malformations.

7. **True** **False** Re-infection is the most common reason sexually transmitted infections recur in a person.

8. **True** **False** Erythromycin ophthalmic ointment will effectively treat chlamydial conjunctivitis in a newborn.

9. **True** **False** Penicillin is the drug of choice for treatment of gonorrhea.

10. **True** **False** If a woman has intra-amniotic infection, the baby is at risk for neonatal sepsis.

11. **True** **False** In general, women with puerperal mastitis may continue to breastfeed as long as antibiotics have been started and an abscess has not formed.

12. All of the following statements about human papillomavirus are correct, *except:*

   A. Women with papillomavirus infection are at increased risk for cervical dysplasia.

   B. Genital papillomas occasionally grow large enough to interfere with vaginal delivery.

   C. Babies born to women with human papillomavirus infection may develop laryngeal papillomas at several years of age.

   D. All genital papillomas should be surgically removed.

13. Which of the following statements about syphilis is *true*?
  A. Babies with congenital syphilis always have a characteristic facial appearance.
  B. Pregnant women with syphilis can pass the infection to their fetuses only during the primary stage of their infection.
  C. Penicillin is the only drug that reliably cures syphilis in the mother and fetus.
  D. Early pregnancy fetal infection rarely results in permanent damage if proper treatment is started soon after birth.

14. Although most babies are born healthy, transplacental infection with parvovirus puts the fetus at risk for
  A. Developing severe anemia
  B. Developing congenital malformations
  C. Becoming a chronic carrier of the virus
  D. Developing thrombocytopenia

15. All of the following statements about group B beta-hemolytic streptococci colonization are correct, *except:*
  A. Neonatal illness is seldom life-threatening.
  B. Risk for postpartum endometritis is increased.
  C. Antibiotics given intravenously to a woman during labor can significantly reduce the likelihood the baby will become infected.
  D. Many women have no symptoms.

16. **True** **False** If an acute toxoplasmosis infection is identified during pregnancy, maternal treatment may reduce transmission to the fetus.

17. **True** **False** Congenital rubella infection in the first trimester frequently causes severe, permanent damage to the fetus.

18. All of the following increase the risk for puerperal endometritis, *except:*
  A. *Chlamydia* infection
  B. Group B beta-hemolytic streptococci colonization
  C. Chorioamnionitis
  D. Hepatitis B infection

19. Which of the following statements about human immunodeficiency virus (HIV) infection is *true*?
  A. All babies born to HIV-positive women will be infected with the virus.
  B. Drug therapy given to an HIV-positive woman during pregnancy and labor, and to the baby after birth, can reduce the number of babies who become infected with the virus.
  C. Women rarely become infected with HIV through injected-drug use and sharing of needles.
  D. Cesarean delivery should be avoided in HIV-positive women.

1. What Are the Risks of Perinatal Infections?

Perinatal infections may cause one or more of the following:

- Maternal illness
  - Permanent damage to one or more organ systems may occur.
  - Chronic disease may develop.
- Maternal death
- Fetal malformations
- Intrauterine growth restriction
- Fetal death
- Premature labor
- Life-threatening neonatal illness

Some infections important in the perinatal period also may cause serious illness in nonpregnant adults and in children. Care should be taken to protect yourself, your coworkers, and other patients from transmission of infectious organisms.

 Observe strict blood and secretion precautions for every delivery.

Standard precautions should be followed at all times, for all patients.

Notify all perinatal personnel (nursing, medical, and support staff) of any suspected or documented maternal infection as soon as it is identified. If the woman or baby will move to another care area after delivery, be sure personnel in that area(s) is aware of the infection, *before* transfer of the mother or the baby.

2. What Factors Govern the Effects of Perinatal Infections?

Fetal effects from maternally acquired infections can vary widely. The following factors work alone, and in combination, to influence the impact an infection has on a fetus or newborn:

- Transmission route
- Gestational age at the time of transmission
- Specific organism
- Individual maternal and/or neonatal resistance
- Degree of maternal illness
- Treatment given
  - A. Transmission Route and Timing
    1. *Transmission Route:* Some infectious agents can be passed from a woman to her fetus or newborn through only one mode of transmission. Other infections can be passed by several routes. Routes of transmission are
       a. *Transplacental:* Organisms in a woman's bloodstream infect the placenta and then enter the fetus's bloodstream. Only a few organisms have the capability of crossing the placenta and infecting the fetus in this way, but those that do often cause devastating effects in the fetus.
       b. *Ascending:* Organisms in a woman's genital tract travel upward, most often after the membranes have ruptured, but occasionally through intact amniotic membranes, and cause infection of the uterus, the membranes (chorioamnionitis), and/or the fetus. This can result in serious fetal and neonatal infection and/or postpartum uterine infection (endometritis).

    c. *Vaginal delivery:* Organisms in the birth canal come in direct contact with the baby and may enter through mucous membranes, breaks in the skin, or the umbilicus.

    d. *Postpartum:* Organisms pass from mother to baby in breast milk or from the mother or other caregivers by any of the ways that infections are passed from person to person (eg, droplet, direct contact).

  2. *Timing of Transmission:* The time during gestation at which infection occurs may influence the effects an organism has on a fetus or newborn. Infection by the same organism at different gestational ages may have different effects.

    Early in pregnancy, when fetal organ systems are forming, transplacental infection may interfere with normal development and result in congenital malformations. Infection with the same organism during late pregnancy may have no effect at all on the fetus, effects that are much less severe, or effects that do not become apparent for months or years.

    Infections acquired at or near the time of delivery (ascending, vaginal delivery, and/or postpartum transmission) will not cause deformities, but may result in life-threatening neonatal sepsis. Neonatal infection in preterm babies is likely to be more severe than infection with the same organism in term babies.

B. Specific Organism and Resistance

  1. *Specific Organism*

    Just as in adults, different organisms cause different illnesses. Fetal or neonatal infection with a specific organism, however, may have manifestations and outcomes that are quite different than adult illness caused by the same organism. Some organisms (particularly viruses) cause mild illness in an adult but may cause congenital malformations and permanent damage to the brain and other organs in a fetus. Other pathogens may be present in a woman's genitourinary tract without causing her to have symptoms, and will not affect fetal development, but may cause life-threatening sepsis in a newborn.

  2. *Immune System Protection*

    a. *Against specific organisms:* During her lifetime, a woman will make antibodies to specific organisms to which she has been exposed. These antibodies may either reduce the severity of or provide protection against subsequent (secondary) infections with the same organism and, therefore, also may protect the fetus if maternal antibodies cross the placenta in sufficient quantities.

    A first-time (primary) maternal infection, during the first trimester, with an organism that can cross the placenta puts the fetus in a particularly hazardous situation. The woman will not have previously developed antibodies against the organism and, therefore, her immune system can offer little protection to herself or her fetus. If fetal infection occurs, it may cause severe, permanent damage, but not all fetuses in this situation become infected. A combination of factors are thought to account for non-infection of some fetuses, including protective properties within the placenta itself.

b. *Passed to the fetus:* Most maternal antibodies cross the placenta during the third trimester, creating some degree of passive immunity for the fetus and newborn. The newborn immune system is not fully functional at birth, with preterm babies having a less effective system than term babies. Maternal antibodies that cross the placenta may help protect the baby during the first 3 to 6 months after birth. By then, the baby's immune system is functioning as effectively as an adult immune system.

Because most maternal antibodies cross the placenta late in pregnancy, babies born before term will not have received maternal antibodies for the same length of time as babies born at term. For these, and other reasons, preterm babies are at higher risk for neonatal infection than term babies (Book III: Neonatal Care, Unit 8, Infections).

C. Maternal Illness

The impact an infection has on a fetus often does not correlate with how sick the pregnant woman is with the infection.

- Serious maternal illness may not affect the fetus, or it may cause indirect effects if the woman has a high fever, becomes dehydrated, or develops systemic complications.
- Mild or asymptomatic viral illness in a woman early in pregnancy may have profound, irreversible effects on the fetus.
- Life-threatening infection in a woman may cause premature labor, even if the infection does not involve the placenta, membranes, or fetus.

D. Treatment Given

Antimicrobial drug therapy is provided for several reasons.

- Treat and cure maternal illness.
- Reduce or prevent maternal signs and symptoms that may affect the fetus.
- Reduce or prevent exposure of the fetus to the infecting organism.
- Minimize effects of infection on the fetus.

Be aware that treatment is *not* available for all perinatal infections. For infections that can be treated, recommendations for specific medications accompany the description of each infection. Medication dosages given in this unit are for use during pregnancy and the immediate postpartum period.

Due to changes in metabolism and expanded blood volume, drug levels are generally lower in pregnant women than in nonpregnant women. All antibiotics cross the placenta to the fetus but in varying amounts, depending on fetal gestational age and the chemical structure of the drug.

Certain antimicrobial medications, or family of drugs, should be *avoided* during pregnancy or lactation, if possible. Use during pregnancy should have individualized consideration of the risks and benefits to the woman and to the fetus. Substitute medications that might provide needed therapy also should be explored. Drugs to avoid are listed in Table 3.1.

Table 3.1. Antimicrobial Medications That Should Be *Avoided* During Pregnancy or Lactation*		
	Possible Adverse Effects	
Drug	**During Pregnancy**	**During Lactation**
Aminoglycosides (especially streptomycin and kanamycin)	May cause eighth cranial nerve damage in fetus (hearing impairment in baby)	Neonatal absorption poor. No known ototoxic effects, but not recommended because drug can affect neonatal GI flora.
Antiviral Amantadine	Association with cardiac defects if given during first trimester	Insufficient data available to make a recommendation.
Ribavirin	Teratogenic and embryotoxic	Insufficient data available to make a recommendation.
Chloramphenicol	May cause "gray baby" syndrome (newborn shock-like state)	Possible bone marrow suppression in baby. Consider discontinuing breastfeeding during maternal therapy.
Fluoroquinolones (ciprofloxacin, etc)	Associated with irreversible arthropathy in animals	Insufficient data available to make a recommendation.
Isoniazid	Acetyl metabolite excreted but no hepatotoxicity reported in babies.	Usually compatible with breastfeeding. Some experts recommend pyridoxine HCl for baby.
Nalidixic acid	Hemolysis in baby with G6PD deficiency	Usually compatible with breastfeeding.
Nitrofurantoin	Hemolysis in baby with G6PD deficiency	Usually compatible with breastfeeding.
Podophyllum	Fetal malformations have been reported	Insufficient data available to make a recommendation.
Sulfonamides	Risk mainly in the third trimester; drug increases the risks of neonatal hyperbilirubinemia by interfering with binding capacity of albumin, thus increasing amount of unbound bilirubin (Book III: Neonatal Care, Unit 7, Hyperbilirubinemia)	Passes into breast milk. Little risk to healthy, term newborns but breastfeeding not recommended for sick or preterm babies until maternal therapy has ended. Caution with G6PD deficiency.
Tetracyclines	Nausea, vomiting, liver disease in woman; stunted growth and (later) teeth stained yellow or brown in child	No restriction to breastfeeding, little or no absorption by baby.
Metronidazole	In vitro mutagen but considered safe during pregnancy.	Discontinue breastfeeding during maternal therapy and for 12-24 hours following single-dose therapy, to allow excretion of drug.

*GI, gastrointestinal; G6PD, glucose-6-phosphate dehydrogenase.

3. How Do You Manage Specific Perinatal Infections?

For sections A and B (that follow), descriptions of specific infections are listed in alphabetical order, according to the most common name of the illness or infecting organism. Infections in section C are listed in chronological order of occurrence (antepartum, intrapartum, postpartum).

A. Sexually Transmitted Infections That May Affect a Fetus

Consider screening *all* pregnant women, even those without symptoms, with cultures or blood tests for common sexually transmitted infections (STIs) (Table 3.3). If an infection is present, maternal treatment may significantly influence neonatal outcome. Be aware that women with one sexually transmitted infection are at high risk for having others.

 If one STI is identified, investigate for others, especially Chlamydia, *gonorrhea, herpes, HIV, and syphilis.*

If an STI that was treated early in pregnancy recurs, take the following steps:
- Reevaluate the treatment that was given.
- Reassess whether all sexual partners were identified.
- Treat or re-treat partners as necessary.
- Re-treat the woman with the same or different medication, depending on your findings, then
  - Retest to see if therapy has been effective.
  - Evaluate the woman for occurrence of nonconsensual sex.

Although failure of treatment does occur (for some infections more often than others), *recurrence of most STIs results most often from reinfection.*

The exceptions are
- *Herpes simplex virus (HSV) or papillomavirus (HPV) infections,* which are likely to recur locally because even optimal treatment does not kill these viruses.

and
- *Human immunodeficiency virus (HIV),* which will persist systemically because treatment may slow progression of the disease but may not eliminate the virus.

Chlamydia

1. *Disease in Women: Chlamydia trachomatis* is the most common reportable STI in the United States. Infected women are often asymptomatic, but may have urethritis or mucopurulent cervical infection. Untreated or recurrent *Chlamydia* infection may lead to premature rupture of membranes (ROM), which significantly increases the risk for preterm birth. Although very unlikely in pregnant women, progression to pelvic inflammatory disease may occur in nonpregnant women, with inflammation and scarring of the fallopian tubes, which may later result in infertility.

2. *Risks for the Fetus and Newborn: C trachomatis* is not known to cross the placenta. About half of the babies born vaginally to infected women will acquire *Chlamydia* organisms during passage through the birth canal. Ascending infection can occur, and some babies born by cesarean delivery with intact membranes will also be infected. Neonatal infection most often takes the form of conjunctivitis, developing at a few days to several weeks of age, but can also present as pneumonia, developing at several weeks or months of age.

Prenatal Considerations
- Consider screening during the first prenatal visit and the third trimester for those women at highest risk, including, but not limited to, women
  - Younger than 25 years, unmarried
  - With new partner or multiple sexual partners
  - With a history of any other STI
- If a woman's *Chlamydia* screen is positive, treat with
  - Azithromycin, 1 g, orally, single dose.

  OR
  - Erythromycin base, 500 mg, orally, every 6 hours for 7 days (or, to reduce gastrointestinal side effects, 250 mg, orally, every 6 hours for 14 days). Retesting 4 to 6 weeks after treatment has ended is recommended.

Note: Erythromycin estolate is contraindicated during pregnancy.

- Test and treat partner(s). Investigate for other STIs.
- Consider retesting by culture 3 weeks after completion of antibiotic therapy.

Intrapartum Considerations
- If antibiotic treatment was started earlier but is not yet complete, continue treatment.

Postpartum Considerations
Maternal
- Reassess maternal treatment, and be sure it is adequate prior to discharge.
- Women with inadequately treated infection have an increased risk for postpartum endometritis. Onset may be soon after delivery or not for 1 to 2 weeks.
- Investigate need to treat partner(s).

Neonatal (See also Book III: Neonatal Care, Unit 8, Infections.)
- Babies born to women with untreated or incompletely treated *Chlamydia* infection should be monitored for development of disease. Prophylactic antibiotics are *not* recommended; neither is cesarean delivery.
- Topical treatment of chlamydial conjunctivitis is ineffective. If chlamydial conjunctivitis or pneumonia develop, systemic antibiotics are needed. Give oral erythromycin 50 mg/kg in 4 divided doses for 14 days.
- Erythromycin is only about 80% effective, so a second course of antibiotics may be needed. Infant follow-up is recommended.

 Routine prophylactic eye treatment with ophthalmic preparations of erythromycin, tetracycline, or silver nitrate used to prevent gonococcal eye infection will not reliably prevent chlamydial conjunctivitis.

Gonorrhea

1. *Disease in Women:* Infection is passed by sexual contact and is highly contagious. Minimal vaginitis or urethritis, with or without discharge, may be the only symptom(s). Untreated maternal infection may lead to premature ROM, which significantly increases the risk for preterm birth. Progression to pelvic inflammatory disease may occur, but is very unlikely during pregnancy. Although rare, systemic disease with arthritis, high fever, and abdominal pain from liver involvement can occur.

2. *Risks for the Fetus and Newborn: Neisseria gonorrhoeae* bacteria do not cross the placenta. Transmission to the baby usually occurs during passage through the vagina. Although rare, ascending infection also can occur through either intact or ruptured membranes, and cause chorioamnionitis. Neonatal infection is usually confined to the eye (if untreated, can cause blindness), but can (rarely) become a life-threatening systemic disease, affecting multiple organs.

Prenatal Considerations
- Consider testing for gonorrhea as a routine part of the first prenatal visit for *all* pregnant women.
- Obtain testing early in pregnancy, and consider testing again during the third trimester, and at delivery, for women at high risk for gonococcal infection or reinfection, especially women who
  – Are 19 years or younger
  – Have recently been diagnosed with another STI.
  – Had early onset of sexual activity or multiple sexual partners
    and/or
  – Are substance users
- Infection with penicillin-resistant organisms is common. Therefore, treatment with an extended spectrum (third generation) cephalosporin is recommended as initial therapy for all patients. Use one of the following:
  – Ceftriaxone, 125 mg, intramuscularly, single dose (preferred because of its effectiveness in treating all infection sites, including the pharynx)
  OR
  – Spectinomycin, 2 g, intramuscularly, single dose (for those who cannot tolerate a cephalosporin)
- When gonorrhea is present, azithromycin or erythromycin treatment for *Chlamydia* is also recommended. (*Chlamydia* infection is common and may be presumed to be present.)
- Although test-of-cure is not routinely done for uncomplicated gonorrhea, it is recommended for pregnant women.
- Test and treat partner(s). Investigate for other STIs.

Intrapartum Considerations
- If the woman is inadequately treated at the time of labor, use internal fetal monitoring judiciously because a scalp abscess may develop at the site the electrode is attached.

Postpartum Considerations
Maternal
- Risk for endometritis is increased if active infection is present at the time of delivery. Give a single dose of ceftriaxone, intramuscularly, soon after delivery.
- Reassess maternal treatment and be sure it is adequate prior to discharge.
- Investigate need to treat partner(s).

Neonatal (See also Book III: Neonatal Care, Unit 8, Infections.)
- Give mandatory prophylactic eye treatment to *all* newborns (whether mother infected or not, whether cesarean or vaginal birth) with ophthalmic preparation of 1% tetracycline, 0.5% erythromycin, or 1% silver nitrate *to prevent* gonococcal ophthalmia neonatorum. Infection can cause blindness.

Do not irrigate eyes after instillation. After 1 minute, excess medication may be wiped away with sterile cotton.

- If maternal gonococcal infection is active at the time of delivery, give the baby a single dose of
  – Ceftriaxone, 25 to 50 mg/kg (not to exceed 125 mg) intravenously or intramuscularly
- If infection develops, topical antibiotic therapy will *not treat* it adequately. Systemic antibiotics are needed for treatment. The baby should be hospitalized for complete evaluation and treatment.

Herpes Simplex Virus (either Type 1 or Type 2 virus)

1. *Disease in Women:* Herpes simplex virus infection is extremely common, with estimates that 16% of adults in the United States are infected, with most unaware of their infection. The virus, once acquired, remains for the person's lifetime. It may be latent and asymptomatic for long periods, broken by episodes of recurrence of symptoms. First infection often causes painful genital vesicles. Recurrent infection is usually less symptomatic. Asymptomatic viral shedding is common in men and women, with most herpes infections transmitted by sexual contact during asymptomatic periods.

2. *Risks for the Fetus and Newborn:* Transplacental transmission is rare, but can occur at any time during pregnancy. Transmission is usually by direct contact with lesions or virus shed from the cervix or lower genital tract during passage through the birth canal, although ascending infection also can occur, even through intact membranes. Risk of transmission to the newborn during vaginal delivery is much lower for recurrent (1% to 2%) than for primary infections (33% to 50%). Neonatal herpes infection carries a high risk of mortality and severe damage, in the survivors, even when antiviral therapy is given. Presentation is split about equally among
   - Disseminated disease involving multiple organs, particularly lungs and liver
   - Disease localized to the central nervous system
   - Disease localized to the skin, eyes, and mouth

Prenatal Considerations

- If symptoms or lesions occur during pregnancy, obtain cultures from the vagina and cervix and, if present, from the lesions.
- Clinical evaluation, viral culture, and type-specific (HSV-1 or HSV-2) serology are important for disease classification and, therefore, patient management. Clinical evaluation alone is frequently unable to detect infection.
- Oral acyclovir or valacyclovir is used to treat initial or recurrent infection. Treatment may be episodic or suppressive therapy. Consultation should be considered.
- Prophylactic treatment with acyclovir in late pregnancy reduces the number of recurrences at term, and reduces the need for cesarean delivery.
- Intravenous (IV) acyclovir is used for patients with complicated or severe infection.
- Treatment with topical acyclovir ointment is ineffective.
- Undertake a discussion of the risks and benefits of vaginal versus cesarean delivery for HSV-positive women, in light of the woman's HSV clinical findings.

Optimal prenatal, intrapartum, and neonatal care depends on identification of maternal infection as primary, nonprimary first episode, or recurrent episode. Consultation with regional center experts is recommended.

Intrapartum Considerations
- Vaginal delivery is recommended, if no active genital lesions can be detected.
- Cesarean delivery is recommended whenever a woman has clinically apparent HSV disease when labor begins.
- If membranes rupture at or near term in a woman with active genital HSV infection, *prompt* cesarean delivery is recommended.
- There is no evidence that there is a duration of rupture of membranes beyond which the fetus does not benefit from cesarean delivery. At any time after rupture of membranes, cesarean delivery is recommended.
- Appropriate management with preterm premature ROM, fetal lung immaturity, and active maternal HSV infection is unclear. Some experts recommend IV acyclovir in this situation. Consult with regional center specialists.
- Avoid internal fetal monitoring whenever possible in women suspected of having active genital herpes.
- If active lesions, genital or nongenital, are present, contact precautions (in addition to standard precautions) should be used during labor, delivery, and postpartum care.

Postpartum Considerations
Maternal
- If maternal lesions are present, the baby may room-in with the mother as long as *good hand-washing* technique is used and maternal lesions are covered with a clean barrier. Educate parents and caregivers about the importance of good hand washing at home.
- If there are no breast lesions, the mother may breastfeed.
- If cold sores are present, the mother should use caution to avoid transmission of the virus to her baby until the lesions have crusted and dried. Such cautions may include not kissing the baby and careful hand hygiene, especially at the time of diaper changing.

Neonatal (See also Book III: Neonatal Care, Unit 8, Infections.)
- Symptoms of systemic or central nervous system infection may be present shortly after birth, or not appear until 4 to 6 weeks of age. Infected babies may or may not develop skin lesions during the neonatal period.
- Because the risk of neonatal HSV infection ranges from less than 5% to more than 50%, depending on whether maternal infection is recurrent or primary, experts disagree about the best neonatal treatment course. Some experts use IV acyclovir to treat all babies, whether symptomatic or not, born to women with active herpes; other experts wait for culture results.

In some situations, determination of maternal HSV serologic status may be helpful in decision making for neonatal management. Consult experts.

- *Immediate IV* acyclovir treatment is generally recommended for
  - Any baby born to an HSV-positive mother who develops symptoms suggestive of HSV infection, such as scalp rashes or vesicles, seizures, respiratory distress, or signs of sepsis
  - Any baby with a positive HSV culture from any site, even if the baby is asymptomatic
- Obtain urine, stool or rectum, mouth or nasopharynx, skin lesions (if present), blood, and eye culture specimens (consider cerebrospinal fluid culture) for HSV 24 to 48 hours after birth from any baby born to a woman with active genital herpes, whether the baby was born vaginally or by cesarean section.
- Isolate any newborn suspected of being infected from all other babies and pregnant women. A private room for the mother, with continuous rooming-in, is one way to accomplish this. Use standard precautions, as well as contact precautions if lesions are present.
- Late-onset HSV can occur. Consider delaying circumcision for a month in boys born vaginally to women with active genital lesions because herpes infection is more likely to occur at a site of skin trauma.
- Teach the parents about signs of late-onset neonatal herpes infection, including rash or skin lesions, respiratory distress, seizures, and/or general signs of illness, and to seek *immediate* care if any signs develop.

Most babies who develop herpes infection are born to women with asymptomatic or unrecognized HSV infection.

Consultation with regional center experts regarding neonatal management of a baby with potential or suspected HSV infection is recommended.

Self-test

Now answer these questions to test yourself on the information in the last section.

A1. In the following list, match each condition or situation on the left with the best choice on the right.

    ____ Mother with *Chlamydia*   a. Ceftriaxone for mother and baby

    ____ Mother with active genital herpes   b. Cesarean delivery

    ____ Mother with active gonorrhea   c. Asymptomatic maternal infection

A2. **True** **False** The risk of premature rupture of membranes and preterm birth is increased when a pregnant woman has gonorrhea.

A3. **True** **False** Neonatal herpes infection is life-threatening.

A4. **True** **False** When a pregnant woman has an infection, any organism in her bloodstream will cross the placenta and also infect the fetus.

A5. **True** **False** Internal fetal heart rate monitoring should be avoided with maternal gonorrhea.

A6. **True** **False** Ascending infection can occur only after rupture of membranes.

A7. **True** **False** Silver nitrate or certain ophthalmic antibiotic ointments are used to treat neonatal gonorrheal ophthalmia.

A8. **True** **False** Women with untreated *Chlamydia* infection have an increased risk for developing endometritis postpartum.

A9. **True** **False** Routine prophylactic eye medications given to prevent gonorrheal ophthalmia will also prevent neonatal chlamydial conjunctivitis.

A10. **True** **False** A newborn suspected of being infected with herpes simplex virus should be isolated from other newborns.

A11. **True** **False** Infection by the *same* organism at different gestational ages may have different effects on the fetus.

A12. **True** **False** The degree of maternal illness corresponds directly with how seriously an infection will affect a fetus.

A13. If maternal gonorrheal infection is present, you should investigate for the presence of

Yes	No	
____	____	Toxoplasmosis
____	____	Syphilis
____	____	*Chlamydia*
____	____	Parvovirus
____	____	Herpes
____	____	HIV

Check your answers with the list that follows the Recommended Routines. Correct any incorrect answers and review the appropriate section in the unit.

Human Immunodeficiency Virus

1. *Disease in Women:* Women with a history of any STI (syphilis, genital herpes, gonor-rhea, and/or *Chlamydia*) are at increased risk for HIV infection for 2 reasons.
   - The occurrence of one STI indicates that either the woman and/or her partner(s) has had an additional partner(s), thus increasing the risk of exposure to HIV.
   - Local inflammation of genital tissue may create a relatively easy portal of entry for the virus.
     Pregnancy itself demonstrates a history of unprotected sexual intercourse. Unprotected intercourse is a common route of HIV transmission to women.

     Sharing of needles by injected-drug users is also a common route of HIV transmission. It accounts for about half of all infections in women.

    Because of the extremely complex, and rapidly changing, management needed for maternal/fetal and neonatal HIV disease, consultation with regional center experts is strongly recommended.

   In addition, refer to recommendations from the Centers for Disease Control and Prevention (www.cdc.gov) and the National Institutes of Health (www.aidsinfo.nih.gov).

2. *Risks for the Fetus and Newborn:* Fetal HIV infection is associated with fetal death, fetal growth restriction, and preterm birth. In addition, HIV-positive women are more likely to have other infections or risk factors that may jeopardize maternal health and/or fetal development. Precise time of transmission from an infected woman to her baby is uncertain, but evidence suggests that (in the absence of breastfeeding), 30% occurs before birth but late in pregnancy and 70% occurs around the time of delivery. The risk of transmission is significantly increased when maternal viral load is greater than 100,000 copies/mL.

   Both antibodies and the virus can cross the placenta. All babies (100%) born to HIV-positive women will test positive for HIV antibodies at birth. Without maternal treatment, 15% to 25% of babies will be infected with the virus.

   Neonatal HIV infection is markedly lower when HIV-positive women receive zidovudine therapy during pregnancy and labor and their babies receive zidovudine treatment after birth. With zidovudine treatment during all 3 perinatal periods (prenatal, intrapartum, and postnatal), the number of babies born to HIV-infected women who become infected is reduced to 5% to 8%.

    Zidovudine therapy for HIV-positive women dramatically reduces the risk of neonatal infection.

   Depending on the viral load, the risk of neonatal infection can be reduced to as low as approximately 2% when cesarean delivery is performed prior to labor or rupture of membranes, whether or not the woman is receiving zidovudine therapy.

Prenatal Considerations
   - Women without known risk factors may be infected with HIV. They may not feel ill and not be aware they are infected until neonatal HIV is diagnosed.

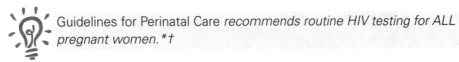

Guidelines for Perinatal Care *recommends routine HIV testing for ALL pregnant women.*†

Extensive pretest counseling and informed consent may be a barrier to universal prenatal HIV testing. The American College of Obstetricians and Gynecologists (ACOG) recommends HIV screening for all pregnant women after they are notified that they will be tested as part of the routine panel of prenatal blood tests unless they decline the test (ie, opt-out screening). The American Academy of Pediatrics (AAP) also endorses the recommendation of the Institute of Medicine for universal (routine) testing, with notification. Know your state's laws because this recommendation may conflict, in some states, with laws governing consent for testing.

- Women at highest risk for HIV infection include, but are *not* limited to
  – Drug users (IV, intramuscular, intradermal routes) or those who exchange sex for money or drugs.
  – Women exposed to contaminated blood. (Blood or blood products after 1983 are *extremely* unlikely to carry HIV, but a minuscule risk still exists.)
  – Women with a history of any other STIs.
  – Women who have had a new or more than one sex partner during this pregnancy.
  – Partners of men who engage in high-risk behaviors (drug use, multiple partners, same-sex partners, etc).
  – Partners of men who are HIV-positive.
- If HIV is found, test for syphilis and other STIs, and for tuberculosis. An HIV-positive individual is at increased risk for other infections, which should be treated immediately and, in some cases, prophylactically.
- Establish gestational age as early and accurately as possible using ultrasound and clinical findings. Avoid amniocentesis at any time during pregnancy.
- Obtain baseline plasma viral-RNA load (number of viral-RNA copies per milliliter of plasma) and again every 3 months during pregnancy.
- Highly active antiretroviral therapy (HAART) used routinely for nonpregnant adults is highly effective in suppressing HIV viral-RNA load. HAART is generally recommended during pregnancy too.
  – Provide zidovudine therapy of 200 mg 3 times a day or 300 mg twice a day, starting at 14 to 34 weeks and continuing throughout pregnancy.
  PLUS
  – Another nucleoside analog, such as zalcitabine, didanosine, stavudine, lamivudine, or abacavir.
  PLUS
  – A protease inhibitor, such as indinavir, ritonavir, or saquinavir — OR — a non-nucleoside analog, such as nevirapine, delavirdine, or efavirenz.

---

*American Academy of Pediatrics, American College of Obstetricians and Gynecologists. Antepartum care. In: Lockwood CJ, Lemons JA, eds. *Guidelines for Perinatal Care*. 6th ed. Elk Grove Village, IL: 2007;84.
†American Academy of Pediatrics. Human immunodeficiency virus infection. In: Pickering LK, Baker CJ, Kimberlin DW, Long SS, eds. *Red Book: 2009 Report of the Committee on Infectious Diseases*. 28th ed. Elk Grove Village, IL: American Academy of Pediatrics; 2009:391.

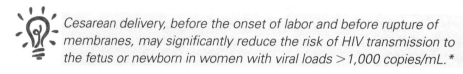
*Cesarean delivery, before the onset of labor and before rupture of membranes, may significantly reduce the risk of HIV transmission to the fetus or newborn in women with viral loads >1,000 copies/mL. ***

- Aggressive antiviral therapy may reduce the risk of HIV transmission to the fetus to as low as 2%. No combination of therapies can guarantee that a newborn will not become infected.
- As early in pregnancy as possible, to allow time for adequate consideration, provide information regarding the risks and benefits of vaginal or scheduled cesarean delivery to all HIV-positive women, whether or not they are taking zidovudine.
  - Maternal morbidity is higher with cesarean delivery than with vaginal delivery, whether or not a woman is HIV-positive. Preoperative maternal health affects the degree of maternal risk associated with surgery.
  - Decision making about delivery route needs to include the woman and to weigh the benefits to the newborn versus maternal health status and risks.
  - HIV-positive women with high plasma viral load (>1,000 copies/mL) are at highest risk for transmission of the virus to their fetuses and newborns. The babies of these women seem to benefit the most from scheduled cesarean delivery. It has not been shown that babies of women with plasma viral load less than 1,000 copies/mL benefit from scheduled cesarean birth.
  - Benefit to the newborn is unknown if cesarean delivery is undertaken after the onset of labor.

Intrapartum Considerations
- If labor starts spontaneously and is allowed to continue, or vaginal delivery is the woman's chosen delivery route,
  - Do not use internal fetal monitoring.
  - Do not perform artificial rupture of the membranes. Rupture of membranes 4 hours or less before delivery has been associated with a significantly lower rate of neonatal HIV infection than when membranes were ruptured for longer than 4 hours.
- Although not as effective as zidovudine therapy started earlier in pregnancy, IV zidovudine during labor has been shown to reduce neonatal HIV infection.
- Intrapartum dosage is the same, regardless of when zidovudine therapy is initiated.
  - Give a 1-hour loading dose of 2 mg/kg intravenously.
  - Follow with a continuous IV infusion of 1 mg/kg per hour until delivery.
- The American College of Obstetricians and Gynecologists recommends that scheduled cesarean deliveries in HIV-positive women be performed at 38 completed weeks of gestation to reduce the likelihood of onset of labor or rupture of membranes before delivery.
  - Provide IV zidovudine prophylaxis, starting 3 hours before surgery to achieve adequate drug levels.
  - Consider giving prophylactic antibiotic therapy to reduce the risk of postpartum maternal infection.

---

*Committee on Obstetric Practice, American College of Obstetricians and Gynecologists. Committee Opinion #234, *Scheduled Cesarean Delivery and the Prevention of Vertical Transmission of HIV Infection.* May 2000.

Postpartum Considerations
Maternal

- Human immunodeficiency virus can be transmitted in breast milk. In the United States, breastfeeding is contraindicated in HIV-positive women, where safe, affordable, and feasible newborn feeding alternatives are available and culturally acceptable. Rooming-in is appropriate.
- Inform neonatal care providers of a mother's HIV status. Know the laws in your state, however, because some states require a mother's written consent before this information can be given to anyone not a part of her own health care team, including neonatal care providers.

Neonatal

- For babies born to mothers with unknown HIV status, rapid HIV antibody testing of the mother and/or baby is recommended as soon as possible after birth, with initiation of infant antiretroviral prophylaxis immediately if the rapid test is positive.
- Continue zidovudine treatment (if mother was treated), or begin treatment of the baby within 8 to 12 hours of birth. Give oral syrup, 2 mg/kg per dose, every 6 hours for the first 6 weeks after birth.

 Even without maternal zidovudine therapy, or scheduled cesarean delivery, zidovudine treatment of the baby can significantly reduce neonatal HIV infection.

- Test babies born to HIV-positive women with HIV RNA or DNA polymerase chain reaction assay during the first 48 hours after birth to try to identify in utero HIV transmission. Test again at 1 to 2 months, although testing at 14 days may aid in decision making about antiretroviral therapy. Early antiviral therapy is indicated for most HIV-infected babies. Consult www.aidsinfo.nih.gov for

  1. Further information about testing and requirements for confirmation of either HIV-positive or HIV-negative status in perinatally exposed babies
  2. Treatment recommendations

- Begin *Pneumocystis carinii* pneumonia prophylaxis at age 4 to 6 weeks for all babies born to HIV-positive women, regardless of the baby's CD4+ T lymphocyte count. Consult www.aidsinfo.nih.gov for additional guidelines for prevention and treatment of other opportunistic infections, such as cytomegalovirus (CMV), *Toxoplasma gondii*, and other organisms.
- Arrange for comprehensive follow-up care for HIV-positive babies, their mothers, and their families.
- ***Information changes rapidly. Consult with regional center experts and refer to www.cdc.gov and www.aidsinfo.nih.gov.***
- The effects of antiviral medications on the fetus and newborn are unknown. Long-term follow-up of babies born to women treated during pregnancy with antiretroviral drugs is recommended, as is reporting of these women and their newborns to the Antiretroviral Pregnancy Registry (800/258-4263 or www.apregistry.com). Follow-up of children with antiretroviral exposure should continue into adulthood.

Human Papillomavirus

1. *Disease in Women:* There are numerous papillomaviruses, several of which cause warts on skin and mucous membranes. The genital variety is called condylomata acuminata. Genital HPV transmission is primarily by sexual contact, with infection being common (up to 40% of sexually active women), and may persist for life or be transient and clear spontaneously. Typically, there are no symptoms with cervical or vaginal HPV infection, but the infection is associated with several cancers. About 90% of cervical cancers and considerable numbers of vulvar, anal, and penile cancers are associated with HPV. Papanicolaou smear can detect the cervical dysplasia typical of HPV infection. Other tests can more specifically detect several types of HPV DNA in cervical cell samples.

   Warty lesions on the perineum may grow rapidly during pregnancy. Occasionally, but rarely, condyloma masses grow large enough to interfere with vaginal delivery. Extensive condylomata also may severely limit distensibility of the vagina and, therefore, carry the risk of vulvovaginal lacerations, with profuse bleeding.

   Current recommendations for HPV vaccination may reduce infection rates in women, and exposure to neonates. Vaccination is recommended outside of pregnancy. If a woman becomes pregnant during the vaccination schedule, it is recommended that she delay completion until after delivery.

2. *Risks for the Fetus and Newborn:* HPV does not cross the placenta. The fetus is unaffected by maternal infection. There is a small risk that, over months or years, a baby exposed to HPV during vaginal delivery may develop laryngeal papillomas as a result of aspiration of infectious secretions.

Prenatal Considerations
- Elimination of the lesions that result from HPV infection is the treatment target, rather than elimination of the virus. Most methods use chemical or physical destruction, but lesions often recur.
- During pregnancy, genital warts may proliferate because of relative immune suppression. Treatment may be delayed until postpartum to evaluate the degree of spontaneous resolution.

Intrapartum Considerations
- Because the risk of laryngeal papillomas is very low, cesarean delivery is not indicated to protect the baby from infection. Cesarean delivery may be necessary, however, if the size or location of condylomas obstruct vaginal delivery or threaten hemorrhage from lacerations.
- Notify pediatric staff of maternal infection so follow-up of the baby for possible laryngeal papillomas can be arranged.

Postpartum Considerations
Maternal
- Provide follow-up for cervical dysplasia. Routine cervical cytologic study (Pap smear) is adequate.

Neonatal (See also Book III: Neonatal Care, Unit 8, Infections.)
- Neonates born to women with HPV do not need to be managed with special precautions in the nursery.

Syphilis

1. *Disease in Women:* In the United States, rates of infection are highest in large urban areas, the rural south, and HIV-infected adults.

   • *Primary Stage:* Chancre (painless ulcer) develops at the site of infection within *weeks* of exposure. While the chancre is present, the disease is highly contagious to sexual partners, or to anyone who comes in direct contact with the lesion. Chancres last 4 to 10 weeks, then heal spontaneously.

   • *Secondary Stage:* Systemic disease with widespread rash (including palms and soles), fever, general malaise, lymphadenopathy, and splenomegaly develops 1 to 2 *months* after the initial infection, and may last for months. The infected person may have several episodes of illness before the disease becomes latent. A flat-appearing condyloma (condylomata lata) may develop on the vulvar-perineal area as a sign of secondary syphilis. Syphilis can be passed to sexual partners at any time, whether the disease is active or latent.

   • *Tertiary Stage:* Involvement of the central nervous system, skin, bones, and visceral organs becomes apparent *years or decades* after the primary infection, and follows secondary stage syphilis and a subsequent asymptomatic latent period of variable duration. Sexual partners can be infected, but the rate of transmission is lower than during the primary stage.

   Transplacental passage of the spirochete *Treponema pallidum* can cause spontaneous abortion, fetal death, or congenital syphilis. During the primary stage, transmission to the fetus occurs in approximately half of infected pregnant women and results in a high rate of fetal loss. Transplacental transmission during the secondary stage is 60% to 100%. Transplacental infection of the fetus declines as the duration of infection lengthens and, during the tertiary stage, occurs in only about 10% of infected pregnant women.

    Transmission to the fetus can occur at any stage of maternal syphilis infection.

2. *Risks for the Fetus and Newborn:* Fetal infection may involve multiple organs as well as cause fetal growth restriction and nonimmune hydrops. It significantly increases the risk of preterm birth. Congenital syphilis can cause varying degrees of damage to heart, spleen, liver, lung, bone, cartilage, skin, and brain tissue. Some consequences of congenital syphilis, such as eighth cranial nerve deafness, may take years to become apparent. The infection may present at birth as rhinitis or more severe respiratory distress, with skin rash, hepatosplenomegaly, anemia, and fever. Some babies will display the characteristic facial appearance (broad, flat face and nose), physical, and x-ray findings of congenital syphilis. Many infected babies, however, have normal appearance and no symptoms.

   Congenital syphilis in an infected but untreated baby may not become apparent for 2 years or longer. During this time, however, serious, irreversible damage may be done to the central nervous system, bones, teeth, eyes, and other organs.

Prenatal Considerations

- Screen *all* pregnant women for syphilis with a nontreponemal serologic test at the first prenatal visit and, among those at high risk again at 28 to 36 weeks. Test and treat partner(s).
- Use Venereal Disease Research Laboratory (VDRL), rapid plasma reagin, or automated reagin test for screening tests. Confirm positive results with a test specific for *Treponema* (florescent treponemal antibody absorption or microhemagglutination test for *T pallidum*).
- If a woman tested positive for syphilis early in pregnancy, or is at high risk for infection/reinfection, rescreen again at 28 weeks' gestation.
- *All* women who have syphilis should be tested for HIV infection and investigated for other STIs.
- Treat with penicillin. (See footnote in Table 3.2.) Treatment with erythromycin is *not* recommended because it does not adequately treat the fetus.
- Wear gloves if lesions are present until 24 hours of treatment have been completed.

 Only penicillin reliably cures syphilis in both the mother and fetus.

Intrapartum Considerations

- If genital lesions are present, the baby may become infected through direct contact during delivery.
- If a woman was not tested prenatally, or is at risk for reinfection, test and begin treatment if results are positive.
- If a woman has a positive test for syphilis, notify pediatrics so treatment of the baby can begin promptly.

Table 3.2. Penicillin Treatment of Syphilis During Pregnancy*	
Disease Stage	**Treatment**
<1-year duration† (primary or secondary stage)	Benzathine Penicillin G 2.4 million units, IM,‡ 1 dose
>1-year or unknown duration (secondary stage)	Benzathine Penicillin G 2.4 million units, IM 1 dose per week for 3 weeks
Neurosyphilis (tertiary stage)	Aqueous Crystalline Penicillin G 3-4 million units, IV every 4 hours for 10-14 days *then give* Benzathine Penicillin G 2.4 million units, IM 1 dose per week for 3 weeks

*If a woman is allergic to penicillin, she should be desensitized to it, then treated with it. Desensitization is complicated, time-consuming, and potentially hazardous. Consult with infectious disease specialists. About 3% to 6% of women allergic to penicillin, and, therefore, at risk for a fatal reaction, are not identified with the usual hypersensitivity testing. Use penicillin cautiously whenever penicillin-allergic status is unknown.

†Some experts recommend 2 doses of benzathine penicillin (2.4 million units, IM), given 1 week apart.

‡IM, intramuscularly.

Postpartum Considerations
Maternal
- Reassess maternal treatment and be sure it is adequate prior to discharge.
- Investigate need to treat partner(s).
- Mother may breastfeed if her infection was adequately treated or she is currently receiving adequate antibiotic therapy.
- Check VDRL titer at 3, 6, 9, 12, and 24 months postpartum. Re-treat if
  - Clinical signs persist or recur.
  - Sustained 4-fold increase in titer occurs.
  - Initially high titer fails to decrease 4-fold within 3 to 6 months.
- Teach the parent(s) that the baby will need to be
  - Evaluated at 1, 2, 4, 6, and 12 months of age.
  - Retested 3, 6, and 12 months after treatment is finished.
  - Depending on the results, re-treatment may be necessary.

Neonatal (See also Book III: Neonatal Care, Unit 8, Infections.)

 No newborn should be discharged from a hospital without determination of the mother's serologic status for syphilis. *

- Testing of cord blood or newborn sera is *not* adequate for syphilis screening because these tests can be nonreactive when the mother is positive.
- False-positive and false-negative test results can occur. Maternal and neonatal test results need to be interpreted jointly. Review the chart in Book III: Neonatal Care, Unit 8, Infections, for comprehensive interpretation guidelines.
- Infected newborns can be severely ill or completely asymptomatic at birth. Even if asymptomatic, consider body fluids infectious until 24 hours after drug therapy has started. Parents, visitors, and health care providers should wear gloves to handle the baby for any reason during that time.
- Treat infected baby with penicillin according to guidelines given in Table 8.4 in Book III: Neonatal Care, Unit 8, Infections.
- Arrange for follow-up examinations and testing.

---

*American Academy of Pediatrics, American College of Obstetricians and Gynecologists. Perinatal infections. In: Lockwood CJ, Lemons JA, eds. *Guidelines for Perinatal Care*. 6th ed. Elk Grove Village, IL: American Academy of Pediatrics; 2007;340.

Table 3.3. Sexually Transmitted Infections That May Affect a Fetus

Infection	Transmission		Isolation	Notes
Recommended Screening	Woman	Fetus/Newborn (delivery = vaginal route)	Standard Precautions (all patients, at all times)	(See Book III: Neonatal Care, Unit 8, Infections, for more details of neonatal care.)
Chlamydia (Chlamydia trachomatis) All high-risk women.	• Sexual contact *Significantly increases risk of preterm birth*	*Transplacental:* no *Ascending:* rarely *Delivery:* yes, direct contact with organisms in genital tract	Isolation not needed for mother or baby.	Routine prophylactic eye treatment used to prevent gonococcal eye infection will *not* reliably prevent chlamydial conjunctivitis. If infection, systemic erythromycin is needed.
Gonorrhea *(Neisseria gonorrhoeae)* All women.	• Sexual contact *Significantly increases risk of preterm birth*	*Transplacental:* no *Ascending:* rarely *Delivery:* yes, direct contact with organisms in genital tract	Isolation not needed for mother or baby.	Give prophylactic eye treatment to all newborns, with tetracycline, erythromycin, or silver nitrate ophthalmic preparation. If maternal infection is active at delivery, give baby single dose of ceftriaxone.
Herpes simplex virus (HSV)	• Sexual contact *Increases risk of preterm birth with primary infection*	*Transplacental:* rarely *Ascending:* rarely *Delivery:* yes, direct contact *Postpartum:* possible.	Isolate baby suspected of infection from babies and pregnant women. Culture 24-48 hours after birth. Breastfeeding OK if no breast lesions. Private room with rooming-in OK.	*High neonatal mortality/morbidity.* *Vaginal* delivery if no lesions present; avoid internal fetal heart rate monitoring. *Cesarean* delivery, preferably before rupture of membranes, if lesions present. *Most newborns with HSV infection have mothers with undetected herpes.*

Infection	Transmission		Isolation	Notes
Human immuno-deficiency virus (HIV) **All women.**	• Sexual contact (common) • Sharing of needles (common) • Broken skin contact with HIV-positive blood/body fluids (rare) • Transfusion of contaminated blood (very rare after 1983) *Increases risk of preterm birth*	*Transplacental:* yes *Ascending:* probably *Delivery:* likely *Postpartum:* virus can be transmitted in breast milk	Isolation not needed for mother or baby. *Information changes rapidly. Consult experts and www.cdc. gov and www .aidsinfo.nih .gov.*	Treatment with zid-ovudine during pregnancy and/or labor, and/or neonatal treatment begun 8-12 hours after birth, significantly reduces neonatal HIV infection. Cesarean delivery also may reduce neonatal HIV infection, especially for women with high viral load. *Most HIV-positive women deliver with their infection undetected.*
Human papil-lomavirus (HPV)	• Sexual contact	*Transplacental:* no *Ascending:* no *Delivery:* yes, aspiration of cervico-vaginal fluid	Isolation not needed for mother or baby.	Neonatal genital warts and laryngeal papilloma are very *rare*.
Syphilis *(Treponema pallidum)* **All women.**	• Sexual contact *Significantly increases risk of abortion, fetal death, and preterm birth*	*Transplacental:* yes, at any stage of maternal illness *Ascending:* no *Delivery:* yes, if maternal genital lesions are present	Body fluids of mother and baby may remain infectious for 24 hours after penicillin started. Visitors, parents, and health care providers should wear gloves to handle baby.	Penicillin is the *only* antibiotic that reliably cures syphilis. If mother allergic, desensitize. *Maternal serologic status should be known before every baby's discharge.* Testing of cord/newborn's blood is not adequate.

Self-test

Now answer these questions to test yourself on the information in the last section.

B1. All babies born to human immunodeficiency virus (HIV)-positive women will

Yes	No	
____	____	Test positive for HIV antibodies
____	____	Be infected with the virus

B2. For each of the following organisms, indicate whether the fetus may become infected during pregnancy or at the time of delivery.

Pregnancy	Delivery	
____	____	Syphilis
____	____	Herpes simplex virus
____	____	Human papillomavirus

B3. **True** **False** In the United States, it is appropriate for a woman with HIV infection to breast-feed her baby.

B4. **True** **False** Sharing of needles by injected-drug users is a common route of HIV transmission to women.

B5. **True** **False** Syphilis infection can pass to the fetus only during the primary stage of maternal infection.

B6. **True** **False** Women with one sexually transmitted infection are at increased risk for having other sexually transmitted infections.

B7. **True** **False** Babies with untreated congenital syphilis may not develop signs and symptoms of the illness until 2 years or longer after birth.

B8. **True** **False** Treatment of HIV-positive women with zidovudine during pregnancy and labor and/or neonatal treatment after delivery significantly reduces the number of babies infected with HIV.

B9. **True** **False** Standard precautions need to be used only for HIV-positive patients.

B10. **True** **False** When maternal human papillomavirus infection is known, neonatal treatment should begin soon after birth.

B11. Indicate whether screening of *all* pregnant women is recommended for these infections.

Yes	No	
____	____	HIV
____	____	Human papillomavirus
____	____	Syphilis
____	____	Gonorrhea
____	____	Herpes simplex virus

Check your answers with the list that follows the Recommended Routines. Correct any incorrect answers and review the appropriate section in the unit.

B. Other Maternal Infections That May Affect a Fetus (Table 3.4)

Cytomegalovirus

1. *Disease in Women:* Diagnosis of primary infection is made by a change in serologic titers. Infection may be asymptomatic or accompanied by non-specific, mild, flu-like symptoms, making it difficult to identify primary cytomegalovirus (CMV) infection in pregnant women. After recovery from the primary infection, the virus may remain latent for years between episodes of recurrent infection. During primary or recurrent

infection, the virus is shed in body fluids and may continue to be shed long after all symptoms of the illness have disappeared.

Cytomegalovirus is widespread, with transmission by sexual contact, or contact with body fluids such as urine (changing diapers) or saliva. Most babies and children are asymptomatic, but most young children excrete the virus, thus exposing child care workers and household members to CMV. Cytomegalovirus-negative women should be counseled about the potential hazards of CMV infection and the particular importance of good hand washing. Routine testing is *not* recommended because there is no treatment. Serial testing of pregnant women suspected of having been exposed to CMV, to establish seroconversion and thus identify a primary infection, may be appropriate.

2. *Risks for the Fetus and Newborn:* Transmission can occur by 3 routes.
   - *In utero,* with primary maternal infection having a significantly higher rate of transmission (approximately 40%) than recurrent illness (<1%)
   - *At birth,* through contact with vaginal fluids containing the virus
   - *After delivery,* through ingestion of CMV-positive breast milk, or from transfusion of blood from a CMV-positive donor *(extremely rare)*

Approximately 1% of all babies are infected in utero and excrete CMV at birth. Transplacental infection, particularly primary maternal infection during the first trimester, can cause varying degrees of damage to the fetus. Babies most severely affected (about 10% of infected fetuses) may show growth restriction, jaundice, and systemic disease, including thrombocytopenia, hepatosplenomegaly, microcephaly, intracerebral calcifications, chorioretinitis, and/or deafness.

Some babies with asymptomatic congenital infection or those infected at birth or soon after (clinical illness is rarely apparent) may be found later in childhood to have hearing loss, learning disability, and/or intellectual disability. Preterm babies are at higher risk for subsequent damage than are term babies.

Prenatal Considerations
- Consult with regional center specialists regarding diagnosis if maternal illness is strongly suspected or documented. Amniotic fluid or fetal blood sampling and ultrasound examination may be used for prenatal diagnosis of congenital CMV infection. There is no cure and current antiviral drugs have limitations, side effects, and unknown safety in pregnancy.
- Discuss pregnancy termination if infection occurs early in pregnancy, particularly if it is a woman's first infection.

Intrapartum Considerations: None specific to CMV infection.
Postpartum Considerations
Maternal
- Notify pediatric staff if maternal infection is suspected so that the baby can be evaluated.
- Cytomegalovirus passed in breast milk usually does not cause neonatal disease in term newborns, probably because of transfer of maternal antibodies. Because preterm newborns may be at increased risk to acquire CMV from breast milk, consultation with regional center specialists regarding breastfeeding by a CMV-positive mother and/or treatment of the milk is recommended.

Neonatal (See also Book III: Neonatal Care, Unit 8, Infections.)
- Determination of infection timing requires a positive viral culture obtained within 3 weeks of birth, unless clinical signs of CMV infection are present, to be certain it is a congenital infection and not acquired during or after birth.
- Consult with regional center specialists regarding neonatal diagnosis, treatment, and long-term follow-up evaluation. Antiviral drugs may be appropriate for babies with certain conditions.
- Evaluate for congenital malformations.

Hepatitis B Virus

1. *Disease in Women:* Infected persons carry the virus in all body fluids, with transmission primarily by intimate (usually sexual) contact and sharing of needles by drug users. Within households, nonsexual transmission occurs adult to child and child to child, although the exact mechanism is unknown. The virus can survive on inanimate objects for a week or longer, but is killed by bleach and commonly used disinfectants. While there is no specific therapy for hepatitis, most adult acute infections are self-limited with complete recovery. Some infected persons develop chronic active hepatitis and others become asymptomatic carriers of the virus and, therefore, are at risk for developing serious liver disease later in life. Hepatitis B virus (HBV) may be transmitted during either acute or chronic infection.

 Since standard precautions and vaccinations were introduced, the number of work-acquired hepatitis infections, and the number of deaths from hepatitis, have declined dramatically in health care workers.

2. *Risks for the Fetus and Newborn:* If untreated, more than half of the babies born to women with hepatitis B infection will become infected, and up to 25% of those babies will eventually develop HBV-related cirrhosis or hepatocellular carcinoma. Transplacental transmission occurs, but is rare. Transmission seems to be mainly through direct contact with the mother's blood at the time of delivery. Rate of transmission is not affected by whether the mother is a chronic carrier or has an acute infection at the time of delivery. There is no evidence to suggest that cesarean delivery reduces the risk of transmission. The risk of transmission during amniocentesis is also low. Immunization of the baby soon after birth, however, reduces the risk of infection almost to zero.

Prenatal Considerations
- It is recommended that all pregnant women be screened with every pregnancy for HBV infection.* More than one-third of infected adults have *no* identifiable risk factor.

 Test all pregnant women for hepatitis B surface antigen (HBsAg) at the first prenatal visit.

- HBV vaccine should be offered to all women of reproductive age. It may be safely given to HBsAg-negative women during pregnancy and lactation. Three doses are needed, with the second dose 1 month and the third dose 6 months after the first dose. Use IM injection into the deltoid muscle. IM injection into the buttocks may not be as effective and is not recommended.

---

*American Academy of Pediatrics, American College of Obstetricians and Gynecologists. Perinatal infections. In: Lockwood CJ, Lemons JA, eds. *Guidelines for Perinatal Care*. 6th ed. Elk Grove Village, IL: American Academy of Pediatrics; 2007;306.

- Screen other children, household contacts, and sexual partner(s) of HBsAg-positive women. HBsAg-negative household members and partners should receive a single dose of hepatitis B immune globulin (HBIG) and begin the HBV vaccine series.
- In late pregnancy, repeat testing of women at high risk for HBV infection.
  - Injected drug users
  - History of any other STI

Intrapartum Considerations

- Test women who were not screened earlier when they are admitted for delivery.
- Route of delivery does not affect the rate of transmission from mother to baby.
- Although it is not clear if internal fetal heart rate monitoring increases the rate of transmission from mother to baby, avoiding internal monitoring is recommended because of the presumed increased risk of transmission it poses.
- Before delivery, notify postpartum and nursery personnel of HBsAg-positive women.

Postpartum Considerations
Maternal

- Breastfed babies of HBsAg-positive mothers should receive hepatitis B vaccine and HBIG.
- Immunization of the baby nearly eliminates the risk of HBV infection by any route of transmission.

Neonatal (See also Book III: Neonatal Care, Unit 8, Infections.)

- Wash maternal blood off baby promptly.

 All newborns should receive hepatitis B vaccine.* Babies born to HBsAg-positive women should also receive HBIG.

- Hepatitis B virus infection can be prevented for approximately 95% of babies born to HBsAg-positive women by administration of HBIG and the hepatitis B vaccine series.
- The first dose of hepatitis B vaccine *and* HBIG should be given within 12 hours of birth for term and preterm babies born to HBsAg-positive women. Hepatitis B vaccine dosage depends on specific preparation used.
- Hepatitis B vaccine and HBIG can be given at the same time, but in different sites. Intramuscular injection into the anterolateral thigh or deltoid muscles are the only recommended sites.
- Babies born to women whose HBsAg status is unknown should be given hepatitis B vaccine within 12 hours of birth. If maternal testing reveals she is HBsAg-positive, HBIG should be given as soon as possible and within 7 days of birth. Hepatitis B vaccine series should be completed.
- Give first dose of hepatitis B vaccine series to *all* babies, according to the protocol given in Book III: Neonatal Care, Unit 8, Infections.

---

*American Academy of Pediatrics, American College of Obstetricians and Gynecologists. Perinatal infections. In: Lockwood CJ, Lemons JA, eds. *Guidelines for Perinatal Care.* 6th ed. Elk Grove Village, IL: American Academy of Pediatrics; 2007;306.

Hepatitis A Virus

1. Fetal effects from these infections are not well-defined.

Hepatitis C Virus

1. In some patient populations, hepatitis C is as common as or more common than hepatitis B. Hepatitis C is usually asymptomatic in early stages. Confirmation of infection is done with recombinant immunoblot assay. People with low serum concentration of hepatitis C RNA who are not coinfected with HIV have a perinatal transmission rate less than 5%. If hepatitis C viral load is high, or the woman is coinfected with HIV, transmission rates may approach 25%. Currently available evidence suggests that cesarean delivery should be performed in HCV-infected women only for standard obstetric indications. Consultation with regional obstetric and infectious disease experts is recommended.

Listeriosis

1. *Disease in Women*: *Listeria monocytogenes* is widespread in the environment but infection is rare and often asymptomatic (about 2,500 reported cases of illness per year in the United States). Pregnant women, however, are roughly 20 times more likely than other healthy adults to become ill with listeriosis. Adult mortality for listeriosis is highly variable, and depends on the patient's underlying immune status and comorbid conditions. Infection is associated with flu-like fever, malaise, headache, backache, intestinal upset or diarrhea, and occasionally more serious findings of endocarditis or encephalitis. Women can have asymptomatic vaginal and fecal reservoirs of the organism. The risk of abortion, fetal death, preterm delivery, and amnionitis is markedly increased with maternal infection.

   Most infections result from eating contaminated food. Pregnant women should avoid foods most likely to harbor *L monocytogenes*, including soft cheeses, raw or unpasteurized cow or goat milk or milk products, including blue-veined or Mexican-style cheeses, unwashed raw vegetables, and undercooked poultry, as well as leftover food or refrigerated smoked fish. Do not eat luncheon meats, bologna, or other delicatessen meats, or prepared meats, such as hot dogs, unless heated until steaming. Avoid the use of a microwave oven for cooking, as uneven heating may occur. Because *L monocytogenes* can grow at refrigerator temperatures of 40°F or colder, all precooked or ready-to-eat foods should be eaten as soon as possible.

   Canned smoked fish and meat; cottage cheese; cream cheese; hard, semi-soft, or *pasteurized* cheeses; and food heated or reheated to steaming hot are safe to eat.

2. *Risks for the Fetus and Newborn*: Transplacental, ascending, and direct contact during delivery are all possible routes of transmission to the baby. Nosocomial outbreaks within nurseries also have been documented. Pneumonia and septicemia are typical of early-onset neonatal disease. Late-onset (after the first postnatal week) illness probably occurs as a result of transmission during delivery, but may result from environmental sources. Meningitis is typical with late-onset illness. Neonatal mortality for listeriosis is high (about 40% to 50%).

Prenatal Considerations

- Diagnosis can only be confirmed by positive culture of blood, amniotic, cerebrospinal, or other body fluid. On microscopic examination *L monocytogenes* can be mistaken for other organisms with similar appearance, so laboratory notification that listeriosis is being considered is important.

- Intravenous antibiotic therapy with ampicillin for 10 to 14 days for maternal infection during pregnancy may prevent infection of the baby. Treatment of severe infection may benefit from the addition of an aminoglycoside, usually gentamicin, and a longer course (14 to 21 days) of therapy. *L monocytogenes* is not responsive to cephalosporins.

Intrapartum Considerations
- Fetal infection is often accompanied by passage of meconium before or during labor.

Postpartum Considerations
Maternal
- Abscesses may be evident within the placenta following delivery.
- Transmission of *L monocytogenes* in breast milk is not known to occur.

Neonatal
- Symptoms are variable and vague and not unlike early and late group B streptococcal (GBS) onset. Granulomatosis infantisepticum or a red rash with scattered, small, pale micro-abscesses can occur in severe neonatal infection.
- Ampicillin is highly effective against *L monocytogenes*, but gentamicin (or another aminoglycoside) is usually added.

Parvovirus B19 (Fifth Disease or Erythema Infectiosum)

1. *Disease in Women:* Parvovirus B19 is widespread, and infection is mainly a disease of school-aged children. While there is no treatment for parvovirus B19, reinfection probably does not occur, and immunity is common. Primary infection may be asymptomatic, but findings are typically mild and include fever, myalgias, arthralgias, headache, and malaise, followed in 7 to 10 days by a rash. The rash is intensely red with a slapped-cheek appearance on the face, but lace-like first on the trunk, then spreading to the arms, buttocks, and thighs. Rash may come and go for weeks or months, and is often less prominent in adults. Arthralgia and arthritis occur frequently in adults, especially women.

   Transmission is thought to be through respiratory secretions and blood. Exposure to infected individuals is difficult to avoid because the rash appears after the contagious period has ended, but good hand washing and proper disposal of used facial tissues, especially by teachers and child care workers, may lessen the rate of transmission. Diagnosis is made by clinical condition and seroconversion from negative to positive antibody status.

2. *Risks for the Fetus and Newborn:* The virus readily crosses the placenta, but transplacental transmission is not known to cause congenital defects, even during early pregnancy infections. Early pregnancy infection may occasionally result in spontaneous abortion, usually 4 to 6 weeks after maternal infection. Infection later in pregnancy may destroy immature red blood cells in the fetus, causing anemia, which may lead to nonimmune hydrops fetalis due to heart failure, and to fetal death. The degree of fetal illness is unpredictable. Most women with prenatal parvovirus B19 infection deliver healthy babies.

Prenatal Considerations
- Consider obtaining a maternal serum alpha-fetoprotein level because an elevated level can be associated with an affected fetus.
- Serial ultrasound examinations should be performed to evaluate for signs of fetal anemia, which may allow intervention before the onset of fetal hydrops. Assessment of middle cerebral artery (MCA) Doppler velocimetry is a reliable tool for screening for fetal anemia. Referral to a maternal-fetal medicine specialist may be necessary for monitoring MCA Doppler values.
- If there is suspicion for fetal anemia based upon MCA Doppler values, or hydrops present, referral to maternal-fetal medicine specialists is strongly recommended. Intrauterine fetal transfusion(s) may be lifesaving.

Intrapartum Considerations: None specific to parvovirus.
Postpartum Considerations
Maternal: None specific to parvovirus.
Neonatal: Check hematocrit soon after birth.

Rubella (German Measles)

1. *Disease in Women:* Before the widespread use of rubella vaccine, rubella was a common, mild illness, especially in children, displaying a typical pattern of rash, fever, and lymphadenopathy. Transmission is by droplet or direct contact with nasopharyngeal secretions. There is no treatment, but infection or immunization confers prolonged, probably lifelong, immunity. Since the introduction of rubella vaccine, the incidence of infection in the United States has dropped 99%. Outbreaks today generally occur only among college students, young adults in military or work settings, and certain under-served groups, such as migrant workers. Approximately 10% of young American adults are currently susceptible to rubella because of lack of vaccination, not declining immunity in those who were vaccinated. Maternal diagnosis is made by clinical condition and serologic testing.

2. *Risks for the Fetus and Newborn:* Likelihood of transplacental transmission of the virus is very high during the first trimester, and somewhat lower later in pregnancy. Maternal infection, especially early during the first trimester, carries a high risk of spontaneous abortion, fetal death, or congenital rubella syndrome, which typically includes serious eye, auditory, cardiac, and neurologic disorders. Intrauterine growth restriction, hepatosplenomegaly, thrombocytopenia, and purpuric skin lesions also may occur. Second trimester infection may be less damaging, but growth restriction, intellectual disability, and/or deafness is possible. Third trimester infection is associated with less risk for fetal damage. Some infected babies will display little or no clinical evidence of their infection at birth, but may show hearing defects, abnormal neuromuscular development, learning deficits, and/or behavioral disturbances later in childhood.

Prenatal Considerations
- Determine immunity at the first prenatal visit for every woman who does not have documented rubella immunity.
- Women should *not* be immunized during pregnancy. However, following accidental maternal vaccination, only 2% of babies had asymptomatic infection and none had evidence of congenital rubella syndrome.
- If a nonimmune pregnant woman is exposed to rubella, test the woman serially to see if seroconversion occurs, indicating infection occurred.

- Routine use of immune globulin for nonimmune pregnant women exposed to rubella early in pregnancy is *not* recommended, but may be considered if termination is not an option. Immune globulin may significantly reduce clinically apparent maternal infection, but does *not* ensure prevention of fetal infection.
- Discuss pregnancy termination if infection occurs early in pregnancy.

Intrapartum Considerations

- Babies with congenital rubella may continue to shed the virus for a year or longer, and can infect others. If congenital infection is suspected, whether or not the baby has clinical evidence of infection, nursery personnel should be notified so appropriate isolation of the baby can be instituted.

Postpartum Considerations
Maternal

- Vaccinate women nonimmune to rubella early during the immediate postpartum period, before discharge.
- Breastfeeding is *not* a contraindication to maternal immunization.

Neonatal (See also Book III: Neonatal Care, Unit 8, Infections.)

- Isolate the newborn from *all* other babies, and from nonimmune pregnant women and health care providers. Contact precautions should be used for at least a year, unless nasopharyngeal and urine cultures are repeatedly negative.
- Evaluate baby for congenital malformations.
- Obtain serology tests to establish the presence or absence of congenital infection (consult with regional center experts regarding appropriate tests and timing of testing) so long-term follow-up and care can be planned. Diagnosis of congenital infection becomes more difficult as time passes and may be impossible to do in children aged 1 year or older.

Self-test

Now answer these questions to test yourself on the information in the last section.

C1. For which of the following maternal infections is the fetus at risk for transplacental infection?

Yes	No	
____	____	Gonorrhea
____	____	Primary parvovirus infection
____	____	Rubella (German measles)
____	____	Cytomegalovirus
____	____	*Chlamydia*
____	____	Listeriosis

C2.	**True**	**False**	Maternal infection with parvovirus may cause severe fetal anemia.
C3.	**True**	**False**	Listeriosis is a food-borne life-threatening infection.
C4.	**True**	**False**	Hepatitis B virus vaccine is recommended for *all* newborns.
C5.	**True**	**False**	Cesarean delivery decreases the rate of transmission of hepatitis B from HBsAg-positive women to their babies.
C6.	**True**	**False**	Primary infection with cytomegalovirus during the first trimester can cause severe, permanent neurologic damage in the fetus.
C7.	**True**	**False**	Breastfeeding by women who are positive for hepatitis B surface antigen should be discouraged because hepatitis B is easily transmitted in breast milk.
C8.	**True**	**False**	Cytomegalovirus rarely crosses the placenta, even during early pregnancy.
C9.	**True**	**False**	When a mother is positive for hepatitis B, treatment of the baby should begin within hours of birth.
C10.	**True**	**False**	When a pregnant woman is diagnosed with parvovirus, acyclovir treatment should be started promptly.
C11.	**True**	**False**	A baby with suspected or proven congenital rubella should be isolated from all other babies.
C12.	**True**	**False**	Hepatitis B virus screening is recommended for *all* pregnant women.
C13.	**True**	**False**	Cytomegalovirus can be transmitted through sexual contact.
C14.	**True**	**False**	First trimester primary maternal cytomegalovirus infection has a high risk of resulting in severe damage to the fetus.
C15.	**True**	**False**	Pregnant women are at much higher risk for listeriosis than are nonpregnant healthy adults.
C16.	**True**	**False**	Maternal postpartum rubella vaccination is a contraindication to breastfeeding.

Check your answers with the list that follows the Recommended Routines. Correct any incorrect answers and review the appropriate section in the unit.

*Group B Beta-Hemolytic Streptococci** (Figures 3.1 through 3.4)

1. *Colonization in Women:* Group B beta-hemolytic streptococci, a gram-positive organism, can colonize the lower gastrointestinal tract, and secondary spread to the genitourinary tract is common. Women with GBS colonization in the lower vagina and/or rectum rarely have symptoms of infection. Approximately 10% to 30% of pregnant women have rectal and/or vaginal GBS colonization. Colonization may be brief, chronic, or intermittent, coming and going with no apparent cause.

   GBS vaginal and/or rectal colonization increases the risk of urinary tract infection (UTI), chorioamnionitis, postoperative infection, and endometritis. Urinary tract GBS infections complicate 2% to 4% of pregnancies. Systemic infection is possible, although rare, in healthy adults.

2. *Risks for the Fetus and Newborn:* Ascending infection can occur through intact membranes, but prolonged rupture of membranes increases the risk. Fetal aspiration of infected amniotic fluid can lead to fetal death, neonatal pneumonia, or sepsis. Babies born to women with GBS colonization may acquire the organisms during vaginal delivery and become colonized themselves, and usually remain asymptomatic. A small number (currently <1%) will develop symptomatic GBS infection. Preterm babies are at greater risk for symptomatic infection. GBS infection in young babies (sepsis or pneumonia, and less often meningitis, osteomyelitis, or septic arthritis) can be life-threatening for term and preterm babies. Mortality and morbidity from GBS infection is high.

3. *Illness and Prevention in Babies:* GBS disease occurs in babies in 2 forms: early onset (within first week after birth) and late onset (most infections are evident within 3 months after birth). The incidence of early onset (most infections) began declining after ACOG and the AAP first issued statements in the early 1990s regarding prevention. Decline in reported cases continued after the Centers for Disease Control and Prevention (CDC) consensus statement was published in 1996, and continued to decline until 1999, at which time a plateau in prevention efforts occurred. New recommendations* are based on research, since these first guidelines were issued and are designed to promote further reduction in neonatal GBS disease. The incidence of late-onset GBS disease is much lower than early-onset illness, and has not changed significantly over the past 20 years.

Prenatal Considerations

- Maternal colonization early in pregnancy is not predictive of neonatal disease. Culture screening in late pregnancy can identify women most likely to be colonized with GBS at the time of delivery and, therefore, at higher risk of transmitting GBS to the fetus.

   Treatment of colonization is not effective in eliminating carriage of GBS and is *not* recommended. Any harm colonization may cause does not occur until the fetus passes through the vagina at birth, or with ascending infection during labor, or after rupture of membranes, with or without labor.

---

*Recommendations for management of GBS and collection of cultures on this and the following pages are based on revised guidelines issued by the Centers for Disease Control and Prevention. Prevention of perinatal group B streptococcal disease. *MMWR Recomm Rep.* 2010;59(RR-10):1-32.

Cultures for GBS taken from the lower vagina and rectum at 35 to 37 weeks' gestation are recommended for every pregnant woman.

Screen each pregnancy, regardless of a woman's GBS status in any previous pregnancy.

- Specimens may be collected by the pregnant woman or by a health care provider by swabbing first the lower vagina (cervical culture is not recommended and a speculum is not needed) and then through the anal sphincter into the rectum.
    - Place the swab(s) into a nonnutritive transport medium. If separate vaginal and rectal swabs were used, both may be put in the same container, because isolation of the colonization site is not important to clinical management and because doing so minimizes laboratory costs.
    - For penicillin-allergic women, specify that clindamycin and erythromycin susceptibility testing is needed if GBS is found.
    - Follow laboratory guidelines to increase the likelihood that GBS, if present, will be identified as well as to determine sensitivity to clindamycin or erythromycin for penicillin-allergic women.
- Except for asymptomatic GBS bacteriuria, antibiotics should *not* be used before the intrapartum period to treat asymptomatic GBS colonization.
- Treat *all* GBS bacteriuria.

GBS UTIs, with or without symptoms, should be treated whenever identified during pregnancy.

Intrapartum Considerations

Intravenous antibiotics should be started when labor begins or membranes rupture for women in the following risk groups:

1. *Women with rectal or vaginal culture positive for GBS at 35 to 37 weeks' gestation during the current pregnancy.* (GBS *colonization* during a previous pregnancy, by itself, is not an indication for intrapartum antibiotics in the current pregnancy.)

2. *Women with either of the following risk factors* should also receive intrapartum antibiotics. Rectal and vaginal cultures do *not* need to be obtained for these women. Antibiotics are recommended in both situations, regardless of culture results, thus making cultures unnecessary.
    - *Previous newborn with GBS infection*
    - *GBS bacteriuria of any concentration during this pregnancy*

3. *Women with the following risk factors and whose culture results are unknown*
    - *Rupture of membranes for 18 hours or longer*
    - *Temperature of 100.4°F (38.0°C) or higher*
    - *Preterm labor* (<37 weeks' gestation)

    Note: Women with any of the 3 risk factors, but whose *culture results are known to have been negative within 5 weeks of delivery*, do *not* require intrapartum GBS antibiotic therapy.

Cesarean Delivery Considerations
- Cesarean birth should *not* be used for GBS-positive women as an alternative to vaginal delivery and intrapartum antibiotic therapy for the prevention of neonatal GBS disease.
- GBS-colonized women with a planned cesarean delivery, and who have not started labor or had rupture of membranes, have a low risk for delivering an infant with early-onset GBS disease, and should *not* routinely receive prophylactic antibiotics during cesarean surgery. Obtain vaginal and rectal cultures at 35 to 37 weeks because onset of labor and rupture of membranes may occur before the planned delivery date.

Antibiotic Choice and Administration
- **Intravenous antibiotics, when appropriate, should be given throughout labor until delivery.**
- *Intravenous administration* is preferred, regardless of the antibiotic used, because higher intra-amniotic concentrations are achieved with IV administration, as compared to IM administration.
  - *Preferred antibiotic is penicillin.* Penicillin G dose is 5 million units intravenously initially, then 2.5 (or 3.0) million units intravenously every 4 hours until delivery.
  - *Alternative antibiotic is ampicillin,* 2 g first dose, intravenously, then 1 g intravenously every 4 hours until delivery.
  - *For penicillin-allergic women,* assess history of allergy and severity of reaction(s) early in prenatal care.
- *Not at high risk for anaphylaxis,* cefazolin is the drug of choice. Cefazolin 2 g initial dose, intravenously, then 1 g intravenously every 8 hours until delivery.
- *At high risk for anaphylaxis,* use prenatal screen culture specimen to test GBS susceptibility to clindamycin. If sensitive, give
  - Clindamycin 900 mg, intravenously, every 8 hours until delivery
  - When GBS is resistant to clindamycin, or susceptibility is unknown, use vancomycin, 1 g, intravenously, every 12 hours until delivery.
- Broad-spectrum antibiotics, including a drug effective against GBS, may be needed to treat chorioamnionitis.

 Appropriate intrapartum maternal antibiotic therapy can significantly reduce the risk that the
- *Baby will become infected with GBS*
- *Woman will develop GBS endometritis*

Onset of Preterm Labor (at 37 weeks or earlier)
- **GBS culture status unknown**
  - Obtain vaginal and rectal cultures.
  - Begin IV penicillin (or alternative for penicillin-allergic women).
- No growth in cultures after 48 hours, stop penicillin (penicillin should be given for at least 48 hours, unless delivery occurs earlier).
- If GBS is identified by culture, manage as for GBS-positive women.

- *GBS-positive women*
  - Give penicillin for 48 hours during tocolysis or until delivery, if labor cannot be stopped.
  - If labor is stopped but recurs within 4 weeks, and is likely to proceed to delivery, begin penicillin and continue antibiotic therapy until delivery.
  - If labor is stopped and does not recur for 4 weeks, repeat vaginal and rectal cultures. Manage during labor as indicated by repeat cultures.
- *GBS-negative women:* There is no indication for intrapartum antibiotic therapy, *unless* they had a previous infant with GBS disease. (See Intrapartum Considerations.)

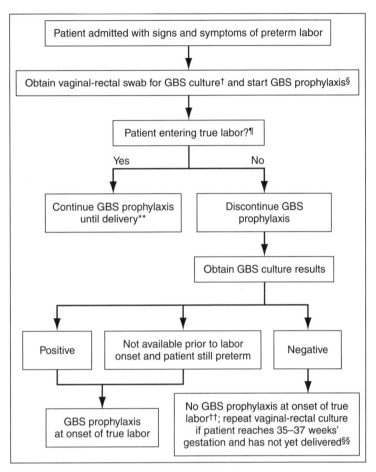

Patient admitted with signs and symptoms of preterm labor

Obtain vaginal-rectal swab for GBS culture† and start GBS prophylaxis§

Patient entering true labor?¶

Yes   No

Continue GBS prophylaxis until delivery**

Discontinue GBS prophylaxis

Obtain GBS culture results

Positive

Not available prior to labor onset and patient still preterm

Negative

GBS prophylaxis at onset of true labor

No GBS prophylaxis at onset of true labor††; repeat vaginal-rectal culture if patient reaches 35–37 weeks' gestation and has not yet delivered§§

* At <37 weeks and 0 days' gestation.

† If patient has undergone vaginal-rectal GBS culture within the preceding 5 weeks, the results of that culture should guide management. GBS-colonized women should receive intrapartum antibiotic prophylaxis. No antibiotics are indicated for GBS prophylaxis if a vaginal-rectal screen within 5 weeks was negative.

§ See Figure 3.3 for recommended antibiotic regimens.

¶ Patient should be regularly assessed for progression to true labor; if the patient is considered not to be in true labor, discontinue GBS prophylaxis.

** If GBS culture results become available prior to delivery and are negative, then discontinue GBS prophylaxis.

†† Unless subsequent GBS culture prior to delivery is positive.

§§ A negative GBS screen is considered valid for 5 weeks. If a patient with a history of PTL is re-admitted with signs and symptoms of PTL and had a negative GBS screen >5 weeks prior, she should be rescreened and managed according to this algorithm at that time.

Figure 3.1. Algorithm for Screening for Group B Streptococcal (GBS) Colonization and Use of Intrapartum Prophylaxis for Women With Preterm* Labor (PTL)

From Centers for Disease Control and Prevention. Prevention of perinatal group B streptococcal disease. *MMWR Morb Mortal Wkly Rep.* 2010;59(RR-10):1-32.

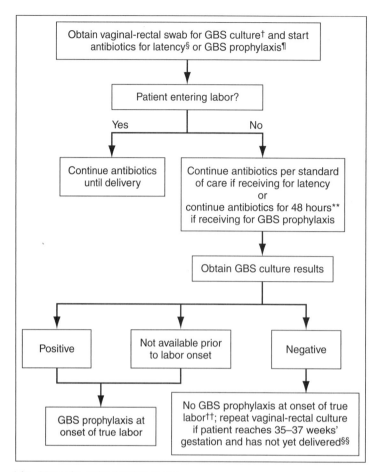

Obtain vaginal-rectal swab for GBS culture† and start antibiotics for latency§ or GBS prophylaxis¶

Patient entering labor?

Yes → Continue antibiotics until delivery

No → Continue antibiotics per standard of care if receiving for latency
or
continue antibiotics for 48 hours** if receiving for GBS prophylaxis

Obtain GBS culture results

Positive

Not available prior to labor onset

Negative

GBS prophylaxis at onset of true labor

No GBS prophylaxis at onset of true labor††; repeat vaginal-rectal culture if patient reaches 35–37 weeks' gestation and has not yet delivered§§

* At <37 weeks and 0 days' gestation.

† If patient has undergone vaginal-rectal GBS culture within the preceding 5 weeks, the results of that culture should guide management. GBS-colonized women should receive intrapartum antibiotic prophylaxis. No antibiotics are indicated for GBS prophylaxis if a vaginal-rectal screen within 5 weeks was negative.

§ Antibiotics given for latency in the setting of pPROM that include ampicillin 2 g intravenously (IV) once, followed by 1 g IV every 6 hours for at least 48 hours are adequate for GBS prophylaxis. If other regimens are used, GBS prophylaxis should be initiated in addition.

¶ See Figure 3.3 for recommended antibiotic regimens.

** GBS prophylaxis should be discontinued at 48 hours for women with pPROM who are not in labor. If results from a GBS screen performed on admission become available during the 48-hour period and are negative, GBS prophylaxis should be discontinued at that time.

†† Unless subsequent GBS culture prior to delivery is positive.

§§ A negative GBS screen is considered valid for 5 weeks. If a patient with pPROM is entering labor and had a negative GBS screen >5 weeks prior, she should be rescreened and managed according to this algorithm at that time.

Figure 3.2. Algorithm for Screening for Group B Streptococcal (GBS) Colonization and Use of Intrapartum Prophylaxis for Women With Preterm* Premature Rupture of Membranes

From Centers for Disease Control and Prevention. Prevention of perinatal group B streptococcal disease. *MMWR Morb Mortal Wkly Rep.* 2010;59(RR-10):1-32.

Neonatal

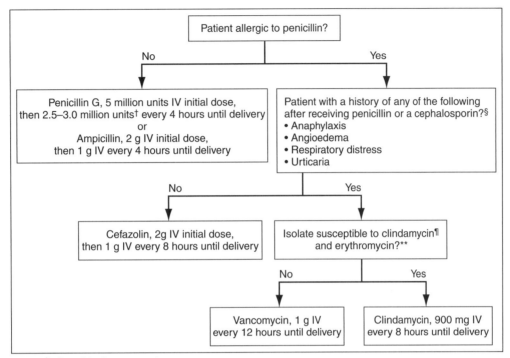

Abbreviation: IV = intravenously.

* Broader spectrum agents, including an agent active against GBS, might be necessary for treatment of chorioamnionitis.

† Doses ranging from 2.5 to 3.0 million units are acceptable for the doses administered every 4 hours following the initial dose. The choice of dose within that range should be guided by which formulations of penicillin G are readily available to reduce the need for pharmacies to specially prepare doses.

§ Penicillin-allergic patients with a history of anaphylaxis, angioedema, respiratory distress, or urticaria following administration of penicillin or a cephalosporin are considered to be at high risk for anaphylaxis and should not receive penicillin, ampicillin, or cefazolin for GBS intrapartum prophylaxis. For penicillin-allergic patients who do not have a history of those reactions, cefazolin is the preferred agent because pharmacologic data suggest it achieves effective intra-amniotic concentrations. Vancomycin and clindamycin should be reserved for penicillin-allergic women at high risk for anaphylaxis.

¶ If laboratory facilities are adequate, clindamycin and erythromycin susceptibility testing should be performed on prenatal GBS isolates from penicillin-allergic women at high risk for anaphylaxis. If no susceptibility testing is performed, or the results are not available at the time of labor, vancomycin is the preferred agent for GBS intrapartum prophylaxis for penicillin-allergic women at high risk for anaphylaxis.

** Resistance to erythromycin is often but not always associated with clindamycin resistance. If an isolate is resistant to erythromycin, it might have inducible resistance to clindamycin, even if it appears susceptible to clindamycin. If a GBS isolate is susceptible to clindamycin, resistant to erythromycin, and testing for inducible clindamycin resistance has been performed and is negative (no inducible resistance), then clindamycin can be used for GBS intrapartum prophylaxis instead of vancomycin.

Figure 3.3. Recommended Regimens for Intrapartum Antibiotic Prophylaxis for Prevention of Early-Onset Group B Streptococal (GBS) Disease*

From Centers for Disease Control and Prevention. Prevention of perinatal group B streptococcal disease. *MMWR Morb Mortal Wkly Rep.* 2010;59(RR-10):1-32.

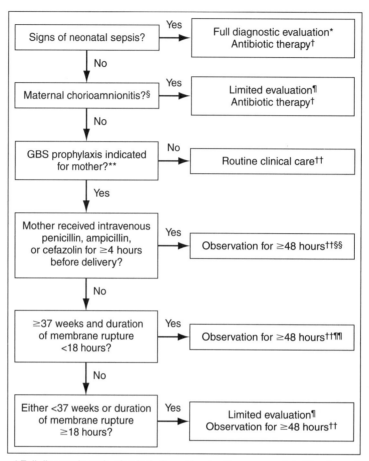

* Full diagnostic evaluation includes a blood culture, a complete blood count (CBC) including white blood cell differential and platelet counts, chest radiograph (if respiratory abnormalities are present), and lumbar puncture (if patient is stable enough to tolerate procedure and sepsis is suspected).

† Antibiotic therapy should be directed toward the most common causes of neonatal sepsis, including intravenous ampicillin for GBS and coverage for other organisms (including *Escherichia coli* and other gram-negative pathogens) and should take into account local antibiotic resistance patterns.

§ Consultation with obstetric providers is important to determine the level of clinical suspicion for chorioamnionitis. Chorioamnionitis is diagnosed clinically and some of the signs are nonspecific.

¶ Limited evaluation includes blood culture (at birth) and CBC with differential and platelets (at birth and/or at 6–12 hours of life).

** See table 3 for indications for intrapartum GBS prophylaxis.

†† If signs of sepsis develop, a full diagnostic evaluation should be conducted and antibiotic therapy initiated.

§§ If ≥37 weeks' gestation, observation may occur at home after 24 hours if other discharge criteria have been met, access to medical care is readily available, and a person who is able to comply fully with instructions for home observation will be present. If any of these conditions is not met, the infant should be observed in the hospital for at least 48 hours and until discharge criteria are achieved.

¶¶ Some experts recommend a CBC with differential and platelets at age 6–12 hours.

Figure 3.4. Algorithm for Secondary Prevention of Early-Onset Group B Streptococcal (GBS) Disease Among Newborns

From Centers for Disease Control and Prevention. Prevention of perinatal group B streptococcal disease. *MMWR Morb Mortal Wkly Rep.* 2010;59(RR-10):1-32.

Toxoplasmosis

1. *Disease in Women:* Toxoplasmosis is a common infection worldwide, caused by the protozoan parasite *T gondii*, with as many as one-third of women in the United States infected. Diagnosis of primary or acute infection is made by documentation of maternal seroconversion. Initial infection almost always confers lifelong immunity. Because toxoplasmosis infection in adults is typically asymptomatic or mild and self-limited, often described as a cold, serologic testing is rarely done and most active infections go undetected. In a pregnant woman with symptoms suggestive of mononucleosis, but a negative heterophile test, toxoplasmosis titers should be considered as part of the diagnostic evaluation. Routine screening of pregnant women is not recommended, except for HIV-positive women. A reference laboratory, such as the Palo Alto Medical Foundation Research Institute's Toxoplasma Serology Laboratory, should be used to confirm acute infection (www.pamf.org).

   T gondii is common to house cats and many other mammals. Transmission of the infection to humans is by exposure to cat feces or by eating raw or undercooked meat containing tissue cysts of the parasite. Except for rare cases of infected donor organs and contaminated blood products, the only person-to-person transmission is by transplacental transfer from a pregnant woman to her fetus.

2. *Risks for the Fetus and Newborn: T gondii* crosses the placenta. Fetal infection early in pregnancy can cause spontaneous abortion or growth restriction and systemic disease, resulting in permanent, severe damage. Typically, hydrocephalus, microcephaly, cerebral calcifications, seizures, deafness, and/or chorioretinitis are present, along with lymphadenopathy, hepatosplenomegaly, jaundice, and/or thrombocytopenia. Most infected fetuses will be asymptomatic at birth, but many of those will go on to demonstrate mental retardation, learning disabilities, impaired vision, or blindness months or years later.

Prenatal Considerations

- Women with negative or unknown *Toxoplasma* serology should avoid
  - Cat litter boxes or gardening in areas cats frequent
  - Cats, especially those with access to wild rodents
  - Eating raw or undercooked meat, especially red meat
- Consider obtaining *preconception* toxoplasmosis titer for women at high risk for contracting the infection. This titer would provide a baseline level in the event an infection is suspected during pregnancy, as well as indicate preexisting immunity if it is positive.
- Consult with regional center specialists if an acute maternal infection is identified. Drug therapy may reduce *T gondii* transmission to the fetus and improve neonatal outcome, but appropriate drugs vary by trimester and some need special authorization.
- Congenital infection is confirmed by *T gondii* found in fetal blood or amniotic fluid.
- When congenital *T gondii* infection is suspected, serial ultrasound examinations are recommended to detect ventricular enlargement in the brain or any other signs of fetal infection.

- Discuss pregnancy termination if infection occurs early in pregnancy.
- Coexisting HIV infection complicates maternal and neonatal evaluation and treatment. Consult with specialists.

Intrapartum Considerations: None specific to toxoplasmosis.
Postpartum Considerations
Maternal

- Notify pediatric staff if maternal infection is suspected.
- Toxoplasmosis has been found in the breast milk of rodents, although there is no information at present regarding human breast milk.

Neonatal (See also Book III: Neonatal Care, Unit 8, Infections.)

- If neonatal diagnosis of *T gondii* is suspected at birth and/or if there is evidence of primary *T gondii* maternal infection during pregnancy, *Toxoplasmosa*-specific tests should be obtained.* It also may be possible to isolate the organism from the placenta, umbilical cord, or baby's blood.
- Treatment with pyrimethamine and sulfadiazine (plus folinic acid) is usually recommended. Treatment is prolonged, often needing a year or longer. Consult with specialists.
- Evaluate for congenital malformations and obtain consultations as indicated for care of the baby and the family.

Tuberculosis

1. *Disease in Women:* Tuberculosis (TB) is an infection of *Mycobacterium tuberculosis* that has progressed over weeks or years to the point that x-ray findings, clinical signs, symptoms, or positive cultures are present. Infection also may be latent, before x-ray and clinical findings develop. Tuberculosis has increased dramatically in the United States, including infections with drug-resistant organisms.

   Treatment recommendations vary according to latent and active phases and primary infection site. Most commonly, the infection is pulmonary, but extrapulmonary infection is possible and can involve bones, joints, uterus, kidneys, etc. Tuberculosis meningitis is also possible.

2. *Risks for the Fetus and Newborn:* Extrapulmonary TB is associated with need for antenatal hospitalization, low Apgar scores, and low birth weight. Also rare is transmission in utero through infected amniotic fluid or at the time of delivery, through aspiration or ingestion of infected maternal fluids. When congenital tuberculosis is suspected, the newborn and mother need prompt evaluation.

   In most cases, transmission is by droplet from the respiratory tract. Droplet is the most common way a mother or household contact with active disease passes the infection to a newborn.

Prenatal Considerations

- All pregnant women at risk for tuberculosis should be screened with a purified protein derivative (PPD) test early in their prenatal care. High-risk factors include
  – Close contact with individual(s) known to have tuberculosis
  – Poverty

---

*For specific recommendations, see American Academy of Pediatrics. *Toxoplasma gondii* infections. In: Pickering LK, Baker CJ, Kimberlin DW, Long SS, eds. *Red Book: 2009 Report of the Committee on Infectious Diseases.* 28th ed. Elk Grove Village, IL: American Academy of Pediatrics; 2009:667.

  – Community settings, such as urban environments; residents and/or employees of correctional or mental institutions, nursing homes, and long-term care facilities
  – Birth in a tuberculosis endemic area
  – Medically underserved group, such as migrant workers
  – Persons with any other systemic disease, such as diabetes mellitus
  – Malnutrition
  – HIV infection, or other immunocompromised medical condition, such as transplant recipient, or chronic immunosuppressant medications, such as glucocorticoids or tumor necrosis factor-alpha inhibitors
  – Substance abuse, including alcohol or injection drug use (Tobacco use also increases the risk of TB infection.)
- If a positive PPD is found for the first time during pregnancy, obtain a chest x-ray and sputum cultures.
- If active disease is found, treat promptly and aggressively with multidrug therapy, in consultation with infectious disease specialists. Management is complex, especially during pregnancy, and must be individualized. Drug resistance can further complicate therapy.
- If infection is latent, with normal chest x-ray and no clinical signs, prompt treatment may be advisable for recent (<2 years) infection or immunosuppression. For all other pregnant women with latent TB, treatment may be delayed until after delivery.
- Arrange for testing and treatment of home contacts. Individuals with tuberculosis also should be tested for HIV, because people who are HIV positive have an increased risk of contracting tuberculosis.

Intrapartum Considerations
- Isolate (respiratory precautions) women with diagnosed or suspected active disease from other pregnant women and all newborns.

Postpartum Considerations
Maternal
- Maintain isolation (respiratory precautions) of the mother.
- In certain situations,* the mother and baby need to be separated until the mother (or sometimes mother and newborn) is receiving appropriate therapy and the mother is considered noncontagious.
- Delay breastfeeding until the mother is noncontagious (usually ≥2 weeks after medication started). If the mother wishes to breastfeed, she may pump her breasts to establish and maintain a milk supply, but the milk should be discarded until the mother becomes noncontagious.
- Several (but not all) antituberculosis medications are considered safe for the fetus and breastfed baby. If a breastfeeding mother and her baby are taking antituberculosis medication, however, excessive drug concentration may occur in the baby. Consult with infectious disease experts.
- Arrange for follow-up of mother and baby. Treatment with antituberculosis drugs can require 18 months of therapy, and compliance with drug regimen can be difficult. Non-adherence is a major problem in providing effective therapy and in limiting the development of drug-resistant strains of *M tuberculosis*.

---

*American Academy of Pediatrics, American College of Obstetricians and Gynecologists. Perinatal infections. In: Lockwood, CJ, Lemons JA, eds. *Guidelines for Perinatal Care*. 6th ed. Elk Grove Village, IL: American Academy of Pediatrics; 2007;337-338.

Neonatal (See also Book III: Neonatal Care, Unit 8, Infections.)
- Treat baby if the mother was incompletely treated or is considered to be contagious at the time of delivery. Consult with infectious disease specialists; maternal and neonatal therapy should be coordinated.
- Consider giving bacille Calmette-Guérin (BCG) vaccine to the baby. BCG action is not to prevent infection but rather to prevent disseminated and life-threatening complications of *M tuberculosis* infection. In the United States, its use is generally confined to noninfected babies who cannot be placed on long-term preventive therapy but who are likely to have prolonged exposure to persistently infectious individuals.
- Reassess testing and treatment of home contacts. Test for HIV.
- Isolate the baby (respiratory precautions) from other newborns and pregnant women until a full evaluation of the baby has been done.

Varicella-Zoster Virus (Chickenpox)

1. *Disease in Women:* Varicella-zoster virus (VZV) infection is characterized by a typical rash, fever, and mild systemic symptoms, although adolescents and adults are likely to be much sicker than children with chickenpox. While rare in children, pneumonia is the most common complication in adults, and can be life-threatening. Pregnant women are more likely to become seriously ill than nonpregnant women. After recovery from the primary infection, the virus remains in latent form. Transmission is usually by direct contact with an infected person, although droplet spread also occurs. Reactivation results in herpes zoster infection (shingles).

2. *Risks for the Fetus and Newborn:* The likelihood of transplacental transmission of the virus is high if maternal infection occurs during the first 20 weeks of pregnancy. First trimester infection carries an increased risk of spontaneous abortion. In a small number of infected fetuses, congenital varicella syndrome will result, which is characterized by limb atrophy and scarring of the skin; neurologic and ophthalmic damage and microcephaly also may occur.

   If a woman delivers while infected, the baby may become infected at delivery and become seriously ill. Neonatal illness may develop between 1 and 16 days after birth, although the usual time from onset of maternal rash to onset of neonatal illness is 9 to 15 days.

 Varicella in the newborn carries a mortality rate as high as 30%.

Prenatal Considerations
- Most women with negative or uncertain history of VZV infection are, in fact, immune. Serologic testing can be used to document immunity. VZV vaccine has been available since 1995 and is widely used to immunize children and susceptible adults.

- Nonimmune women should *not* be immunized during pregnancy because the possible effects of vaccine on the fetus are not completely known. The VARIVAX Pregnancy Registry has reported no occurrences of congenital varicella syndrome or other birth defects with inadvertent exposure to varicella immunization during pregnancy. The registry has been active since 1995 (800/986-8999). Immunization of nonimmune women should be done *at least* 1 month before conception or delayed until after delivery.
- The administration of VariZIG* or immune globulin intravenous (IGIV) to nonimmune pregnant women has been recommended within 96 hours of exposure to VZV during pregnancy. This was intended to prevent or reduce the severity of maternal disease, but is not thought to have effectiveness after the disease has become established. Whether it will protect the fetus is unknown. Varicella-zoster immune globulin is no longer available, as the only manufacturer ceased production.
- Acyclovir antiviral therapy for VZV infections during pregnancy may be appropriate for some women. Consult with infectious disease specialists.
- Discuss pregnancy termination if infection occurs early in pregnancy.

Intrapartum Considerations
- Administer VariZIG or IGIV to nonimmune pregnant women if exposed to varicella within 96 hours of delivery.
- Women with active disease should be isolated from other pregnant women and all newborns. Those who receive VariZIG should be isolated until 28 days after exposure to varicella. Use standard, contact, and airborne precautions.
- Notify pediatrics if the mother was recently exposed to chickenpox or develops a rash between 5 days before and 2 days after delivery.

Postpartum Considerations
Maternal
- Review intrapartum guidelines. Institute isolation precautions, as appropriate.
- Breastfeeding is not a contraindication to postpartum immunization of a nonimmune woman. Lactating women susceptible to VZV infection should be vaccinated.
- Women without evidence of immunity to varicella should receive the first dose of VZV vaccine before hospital discharge, with the second dose given 4 to 8 weeks later.

Neonatal (See also Book III: Neonatal Care, Unit 8, Infections.)
- If a woman develops a rash within 5 days before and 2 days after delivery, give VariZIG to the baby as soon as possible. Prevention and/or reduction in severity is important because neonatal varicella infection carries a high mortality rate.
- A term baby who is more than 2 days old when first exposed to varicella (including one whose mother developed a rash >48 hours after delivery) does not need VariZIG because the risk of complications from infection is no greater than for older children. VariZIG is indicated, however, for some preterm babies. Consult specialists regarding individual babies.

---

*Available under an investigational new drug protocol and can be requested by calling 800/843-7477. See American Academy of Pediatrics. Varicella-zoster infections. In: Pickering LK, Baker CJ, Kimberlin DW, Long SS, eds. *Red Book: 2009 Report of the Committee on Infectious Diseases*. 28th ed. Elk Grove Village, IL: American Academy of Pediatrics; 2009:719.

- If hospitalized, isolate the baby from birth until 21 days of age, unless VariZIG was given, in which case isolate the baby for 28 days.
- Newborns with VZV infection should be isolated with standard, airborne, and contact precautions for the duration of their illness. Babies born with congenital VZV infection contracted earlier in gestation do not need isolation.
- Consult with regional center specialists regarding treatment of individual babies.
- Pregnancy within a household is not a contraindication for immunization of a child within the household. Children susceptible to VZV infection should be immunized just as they would be if not in contact with a pregnant woman.

Table 3.4. Other Maternal Infections That May Affect a Fetus*				
Infection	Transmission		Isolation	Notes
Recommended Screening	Woman	Fetus/Newborn	Standard Precautions (all patients, at all times)	(See Book III: Neonatal Care, Unit 8, Infections, for more details of neonatal care.)
Cytomegalovirus (CMV)	• Sexual contact • Casual contact with infected fluids, including urine and saliva • Transfusion of contaminated blood (rare)	*Transplacental:* yes *Ascending:* no *Delivery:* yes, direct contact with organisms in birth canal *Postpartum:* CMV can be transmitted in breast milk (preterm baby at higher risk)	Isolation not needed for mother or baby. CMV passed in breast milk but does not cause neonatal disease in term babies, probably due to passage of maternal antibodies.	Approximately 1% of all newborns are infected and excrete CMV at birth. Most babies are asymptomatic. Consult experts regarding breastfeeding of preterm baby by CMV-positive mother and antiviral therapy for neonatal CMV.
Hepatitis B virus (HBV) *All women at first prenatal visit.*	• Intimate contact, usually sexual (most common) • Sharing of needles by injected-drug users • Transfusion of contaminated blood (very rare)	*Transplacental:* rare *Ascending:* no *Delivery:* yes, through direct contact with mother's blood *Postpartum:* yes, close personal contact HBsAg-positive adult and child, unless baby immunized	Isolation not needed for mother or baby. Breastfeeding is not contraindicated, but breast-fed babies should receive both HBIG and HBV vaccine.	HBV vaccine may be given to HbsAg-negative women during pregnancy or lactation. Delivery route does not alter transmission rate. *All newborns should receive HBV vaccine, with first dose given within 12 hours of birth.* Babies born to HBsAg-positive women also should receive HBIG.

Table 3.4. Other Maternal Infections That May Affect a Fetus* (continued)

Infection	Transmission		Isolation	Notes
Listeriosis (*Listeria monocytogenes*)	• Eating contaminated food ***Significantly increases risk of abortion, fetal death, preterm birth, and amnionitis***	*Transplacental:* yes *Ascending:* yes *Delivery:* yes, through direct contact with mother's blood *Postpartum:* yes, nosocomial outbreaks have occurred	Isolation not needed for mother or baby. Transmission in breast milk is not known to occur.	Provide prenatal instruction about foods to avoid and proper heating of prepared foods. Organism is common but recognized infection is rare. Pregnant women, however, are at high risk for serious illness after contracting listeriosis. Maternal and neonatal mortality is high.
Parvovirus B19 (fifth disease or erythema infectiosum)	Contact with respiratory secretions or blood	*Transplacental:* yes *Ascending:* no *Delivery:* no	Isolation not needed for mother or baby.	Most babies are born healthy, but a few may have fetal anemia, heart failure from nonimmune hydrops. Affected fetuses may benefit from fetal transfusion.
Rubella Virus (German measles) **See notes at right.**	• Droplet • Direct contact with nasopharyngeal secretions	*Transplacental:* yes *Ascending:* no *Delivery:* no	Babies with congenital rubella may shed virus for 1 year or longer. Isolate newborn from all babies and non-immune adults.	***Measure rubella antibodies at first visit for every woman without documented immunity.*** If nonimmune, vaccinate postpartum. Breastfeeding does not contraindicate maternal immunization.
Streptococci (group B beta-hemolytic streptococci [GBS]) **All women, every pregnancy at 35-37 weeks' gestation.**	• Sexual or direct contact Systemic maternal infection is rare. Colonization is common and increases risk of bacteriuria, chorioamnionitis, endometritis, preterm labor, and neonatal infection.	*Transplacental:* no *Ascending:* yes *Delivery:* yes, direct contact with organisms in birth canal	Isolation not needed for mother or baby.	***Treat all bacteriuria, whether symptoms or not.*** Appropriate intrapartum maternal antibiotic therapy can dramatically reduce risk 1. Baby will become infected with GBS (neonatal infection is life-threatening). 2. Woman may develop GBS endometritis. ***See Figure 3.1.***

Table 3.4. Other Maternal Infections That May Affect a Fetus* *(continued)*

Infection	Transmission		Isolation	Notes
Toxoplasmosis *(Toxoplasma gondii)* **All HIV-positive women.**	• Cats or cat feces (most common) • Raw or under-cooked meat (rare) • Contaminated blood products or infected donor organs (rare)	*Transplacental:* yes *Ascending:* no *Delivery:* no	Isolation not needed for mother or baby. No information is available about human breast milk.	If infection suspected during pregnancy, consult specialists because treatment may reduce transmission to the fetus. Consult specialists regarding neonatal diagnosis, treatment, and long-term follow-up evaluation.
Tuberculosis (TB) **All high-risk women.**	• Droplet	*Transplacental:* rare *Ascending:* no *Delivery:* aspiration or ingestion of infected maternal fluids (rare) *Postpartum:* droplet	Isolate (respiratory precautions) women diagnosed or suspected of having TB. In certain situations, mother and baby may need to be separated temporarily. Delay breastfeeding (pump and discard milk) until noncontagious (2 weeks or longer, depending on therapy). Isolate baby (respiratory precautions) until fully evaluated.	• Treat baby if mother considered to be contagious at time of delivery. • Test mother and baby for HIV. • Consider BCG vaccine for baby. • Consult with infectious disease specialists because prenatal and neonatal therapy is complicated. • Arrange for long-term follow-up because treatment may take 18 months for mother and baby.
Varicella-zoster virus (VZV) (chickenpox)	• Direct contact with infected person (most common) • Droplet (uncommon)	*Transplacental:* yes *Ascending:* no *Delivery:* yes, if mother infected at time of delivery *Postpartum:* yes, if mother develops a rash between 5 days before and 2 days after delivery	Isolate (contact, airborne, standard) women with active disease. Isolate women who receive VariZIG for 28 days. If hospitalized, isolate baby from birth until 21 days of age, unless VariZIG was given, in which case isolate baby for 28 days.	Consider giving VariZIG to nonimmune pregnant women within 96 hours of exposure. If a woman develops a rash within 5 days before and 2 days after delivery, give VariZIG to the baby as soon as possible. A term baby more than 2 days old when exposed to varicella does not need VariZIG because risk of complications from infection is no greater than for older children.

*HbsAg, hepatitis B surface antigen; HBIG, hepatitis B immune globulin; BCG, bacille Calmette-Guérin; VariZIG, varicella-zoster immune globulin.

Self-test

Now answer these questions to test yourself on the information in the last section.

D1. True   False   Maternal vaginal colonization with group B beta-hemolytic streptococci can lead to neonatal sepsis.

D2. True   False   A woman with varicella-zoster virus at the time of delivery should be isolated from all pregnant women and newborns.

D3. True   False   It is safe for a woman with active tuberculosis to breastfeed her baby as soon as her treatment is started.

D4. True   False   A woman with diagnosed or suspected active tuberculosis at the time of delivery should be isolated from all pregnant women and newborns.

D5. True   False   When a woman has active tuberculosis at the time of delivery, 18 months of therapy with antituberculosis drugs may be needed for adequate treatment of the mother and the baby.

D6. True   False   When a woman develops a rash from varicella-zoster virus infection within 5 days before delivery, administration of VariZIG to the newborn is indicated.

D7. True   False   Neonatal varicella-zoster (chickenpox) infection at 2 days of age or less is usually much less severe than in older children.

D8. For each of the following organisms, indicate how the fetus may become infected:
   a. Transplacental   _____ Gonorrhea
   b. Ascending   _____ Toxoplasmosis
   c. At delivery   _____ Varicella-zoster (chickenpox)

D9. A woman's group B beta-hemolytic streptococci culture results are unknown. Which of the following are indications for antibiotics during labor for the prevention of neonatal group B beta-hemolytic streptococci infection?

Yes	No	
____	____	Maternal fever of 38°C (100.4°F)
____	____	Rupture of membranes for 20 hours
____	____	Post-term labor
____	____	Maternal thrombocytopenia
____	____	Previous baby with group B beta-hemolytic streptococci infection
____	____	Group B beta-hemolytic streptococci bacteriuria early in pregnancy

D10. Which of the following is the *most common* way for a newborn to acquire group B beta-hemolytic streptococci infection?
   A. Direct contact with organisms during passage through the birth canal
   B. Transplacental passage from organisms in the mother's blood to the fetus, near term
   C. Direct contact with organisms on the skin of caregivers, soon after birth
   D. Through breastfeeding, from organisms on the mother's skin and in the breast milk

Check your answers with the list that follows the Recommended Routines. Correct any incorrect answers and review the appropriate section in the unit.

C. Sites of Maternal Infection With a Variety of Causative Organisms

Bacterial Vaginosis

1. *Condition in Women:* This is not an infection in the usual sense, but rather an abnormal distribution of organisms that occur normally in the vagina. Hormonal changes (including pregnancy) or antibiotic administration are thought to cause an imbalance in the normal vaginal flora, with the usual lactobacilli organisms largely replaced by other organisms. *Gardnerella vaginalis* is the organism most often associated with bacterial vaginosis (BV). A woman with BV may be asymptomatic or may have a foul-smelling white or yellowish vaginal discharge. The odor is often described as "fishy" and may be accentuated after sexual intercourse (due to the pH of semen). BV may increase the risk of chorioamnionitis, preterm delivery, and postpartum endometritis.

2. *Risks for the Fetus and Newborn:* The risks to the fetus and newborn are those associated with preterm birth, premature ROM, and/or chorioamnionitis, if any of those conditions develop.

Prenatal Considerations

- Pregnant women with symptoms of BV should be treated.
- Treatment recommendations include
  - Metronidazole, 250 mg, orally, 3 times/day for 7 days
  OR
  - Clindamycin, 300 mg, orally, 2 times/day for 7 days
- Sexual transmission does not seem to play a role in this condition because treating sexual partners does not reduce recurrence.
- Screening for BV is not currently recommended as a strategy to reduce the incidence of preterm birth.

Intrapartum Considerations: None specific to BV.

Postpartum Considerations

Maternal

- Risk of endometritis is increased, particularly with cesarean delivery.

Neonatal: None specific to BV.

Urinary Tract Infection and Acute Pyelonephritis

1. *Disease in Women:* Asymptomatic bacteriuria and symptomatic UTI are more common during pregnancy because of the anatomic and physiologic changes that lead to urinary stasis. In addition, bacteriuria and UTI are significantly more likely to progress to pyelonephritis during pregnancy than at any other time. Pyelonephritis can cause serious maternal illness (systemic infection and/or kidney damage). Symptomatic or asymptomatic UTI also increases the risk for postpartum endometritis.

2. *Risks for the Fetus and Newborn:* Maternal UTI is associated with increased risk of preterm labor and of premature ROM.

Prenatal Considerations

Bacteriuria (symptomatic or asymptomatic)

- Obtain urine culture or other test for asymptomatic bacteriuria routinely for *all* women at the first prenatal visit.
- Positive screening test result should be confirmed with a urine culture.

- Treat positive cultures, with or without UTI symptoms (burning, frequency, urgency), promptly with appropriate antibiotics. Recommended antibiotics, until sensitivities are known, include trimethoprim-sulfamethoxazole, nitrofurantoin, and cephalexin.
- A 3-day course of antibiotic therapy is adequate for most women.
- *Escherichia coli* is most commonly the infecting organism and is often resistant to ampicillin. Treatment with ampicillin or amoxicillin is not recommended unless culture and antibiotic sensitivity results are known.
- Obtain follow-up urine culture 10 to 14 days after completion of antibiotic therapy.
- For women treated for bacteriuria, periodically rescreen during pregnancy. If it recurs, antibiotic suppressive therapy for the remainder of the pregnancy is generally recommended.

 Screen all pregnant women for bacteriuria. If found, whether symptomatic or asymptomatic, treat bacteriuria promptly and aggressively.

Acute Pyelonephritis
- Women with fever of 38°C (100.4°F) or higher, with flank pain (usually right side) and urinary symptoms should be evaluated without delay. Clumps of white blood cells in the urine indicate the need for hospitalization. Treatment includes
  - IV fluid infusion
  - IV antibiotics, followed by oral antibiotics after hospital discharge
  - Investigation for presence of renal stones, especially in patients with recurrent urinary infections or history of stones
- If pyelonephritis and/or lower UTI recurs, consider antimicrobial suppressive therapy for the remainder of the pregnancy.

Intrapartum Considerations
- Continue antibiotic therapy if started earlier and course not yet completed.

Postpartum Considerations
Maternal
- Risk of endometritis is somewhat increased, particularly if delivery was by cesarean section.

Neonatal
- If maternal infection is active at the time of delivery
  - Obtain blood cultures.
  - Check complete blood count with differential.
  - Consider starting antibiotics.
  - Observe closely for evidence of respiratory distress and/or sepsis. If any signs of illness develop, treat promptly with antibiotics.

Intra-amniotic Infection or Chorioamnionitis: Infection of the amniotic membranes is a serious infection that puts a woman at risk for sepsis and postpartum endometritis and a fetus at risk for preterm birth and/or neonatal sepsis. Management is presented in Book II: Maternal and Fetal Care, Unit 6, Abnormal Rupture and/or Infection of the Amniotic Membranes.

Puerperal Endometritis

1. *Maternal Illness:* "Childbed fever" or infection of the endometrium (lining of the uterus) following delivery was once a major cause of maternal mortality, but is rarely fatal today. The likelihood of infection is increased after cesarean delivery. It can occur in any woman, but those with premature ROM, untreated or inadequately treated gonorrhea or *Chlamydia* infection, GBS colonization, or UTI are at highest risk.

   Infection of the endometrium may extend into the myometrium, and possibly on into the pelvic veins and even the inferior vena cava. When found in the pelvic veins, it is termed septic pelvic thrombophlebitis. Septic pelvic thrombophlebitis may be life-threatening if untreated, due to the possibility of pulmonary embolism and overwhelming sepsis. Treatment involves heparin infusion and IV antibiotic therapy.

2. *Risks for the Newborn:* The reason the mother developed endometritis may also pose a serious risk for neonatal infection.

Signs and Symptoms
- Fever 38°C (100.4°F) or higher more than 24 hours after delivery
- Abdominal cramping pain
- Foul-smelling lochia
- Leukocytosis (elevated white blood cell count)

Diagnosis
- Uterine tenderness (diagnosed by bimanual examination of the uterus and adnexa)
- Foul-smelling lochia
- No indication of other infections
  - No mastitis
  - No pneumonia (consider obtaining a chest x-ray)
  - No pyelonephritis (check urinalysis and culture)

Treatment
Initial
- Begin IV antibiotic therapy.
  - *Vaginal delivery*
- Penicillin plus an aminoglycoside
  OR
- Extended-spectrum penicillin or cephalosporin
  - *Cesarean delivery*: Anaerobic organisms are more likely to be involved; consider treatment with gentamicin 1.5 mg/kg plus clindamycin 900 mg every 8 hours.
- Continue treatment until the woman has been afebrile and symptom-free for 24 to 48 hours.

If fever is present 48 hours after antibiotics started,
- Suspect *Bacteroides* or enterococci infection, or drug-resistant organisms.
- Repeat pelvic examination to evaluate for pelvic abscess.
- Consider vaginal probe ultrasound examination to search for retained placental tissue or abscess.
- Review antibiotic regimen
  - If using an extended-spectrum penicillin or cephalosporin, consider switching to penicillin (or ampicillin) plus gentamicin and clindamycin (or metronidazole).

OR
- – If using gentamicin and clindamycin, consider adding ampicillin for coverage of enterococcus. Consider substituting metronidazole for clindamycin. If an abscess is suspected, aztreonam may be more effective than gentamicin.
- If metronidazole is used, recommend discontinuing breastfeeding during therapy, and for 12 to 24 hours following the end of therapy, to allow maternal excretion of the drug. During this time, the mother may pump her breasts to establish and maintain her milk supply, but the milk should be discarded, due to the high concentration of metronidazole in breast milk.

If fever persists for an additional 48 hours,
- Consider pelvic ultrasound examination, if not done earlier.
- Repeat pelvic examination, looking for pelvic abscess or induration of the parametrium (area between the layers of the broad ligament).
  - – If abscess found, consult with experts regarding surgical drainage.
  - – Begin heparin therapy (pelvic thrombophlebitis is likely to be present).
- Consult with regional center specialists; consider transfer of the patient.

Puerperal Mastitis
1. *Maternal Illness:* Postpartum inflammation of the breast(s) rarely develops while the mother is still hospitalized, but can become a significant problem for the woman after she goes home. Proper breastfeeding technique that encourages milk drainage from all areas of the breast decreases the likelihood of mastitis developing.

2. *Risks for the Newborn:* Infectious mastitis does not pose a threat to a healthy newborn unless an abscess has formed. If an abscess is present, breastfeeding with the affected breast will need to be interrupted temporarily.

Signs and Symptoms
- Breast (usually only one is affected) is swollen, reddened, tender, and hot.
- Red streaks (infected lymph vessels) may lead away from the tender area.

Treatment
- Begin penicillinase-resistant penicillin, or erythromycin if the woman is sensitive to penicillin.
- Consider obtaining a culture of the milk. This may be done by the mother expressing a sample of milk, after careful cleansing of her breast.
- Breastfeeding may continue and is encouraged at frequent intervals to ensure emptying the affected breast. Mastitis usually resolves with antibiotic therapy and continued lactation. Pain medication may be needed for several days to allow breastfeeding.
- Breast abscess is rare. If one occurs,
  - – Drain the abscess as soon as it becomes fluctuant.
  - – Rupture of an abscess into the ductal network of the breast can release large numbers of organisms into the breast milk. For this reason, nursing with the affected breast is not recommended when an abscess is present (nursing on the unaffected side may continue). A breast pump, with the milk discarded, may be used on the affected side to empty the breast and facilitate lactation.
  - – Nursing with the affected breast may resume after the abscess has been surgically drained and antibiotic therapy instituted.

Self-test

Now answer these questions to test yourself on the information in the last section.

E1.	True	False	*All* pregnant women should be screened for asymptomatic bacteriuria.
E2.	True	False	Bacterial vaginosis may increase the risk for maternal complications *and* preterm delivery.
E3.	True	False	Only women with symptomatic urinary tract infection should be treated with antibiotics.
E4.	True	False	Postpartum endometritis can progress to septic pelvic thrombophlebitis.
E5.	True	False	Sexual contact seems to be the way bacterial vaginosis is spread.
E6.	True	False	When mastitis is present, breastfeeding must stop completely to avoid infection of the baby.
E7.	True	False	Acute pyelonephritis in a pregnant woman requires hospitalization, intravenous antibiotics, and fluid infusion.
E8.	True	False	Physiologic changes during pregnancy increase the risk of urinary tract infection, even for women who have never had a urinary tract infection.
E9.	True	False	Urinary tract infection, whether it is symptomatic or asymptomatic, increases the risk of premature rupture of membranes and preterm labor.
E10.	True	False	Antibiotic treatment for puerperal mastitis is penicillinase-resistant penicillin or erythromycin.
E11.	True	False	Initial treatment of puerperal endometritis includes intravenous administration of antibiotics.
E12.	True	False	Bacterial vaginosis is often associated with a "fishy" odor.
E13.	List at least 3 signs of postpartum endometritis.		

_____

_____

_____

Check your answers with the list that follows the Recommended Routines. Correct any incorrect answers and review the appropriate section in the unit.

Perinatal Infections

Recommended Routines

All the routines listed below are based on the principles of perinatal care presented in the unit you have just finished. They are recommended as part of routine perinatal care.

Read each routine carefully and decide whether it is standard operating procedure in your hospital. Check the appropriate blank next to each routine.

Procedure Standard in My Hospital   **Needs Discussion by Our Staff**

_____   _____   1. Establish a system to ensure use of standard precautions by all staff members.

_____   _____   2. Establish a written protocol to obtain lower vagina and rectal cultures for group B beta-hemolytic streptococci from all women at 35 to 37 weeks' gestation (unless a woman had an earlier baby with group B beta-hemolytic streptococci infection or had group B beta-hemolytic streptococci bacteriuria in current pregnancy).

_____   _____   3. Establish a written protocol for prenatal and intrapartum management for the prevention of neonatal group B beta-hemolytic streptococci infection.

_____   _____   4. Establish a policy to screen *all* women with culture, serology, and/or other test as early in pregnancy as possible, for
- Bacteriuria
- Gonorrhea
- Hepatitis B virus
- Human immunodeficiency virus
- Syphilis

_____   _____   5. Establish a protocol for treatment of bacteriuria, whether symptomatic or asymptomatic.

_____   _____   6. Establish a system for timely transfer of information about possible or proven maternal infections to neonatal providers.

_____   _____   7. Establish written guidelines for isolation of
- Women with active genital herpes and their babies
- Babies with congenital rubella
- Women with active tuberculosis and their babies
- Women with varicella-zoster infection, or recent exposure, and their babies

_____   _____   8. Establish written guidelines for
- Prophylactic eye care of all newborns
- Newborns at risk for chlamydial conjunctivitis

_____   _____   9. Establish a system to ensure administration of
- Hepatitis B virus vaccine to *all* babies, with first of 3-dose series given soon after birth (Book III: Neonatal Care, Unit 8, Infections)
- Hepatitis B virus vaccine (first dose) and hepatitis B immune globulin to preterm and term babies born to women positive for hepatitis B surface antigen, given within 12 hours of birth

_____   _____   10. Establish a system to ensure maternal serologic status for syphilis is known for *every* newborn before discharge.

Self-test Answers

These are the answers to the self-test questions. Please check them with the answers you gave and review the information in the unit wherever necessary.

A1. c. Asymptomatic maternal infection = mother with *Chlamydia*
     b. Cesarean delivery = mother with active genital herpes
     a. Ceftriaxone for mother and baby = mother with active gonorrhea

A2. True

A3. True

A4. False. Most organisms *cannot* cross the placenta and infect the fetus. The ones that can, however, are often capable of causing serious damage to the fetus.

A5. True

A6. False. Ascending infection is more likely to occur after the membranes have ruptured, but can occur through intact membranes.

A7. False. Prophylactic eye treatment with silver nitrate or antibiotic ointment is used to *prevent* neonatal gonorrheal ophthalmia. If an infection develops, topical treatment is not adequate. *Systemic antibiotics* must be used to *treat* it.

A8. True

A9. False. Routine prophylactic eye treatment with silver nitrate, erythromycin, or tetracycline will *NOT* reliably prevent neonatal chlamydial conjunctivitis. Some experts advise that all babies born to women with untreated *Chlamydia* infection receive oral erythromycin for 14 days.

A10. True

A11. True

A12. False. A woman may have a mild or asymptomatic viral illness that causes serious fetal illness or damage. Likewise, certain serious maternal illnesses may not affect the fetus at all.

A13. The presence of any one sexually transmitted infection should prompt investigation for other sexually transmitted infections.

Yes	No	
	X	Toxoplasmosis
X		Syphilis
X		*Chlamydia*
	X	Parvovirus
X		Herpes
X		HIV

B1.

Yes	No	
X		Test positive for HIV antibodies
	X	Be infected with the virus

B2.

Pregnancy	Delivery	
X	X	Syphilis
X	X	Herpes simplex virus
	X	Human papillomavirus

B3. False. HIV can be passed from an infected woman to her newborn in her breast milk.

B4. True

B5. False. Syphilis infection can pass to the fetus during *any* stage of maternal infection. Transplacental transfer rates are: primary stage = approximately 50%, secondary stage = approximately 100%, tertiary stage = approximately 10%.

B6. True

B7. True

133

B8. True

B9. False. Standard precautions need to be used for *all patients at all times*. Use of these precautions has dramatically lowered the incidence of work-acquired hepatitis infections in health care workers.

B10. False. There is no treatment for neonatal human papillomavirus (HPV). Only a very small number of babies born to women with HPV become infected, but if infection occurs at the time of delivery, symptoms may not be evident for months or years.

B11.

Yes	No	
X	___	HIV
___	X	Human papillomavirus
X	___	Syphilis
X	___	Gonorrhea
___	X	Herpes simplex virus

C1.

Yes	No	
___	X	Gonorrhea
X	___	Primary parvovirus infection
X	___	Rubella (German measles)
X	___	Cytomegalovirus
___	X	*Chlamydia*
X	___	Listeriosis

C2. True

C3. True

C4. True

C5. False. The route of delivery does not affect the rate of transmission of hepatitis B virus from women positive for hepatitis B surface antigen to their babies. Cesarean delivery should be used only for obstetric reasons.

C6. True

C7. False. Breastfeeding by women positive for hepatitis B surface antigen does not increase the risk of infection for the baby. Vaccination of the baby eliminates nearly all risk. Administration of hepatitis B virus vaccine and hepatitis B immune globulin is recommended for breastfed babies of women positive for hepatitis B surface antigen.

C8. False. Cytomegalovirus, particularly during a primary infection, easily crosses the placenta in early pregnancy. Because maternal illness is mild, such infections are rarely detected.

C9. True

C10. False. Acyclovir is used in the treatment of herpes simplex infection, but systemic therapy should be avoided during pregnancy. There is no treatment for parvovirus B19. If maternal parvovirus infection is identified during pregnancy, the fetus should be monitored for possible (although uncommon) serious complications.

C11. True

C12. True

C13. True

C14. True

C15. True

C16. False. Breastfeeding is not a contraindication to postpartum rubella vaccination of a nonimmune mother.

D1. True

D2. True

D3. False. A woman with active tuberculosis needs to maintain respiratory precautions and delay breastfeeding until she is noncontagious. Depending on the specific therapy and strain of tuberculous bacilli, this will take 2 weeks or more after appropriate medications are started.

D4. True

D5. True

D6. True

D7. False. The reverse is true. Neonatal varicella-zoster (chickenpox) infection at 2 days of age or younger is usually much more severe than in older children.

D8. a. Transplacental   <u>b, c</u>   Gonorrhea
    b. Ascending   <u>a</u>   Toxoplasmosis
    c. At delivery   <u>a, c</u>   Varicella-zoster (chickenpox)

D9.

Yes	No	
X	___	Maternal fever
X	___	Rupture of membranes for 20 hours (18 hours or longer)
___	X	Post-term labor
___	X	Maternal thrombocytopenia
X	___	Previous baby with group B beta-hemolytic streptococci infection
X	___	Group B beta-hemolytic streptococci bacteriuria early in pregnancy

D10. A. Direct contact with organisms during passage through the birth canal

E1. True

E2. True

E3. False. Women with asymptomatic bacteriuria, as well as women with symptomatic urinary tract infection, should be treated with antibiotics. All women should be checked routinely at the first prenatal visit for asymptomatic bacteriuria. Positive cultures, with or without symptoms, should be treated promptly and aggressively with appropriate antibiotics.

E4. True

E5. False. Sexual transmission does not appear to play a role in bacterial vaginosis. Treating sexual partners does not reduce recurrence.

E6. False. There is no reason to stop breastfeeding when mastitis is present, unless an abscess develops (which rarely happens). If an abscess develops, breastfeeding from the affected breast should be temporarily interrupted.

E7. True

E8. True

E9. True

E10. True

E11. True

E12. True

E13. Any 3 of the following:
- Maternal fever 38°C (100.4°F) or higher more than 24 hours after delivery
- Elevated white blood cell count
- Abdominal cramping
- Foul-smelling lochia

135

Unit 3 Posttest

If you are applying for continuing education credits, a posttest for this unit is available online. Completion of unit posttests and the book evaluation form are required to achieve continuing education credit. For more details, visit www.cmevillage.com.

Unit 4: Various High-Risk Conditions

Objectives

In this unit you will learn

A. What medical conditions place a pregnant woman and/or her fetus at risk

B. How to evaluate and monitor medical risk factors during pregnancy, labor, and the post-partum period

C. What implications maternal medical conditions have for the baby after birth

D. How to evaluate and monitor the baby for possible complications from maternal medical conditions

E. What obstetric conditions (either factors identified in a previous pregnancy or present in the current pregnancy) place a woman and/or her fetus at risk

F. How to evaluate and monitor obstetric risk factors during pregnancy, labor, and the post-partum period

G. What implications obstetric conditions have for the baby after birth

H. How to evaluate and monitor the baby for possible complications from obstetric conditions

Note: Not all management and treatment details are presented in this unit. For some conditions (obstetric hemorrhage, preterm labor, etc), detailed care descriptions are presented in other units in this book. For other, extremely high-risk conditions, consultation with and/or referral to maternal-fetal medicine specialists is strongly recommended. Some extremely high-risk conditions pose significant risk to the woman's health during pregnancy, and pregnancy may result in permanent damage to the most affected organ (heart or kidneys, etc). These conditions also may pose significant risk to fetal health and well-being. A woman needs to have specific, detailed, and up-to-the-moment information about the risks and the management options to make informed decisions. If pregnancy continues, management is often complex.

Unit 4 Pretest

Before reading the unit, please answer the following questions. Select the *one* **best** answer to each question (unless otherwise instructed). Record your answers on the test and check them against the answers at the end of the book.

1. Assuming the only risk factors are those stated, which situation represents the *lowest* risk?

    A. 13-year-old high school girl whose parents are very wealthy

    B. 32-year-old woman who has severe, but well-controlled, asthma

    C. 24-year-old woman who is pregnant with twins

    D. 28-year-old woman who had rubella (German measles) 2 years ago

2. True   False Women who are heavy smokers are much more likely to deliver large-for-gestational-age babies.

3. True   False A woman who delivered one stillborn baby has an increased risk of delivering another stillborn baby.

4. True   False Placental function declines in post-term gestations, significantly increasing the risk for non-reassuring fetal monitoring during labor.

5. True   False Maternal immune thrombocytopenic purpura may place the fetus and newborn at risk for internal or intracranial hemorrhage.

6. True   False Women with antiphospholipid antibody syndrome should use only estrogen-containing oral contraceptives.

7. Which of the following are recommended for a 26-year-old woman pregnant with twins?

Yes	No	
___	___	Prenatal visit every week during the third trimester
___	___	Extra iron and folic acid supplementation
___	___	Amniocentesis for chromosomal analysis
___	___	Serial ultrasound evaluations of fetal growth

8. Which of the following are associated with fetal growth restriction?

Yes	No	
___	___	Hydramnios
___	___	Systemic lupus erythematosus
___	___	Severe maternal hypertension
___	___	Multifetal gestation
___	___	Placenta previa

9. True   False The dosage of an anticonvulsant medication to a woman with a seizure disorder should *not* be readjusted during pregnancy.

10. True   False Twins in nonvertex-vertex presentation are generally delivered vaginally.

11. True   False A fetus may develop goiter if maternal hyperthyroidism was treated during pregnancy.

12. True   False Growth-restricted fetuses are at increased risk for non-reassuring testing during labor.

13. Which of the following is *most* likely to be associated with oligohydramnios?
A. Fetal growth restriction
B. Fetal gastrointestinal tract abnormality
C. Maternal diabetes mellitus
D. Multifetal gestation

14. Which of the following is *most* likely to be associated with a post-term pregnancy?
A. Decreased volume of amniotic fluid
B. Cardiac defect in the fetus
C. Woman with 4 or more previous pregnancies
D. Congenital infection

15. Vaginal birth after a cesarean delivery is usually contraindicated when
A. Estimated fetal weight is greater than 2,500 g
B. Epidural anesthesia is planned
C. A classical (vertical) uterine incision was used for the previous cesarean delivery
D. Previous birth was preterm

16. Hydramnios is associated with an increased risk for
A. Umbilical cord compression
B. Anencephaly
C. Maternal hypertension
D. Congenital infection

17. All of the following are accurate statements regarding severe maternal anemia, *except:*
A. Non-iron deficiency anemia may be due to chronic medical illnesses.
B. If postpartum hemorrhage occurs, it is more likely to be fatal.
C. A fetus generally adapts better to chronic maternal anemia than to acute blood loss.
D. Non-iron deficiency anemia should be treated with vitamin B_{12}.

18. In general, pregnant teenagers are at increased risk for all of the following, *except:*
A. Sexually transmitted infections
B. Precipitate labor
C. Pregnancy-specific hypertension
D. Preterm delivery

19. **True   False**   Heparin use is contraindicated in women with antiphospholipid antibody syndrome.

20. **True   False**   Hydramnios is associated with congenital infection.

Medical Risk Factors and Their Implications

For each condition presented in this unit, sections are given for *prenatal considerations, intrapartum considerations,* and *postpartum considerations: maternal* and *neonatal.* Lists within each section identify the procedures or tests that comprise the minimum, basic evaluation for all women, fetuses, and babies with that particular risk factor. Women and their babies may each have several risk factors that may be the same or may be different from each other. Tests or procedures beyond those listed also may be needed. In addition, the lists do not include routine evaluation and care measures.

1. What Are Medical Risk Factors?

A preexisting medical illness may adversely affect the outcome of pregnancy and/or pregnancy may affect the underlying medical condition. These effects may be heightened as the pregnancy progresses. Care requires a balance between treatment of the medical condition and management of the pregnancy, and between fetal and maternal considerations.

If possible, there should be planning for pregnancy *before* conception, with discussion of the

- Risks to the fetus from maternal disease
- Long-term risks to the woman's health if there is worsening of a medical condition with pregnancy
- Probable medical management during pregnancy
- Risks and benefits of medications that may be needed during pregnancy

While any medical condition can affect pregnancy, the following are especially likely to place a pregnant woman and/or her fetus at risk. Some significant risk factors, such as hypertension and infectious diseases, are not presented here because other units within this book are devoted to those topics.

A. Cardiovascular Disease

As pregnancy progresses, oxygen consumption, blood volume, heart rate, and cardiac output all increase. Women with heart disease may have difficulty responding to the stress these changes place on heart function. Evaluation and treatment will vary depending on the specific heart disease and its severity. Consultation with cardiac, maternal-fetal, and pediatric specialists is recommended for the care of the woman and her fetus, especially if there is any evidence of maternal cardiac decompensation (edema, shortness of breath, rales and rhonchi on auscultation of the lungs).

 The effect of pregnancy on a woman with heart disease is closely related to her prepregnancy clinical status.

New York Heart Association Classification of Heart Disease: This system uses symptoms with physical activity to classify the relative severity of heart disease. The categories are

Class I.   Patients with cardiac disease but without resulting limitation of physical activity. Ordinary physical activity does not cause undue fatigue, palpitation, dyspnea, or anginal pain.

Class II.   Patients with cardiac disease resulting in slight limitation of physical activity. They are comfortable at rest. Ordinary physical activity causes fatigue, palpitation, dyspnea, or anginal pain.

Class III.   Patients with cardiac disease resulting in marked limitation of physical activity. They are comfortable at rest. Less than ordinary activity causes fatigue, palpitation, dyspnea, or anginal pain.

Class IV. Patients with cardiac disease resulting in inability to carry on any physical activity without discomfort. Symptoms of heart failure or the anginal syndrome may be present even at rest. If any physical activity is undertaken, discomfort increases.

1. **Class I and Class II** (New York Heart Association classification). Although patients usually tolerate pregnancy well, this degree of heart disease poses a risk to a woman and her fetus. Limitation of physical activity may be needed, especially for women with Class II heart disease. Medical management of cardiac decompensation may be required during the second and third trimesters, and invasive hemodynamic monitoring during labor and the postpartum period may be necessary.

Prenatal Considerations
- Be aware of the possible influence of maternal medications on fetal condition.
  - Oral anticoagulants are hazardous to fetal development and should be replaced with heparin therapy, either unfractionated or low-molecular weight heparin (if possible, before conception).
  - Diuretics may interfere with placental perfusion, although much less likely in women chronically treated with diuretics prior to conception.
- If a woman has congenital heart disease, consider obtaining a fetal echocardiogram because there is an increased risk that the baby also will have congenital heart disease, although not necessarily the same type as the mother.
- Counsel the woman to avoid excessive weight gain, as appropriate for her initial body mass index (BMI).
- Encourage daily rest periods and reduction in usual activities and work schedule.
- Schedule frequent prenatal visits (every 2 weeks or more often). Watch for evidence of congestive heart failure (CHF)—question the woman specifically about changes in activity and work tolerance, dyspnea, orthopnea; auscultate her lungs thoroughly; assess whether weight gain is normal (weight gain from retained fluid may indicate CHF); and consider chest x-ray and/or pulmonary function tests if there is uncertainty regarding cardiac status.

Intrapartum Considerations
- Use cesarean delivery only for obstetric indications (for most patients with heart disease, anesthesia and surgery pose a greater risk than labor).
- Consider antibiotics.
  - The American Heart Association does *not* recommend prophylactic antibiotic therapy with either vaginal or cesarean delivery, *except* for women with heart disease who are *febrile* at the time of delivery. Mitral-valve prolapse typically is not considered an indication for prophylactic antibiotics.
  - For women with heart disease or a history of endocarditis, who show no signs of infection at the time of delivery, antibiotic prophylaxis is individualized. Consult with the woman's cardiologist and/or maternal-fetal medicine specialist.
  - If a woman with heart disease has a fever at the time of delivery, the recommended prophylactic antibiotic regimen is
- Ampicillin, 2 g intramuscularly or intravenously, plus gentamicin, 1.5 mg/kg (not to exceed 120 mg) within 30 minutes of delivery, followed 6 hours later by ampicillin 1 g, intramuscularly or intravenously, or amoxicillin, 1 g, orally.
- If a woman is allergic to ampicillin, use vancomycin, 1 g, intravenously, given over 1 to 2 hours and completed within 30 minutes of delivery; no postpartum dose is needed.

- Keep intravenous (IV) fluid intake to a minimum (<1,000 to 1,500 mL/day).
- Minimize cardiac workload.
  - Minimize pain (increased heart rate due to reaction to pain may lead to heart failure).
  - Use narcotic analgesia or regional anesthesia as needed for pain relief.
  - Consider epidural anesthesia, which is appropriate for most patients, once normal labor has been achieved.
- Watch for CHF during the second stage of labor and the first few days after delivery.

Postpartum Considerations

Maternal

- If antibiotic prophylaxis was given, provide follow-up dose after delivery, as appropriate, to complete the course of antibiotics. (See Intrapartum Considerations.)
- Continue to monitor for deterioration of cardiac function.

Neonatal

- Recommended actions depend on fetal response to labor and delivery.
- If mother has congenital heart disease, evaluate newborn for evidence of congenital heart disease.
- If mother has been on thiazide diuretics and the baby has petechiae or otherwise shows evidence of bleeding, consider evaluation of platelet levels, because neonatal thrombocytopenia has been reported.

2. **Class III and Class IV** (New York Heart Association classification). Because of considerable risk to maternal health from heart failure during pregnancy, labor, or delivery, prompt consultation with a cardiologist and/or maternal-fetal medicine specialist is needed.

 Women with Class III or IV heart disease have a significant risk of decompensation during pregnancy or postpartum. Care by specialists at a regional medical center is strongly advised.

B. Metabolic/Endocrine Disease

Thyroid Disease

1. **Hyperthyroidism:** Consultation with specialists trained and experienced in the treatment of this disease during pregnancy is recommended. If a woman's disease is not stable prepregnancy, management can be especially complex. Even if hyperthyroidism is well-controlled, it may worsen dramatically during pregnancy. Initial diagnosis during pregnancy can be difficult because serum levels of certain thyroid hormones normally change with pregnancy, and the use of radioactive iodine is contraindicated.

Prenatal Considerations

- Thyroid-stimulating hormone (TSH) and free thyroxine levels may need to be followed and medication adjusted accordingly.
- Monitor for pregnancy-specific hypertension because the risk is increased. If found, manage according to guidelines in Unit 1, Hypertension in Pregnancy, in this book.
- Monitor fetal well-being and growth because there is an increased risk for growth restriction.
- Consider assessing for fetal goiter by ultrasound at term. Large fetal goiters can cause hyperextension of the head, which may require cesarean delivery.

- If signs of thyroid storm develop (maternal heart rate above 130, sweating, fever, eye abnormalities, and shortness of breath), the woman will need intensive care. Treatment with propranolol, saturated solution of potassium iodide, and antipyretics may be necessary.

 Thyroid storm can be life-threatening. Consultation with endocrinologists and maternal-fetal medicine specialists is strongly recommended.

Intrapartum Considerations
- In stable patients, continue the same dosage of autonomic drugs (eg, propranolol) and antithyroid medication during the intrapartum period.
- Although rare, sudden development of thyroid storm can occur, particularly in poorly controlled hyperthyroid women.

Postpartum Considerations
Maternal
- Hyperthyroidism may become unstable. Monitor the woman carefully for several weeks postpartum for tachycardia, palpitations, increased sweating, and/or unexplained diarrhea.
- Mother may breastfeed if she requires treatment with methimazole.
- Propylthiouracil is considered compatible with breastfeeding. Periodic evaluation of the baby's thyroid function may be prudent.

Neonatal
- Consultation with pediatric specialists is recommended.
- Evaluate for hypothyroidism, hyperthyroidism, or goiter because any of these conditions may be present.
- Initially, the baby may develop transient hypothyroidism from placentally transferred propothiouracil (given as therapy to the mother) or from antithyroid antibodies that may cross the placenta.
- After several weeks, the baby may develop hyperthyroidism from thyroid-stimulating immunoglobulins, which also cross the placenta.
- Monitoring and/or treatment may be needed for weeks or months.

2. **Hypothyroidism:** A woman may be stable on thyroid replacement therapy, with her serum TSH within the normal range throughout pregnancy. If her condition is unstable, consultation with specialists trained and experienced in the treatment of this disease during pregnancy is recommended.

   Note: Women with untreated hypothyroidism are more likely to be anovulatory or have recurrent first trimester losses. Pregnancy can occur unexpectedly during early treatment of the disease.

Prenatal Considerations
- Check TSH levels at first prenatal visit and each trimester.
- Continue thyroid replacement throughout pregnancy to maintain TSH levels within normal range. For most women, drug dosage may need to be increased.
- Monitor fetal well-being because there is an increased risk for adverse events, including preeclampsia, placental abruption, low birth weight (secondary to preterm delivery due to preeclampsia), perinatal mortality, and neuropsychological impairment.

Intrapartum Considerations: None specific to hypothyroidism
Postpartum Considerations
Maternal

- Monitor TSH levels and readjust thyroid replacement dosage as necessary.
- Mother may breastfeed as long as she is euthyroid on thyroid replacement medication.

Neonatal

- Baby is usually unaffected; however, evaluate for hypothyroidism, hyperthyroidism, or goiter because any of these complications may occur.
- Consultation with pediatric specialists is recommended.

Self-test

Now answer these questions to test yourself on the information in the last section.

A1.	**True**	**False**	Oral anticoagulants, rather than heparin, should be used during pregnancy.
A2.	**True**	**False**	Thyroid storm can be life-threatening.
A3.	**True**	**False**	A woman with congenital heart disease was treated for congestive heart failure and pulmonary edema early in pregnancy. Near term, she is stable, without symptoms, and has a clear chest x-ray. You can anticipate her labor and delivery will be uncomplicated.
A4.	**True**	**False**	Thyroid storm may develop in a woman with hypothyroidism.
A5.	**True**	**False**	Cesarean delivery is usually less of a risk for a woman with heart disease than labor would be.
A6.	**True**	**False**	Antibiotics are recommended during labor and for 6 hours postpartum for all women with Class I or II heart disease.
A7.	**True**	**False**	With maternal hyperthyroidism, postpartum monitoring and treatment of the woman *and* her baby may be needed for months.
A8.	**True**	**False**	A woman with congenital heart disease is at increased risk for delivering a baby with congenital heart disease.

A9. Which of the following are appropriate care measures for a woman with Class II heart disease?

Yes	No	
____	____	Plan to deliver by cesarean section.
____	____	Evaluate frequently for evidence of congestive heart failure.
____	____	Keep intravenous fluids during labor to a minimum amount.

A10. Which of the following may be signs of thyroid storm?

Yes	No	
____	____	Maternal heart rate of 60 beats per minute
____	____	Sweating
____	____	Shortness of breath
____	____	Fever
____	____	Dry skin
____	____	Deep, labored breathing
____	____	Maternal heart rate of 150 beats per minute

Check your answers with the list that follows the Recommended Routines. Correct any incorrect answers and review the appropriate section in the unit.

C. Hematologic Disease

1. **Severe Anemia**

   Prenatal Considerations

   - Generally, a fetus can adapt better to chronic maternal anemia than to sudden maternal blood loss.
   - Investigate the cause of the woman's anemia.

    Accurate identification of the cause of severe anemia is the most important aspect of care.

   - Rule out chronic gastrointestinal blood loss with stool guaiac test. If stool guaiac is positive, investigate likely causes (ulcers, hemorrhoids, etc) and treat the underlying condition.
   - If the cause is iron deficiency, prescribe iron, folic acid, and vitamin supplements. Provide nutritional counseling.
   - Non-iron deficiency anemia may be due to chronic medical conditions, particularly renal failure. Check urinalysis and renal function tests.
   - Non-iron deficiency anemia also may be due to a maternal hemoglobinopathy.

   Intrapartum Considerations

   - ***If obstetric hemorrhage occurs, it is more likely to be fatal for a severely anemic woman.*** Hemoglobin below 6 g/dL represents a greatly diminished number of red blood cells and, therefore, a greatly reduced oxygen carrying capacity. In the face of severe anemia, bleeding does not need to be massive for a critical volume of red cells to be lost, resulting in an irretrievable lack of oxygen delivery to all body cells.

   Postpartum Considerations

   Maternal

   - Check hematocrit and hemoglobin.
   - Reassess or begin treatment, accordingly to the cause.
   - Monitor carefully for postpartum hemorrhage.

   Neonatal

   - Evaluate for neonatal anemia.

2. **Hemoglobinopathies (Sickle Cell Disease [SS, SC, and Sβ-Thalassemia]):** Sickle cell *disease* (SS Hgb) is a serious, painful, and debilitating disease. Sickle cell *trait* (SA Hgb) may be asymptomatic, have mild symptoms intermittently, or cause symptoms only in specific circumstances (eg, at high altitude). Women of African, Mediterranean, or Asian descent are at increased risk for abnormal hemoglobin.

    Hemoglobinopathies can be quite unstable during pregnancy, seriously jeopardizing the health of both a woman and her fetus. Consultation with, and/or referral to, maternal-fetal medicine specialists and hematologists at a regional medical center is strongly recommended.

   Prenatal Considerations

   - For a fetus to have SS Hgb, *both* parents must either have SS Hgb or SA Hgb. If both parents have SS Hgb, the fetus will have SS Hgb. If both parents have either the disease (SS Hgb) or the trait (SA Hgb), the fetus can inherit either the disease or the trait. Carrier state of an adult can be detected through a blood test (hemoglobin electrophoresis). If the fetus is at risk for the disease, prenatal diagnosis is possible, usually through amniocentesis or chorionic villus sampling (CVS). Consult with maternal-fetal medicine staff regarding recommended procedures and laboratory tests needed.

- Maternal disease (SS Hgb) significantly increases the risk for fetal growth restriction, fetal death, premature rupture of membranes, and preterm labor. Fetal well-being and growth need extremely close monitoring.
- Maternal crises of sickle cell disease (SS Hgb) may occur more frequently during pregnancy and may be life-threatening due to thrombosis, emboli, infection, or heart failure.
- Urinary tract infections are especially likely in women with either SA Hgb or SS Hgb. Treat all infections aggressively with antibiotics. Screen women at least once per trimester for asymptomatic bacteriuria.

Intrapartum Considerations
- Women with SA Hgb (sickle cell trait) generally require no special treatment during labor. If they are anemic, oxygen by mask may be helpful. Use pulse oximetry to monitor maternal oxygenation.
- Intrapartum management of women with SS Hgb (sickle cell disease) is complex. The disease can worsen dramatically during labor. Labor and delivery at a regional medical center is strongly recommended.

Postpartum Considerations
Maternal
- There are no special postpartum considerations for women with SA Hgb.

Neonatal
- Many states include testing for hemoglobinopathies as part of the routine newborn screen. Know the requirements of your state.
- Obtain a blood sample and place on State screen filter paper for subsequent electrophoresis to determine if a baby has sickle cell disease, sickle cell trait, or is not affected. If affected, a baby will not show signs of illness for several months.
- Provide
  - Counseling for the parents regarding future pregnancies
  - Treatment for the baby, as appropriate, early in infancy

3. **Thrombocytopenia:** Two forms of thrombocytopenia are commonly recognized.

Gestational Thrombocytopenia
This is a benign condition that occurs only during pregnancy. It is fairly common but has no maternal symptoms and does not result in fetal or neonatal thrombocytopenia. Gestational thrombocytopenia is important only to distinguish it from immune thrombocytopenic purpura (ITP).

Gestational thrombocytopenia is characterized by
- No history of easy bruising or bleeding
- Normal or slightly low platelet count in early pregnancy
- Low platelet count, generally between 75,000/mm³ and 150,000/mm³, in late pregnancy
- Normal platelet count between pregnancies

Immune Thrombocytopenic Purpura

This disease is not related to pregnancy and is usually diagnosed when a nonpregnant woman is found to have easy bruising and abnormal bleeding. If thrombocytopenia is found for the first time when a woman is pregnant, gestational thrombocytopenia needs to be distinguished from ITP, which is characterized by

- History of easy bruising and bleeding
- Medical records that show a previously low platelet count (nonpregnant state)
- Low platelet count, below 150,000/mm^3, in early pregnancy
- Low platelet count, generally less than 75,000/mm^3, in late pregnancy

If previous (nonpregnant) platelet counts are not available, it may not be possible to make the distinction between gestational thrombocytopenia and ITP. Platelet counts below 75,000/mm^3 are usually, but not always, associated with ITP rather than gestational thrombocytopenia.

With ITP, maternal platelet counts sometimes drop to extremely low levels. Treatment for symptomatic ITP is complex. Consultation with maternal-fetal medicine specialists is recommended.

In addition, some women with ITP have antiplatelet antibodies that cross the placenta. These maternal antibodies attack the proteins on the surface of the fetus's platelets, destroying the fetal platelets. Currently available tests cannot differentiate between antibodies in the pregnant woman's blood that will attack fetal platelets and antibodies that will not. Estimates of the risk of neonatal thrombocytopenia vary widely; a summary of case series suggests a 10% chance of platelet count less than 50,000, and 5% chance of platelet count less than 20,000. Platelet counts of babies born to women with ITP may drop sharply in the days immediately *after* birth, due to increase in neonatal splenic function.

Prenatal Considerations

- It is especially important to instruct the woman with low platelet counts (from ITP or gestational thrombocytopenia) not to use aspirin or aspirin-containing medications, which inhibit the ability of platelets to stick together to stop bleeding.
- Route, location, and timing of delivery is controversial. Percutaneous umbilical blood sampling (PUBS) is no longer recommended to determine fetal platelet count because it carries an approximate 2% risk of fetal hemorrhage and death, which is greater than the risk of significant neonatal intracerebral hemorrhage (<1%).

 Consultation with and/or referral to maternal-fetal medicine specialists for consultation is recommended. Maternal status may influence preferred delivery location.

Intrapartum Considerations

- Current recommendations are to manage labor and delivery in the usual fashion, without fetal platelet count assessment, and to reserve cesarean delivery for the usual obstetric indications.

Postpartum Considerations
Maternal

- Monitor for excessive bleeding.

Neonatal
- Check platelets; level may drop so monitor daily for several days.
- Consider cranial ultrasound or computed tomography to check for intracranial hemorrhage if neonatal platelet count is low.

D. Immunologic Disease

1. **Antiphospholipid Antibody Syndrome (APS):** This is an autoimmune disease characterized by certain clinical findings, especially recurrent spontaneous abortion, unexplained fetal death, and/or venous or arterial thrombosis, as well as the presence of specified levels of antiphospholipid antibodies. Because inconsistency in determining antibody levels exists in many laboratories, repeated results from a reliable laboratory are recommended. Lupus anticoagulant and anticardiolipin antibodies are 2 of numerous antiphospholipid antibodies (APLAs). The clinical significance, particularly during pregnancy, of the other APLAs has not been clearly identified. Women with APLAs at lower titers than required to meet the definition of APS may have APLA-related disorders, but are generally at lower risk for the complications associated with APS.

   The most significant complication associated with APS is thrombosis. Most thrombotic events are venous and most commonly appear as a blood clot in a lower extremity or as a pulmonary embolism. Arterial thrombosis is also possible, with stroke being the most common clinical picture. Venous and arterial thrombosis due to APS can appear in uncommon locations, and a clot found in such a site should prompt investigation for APS. Pregnancy and the use of estrogen-containing oral contraceptives are associated with thrombosis in women with APS.

   While women with systemic lupus erythematosus (SLE) also may have antiphospholipid antibodies, most women with APLAs do not have SLE. Women with APLAs but without SLE may be asymptomatic. Women with APS or APLA-related disorders are often first identified as having antiphospholipid antibodies when evaluated for repeated pregnancy losses.

    Women with APS require complex therapy during pregnancy. Consultation with and/or referral to maternal-fetal medicine specialists at a regional medical center is recommended.

   Prenatal Considerations
   - Certain APLAs cause a false-positive reaction on maternal and newborn nontreponemal tests for syphilis. Use treponemal tests for women with APLAs.
   - Women with APS or APLA-related disorders are at increased risk for
     - Spontaneous abortion
     - Fetal growth restriction
     - Second and third trimester fetal death
     - Non-reassuring fetal heart rate patterns (often preceding second or third trimester fetal death)
     - Early-onset preeclampsia (often before 34 weeks' gestation).
     - Preterm delivery, usually iatrogenic, due to pregnancy complications such as preeclampsia.

Several theories exist as to the mechanism of fetal loss and growth restriction, but none fully explain the clinical findings.

- Heparin, either unfractionated or low-molecular weight, and low-dose aspirin is the recommended therapy for women with APS. Dosage and timing of initiation of therapy needs to be individualized.
- Appropriate treatment for women with low levels of APLAs is not clearly identified.
- Frequent antenatal testing of fetal status should start at approximately 28 weeks.

Intrapartum Considerations
- Careful monitoring of maternal and fetal status

Postpartum Considerations
Maternal
- Rarely, the course of APS becomes life-threatening. A small number of women with APS develop fever, multiple thromboses, and renal and cardiopulmonary failure postpartum.
- Estrogen-containing oral contraceptives should *not* be used.
- Women with a previous thrombotic event should be treated for lifelong anticoagulation. Coumarin is usually the anticoagulant medication used, except during a subsequent pregnancy. During pregnancy, low molecular heparin should be used for women with a history of thrombosis. It is not clear whether or not women with APS, but without a history of thrombosis, should have long-term anticoagulation therapy.

Neonatal
- Anticipate possible need for neonatal resuscitation.
- Baby may be preterm and small for gestational age. Screen for corresponding risk factors. Provide care appropriate for size and gestational age. (See Book I: Maternal and Fetal Evaluation and Immediate Newborn Care, Unit 6, Gestational Age and Size and Associated Risk Factors.)

2. **Systemic Lupus Erythematosus:** This is an autoimmune disease that most often affects women of child-bearing age. It is a multisystem, progressive disease characterized by periods of exacerbation and remission. The severity of SLE varies widely. Whether SLE is active or in remission is likely to affect maternal (and fetal) status during pregnancy.

Autoimmune antibodies are produced that can affect nearly every organ system, causing an inflammatory immune response. Signs and symptoms are typically variable and may be vague and subtle or pronounced and severe. They may include joint and/or muscle pain (vague or severe), nephritis, hypertension, low white blood cell or platelet counts, anemia, rash over nose and cheeks, pneumonitis, pleurisy, intermittent low-grade fever, pericarditis, myocarditis, and/or central nervous system involvement with seizures, irritability, headaches, inattentiveness, difficulty coping with small problems, and/or psychosis.

Antinuclear antibodies (ANA) can be detected in about 95% of patients with SLE. Antiphospholipid antibodies occur in approximately 30% of patients with SLE, with lupus anticoagulant and anticardiolipin antibodies being 2 of particular significance. Lupus anticoagulant antibodies (contrary to what the name may seem to imply) increase the risk for thrombi and emboli formation, which can affect maternal organ systems, as well as the placenta.

Certain maternal antibodies may cross the placenta during pregnancy and damage the conduction system of the fetal heart, causing fetal heart block.

Medication therapy for a woman with SLE may be simple or extraordinarily complex, especially during pregnancy. Consultation with maternal-fetal medicine specialists is essential.

Prenatal Considerations

- Certain APLAs cause a false-positive reaction on maternal and newborn non-treponemal tests for syphilis. Use treponemal tests for women with SLE.
- The women with SLE who are most likely to have a good pregnancy outcome are those with
  - A planned pregnancy that occurs when the disease has been in remission for at least 6 months
  - Adequate renal function (serum creatinine ≤1.5 mg/dL, creatinine clearance of ≥60 mL/min, proteinuria of <3 g/day)
- *Effects of pregnancy on SLE:* Pregnancy probably does not affect the long-term prognosis for SLE, but "flares" or periods of exacerbation seem to occur more often during pregnancy. Some presumed SLE flares may not reflect antigen-antibody reactions of SLE, but rather indicate other processes, such as preeclampsia; eclampsia; or hemolysis, elevated liver enzymes, and low platelets (HELLP) syndrome. Although sometimes difficult to distinguish between worsening SLE and pregnancy-specific hypertension, worsening proteinuria, hypertension, or thrombocytopenia, and/or the onset of seizures, can be presumed to represent superimposed preeclampsia or eclampsia and should be treated accordingly.
- *Effects of SLE on pregnancy*
  - *Spontaneous abortion and fetal death during early pregnancy*: Risk is increased significantly, particularly if APLAs are present.
  - *Fetal growth restriction, non-reassuring fetal status, or fetal death during late pregnancy*: Risk is increased significantly if maternal hypertension and renal compromise are present. Fetal death also can result from cardiac failure in association with heart block.
  - *Preterm delivery*: Risk of preterm birth is increased with SLE, and may be due to spontaneous onset of labor or to maternal and/or fetal indications for preterm delivery.
- Consider delivery at a regional center, even for stable women, because SLE can worsen suddenly during labor or immediately postpartum.
- In addition to obstetric and medical care, physical therapy, exercise and dietary planning, psychiatric care, pain management, and/or the assistance of social services may be needed for the pregnant or postpartum woman.
- Frequent antenatal testing of fetal growth and well-being should start at approximately 28 weeks and may include Doppler study of umbilical blood flow, as well as serial ultrasound examinations, nonstress test (NST), biophysical profile (BPP), and amniotic fluid index (AFI) testing.
- Fetal arrhythmia is rare. If present (heart block is most common), referral to regional center specialists for evaluation is recommended. Anticipate the likely need for neonatal intensive care immediately after birth.

Surveillance and care of maternal and fetal health during pregnancy in a woman with SLE is often extremely complex. Consultation with and/or referral to maternal-fetal medicine specialists is strongly recommended.

Intrapartum Considerations
- Care depends on the woman's condition. Deterioration in maternal condition can occur suddenly.
- Fetal health is likely to be threatened by preterm labor, iatrogenic or spontaneous, and/or intrauterine growth restriction.
- If the conduction system of the fetal heart was affected, arrhythmias (particularly heart block) may be seen on the fetal heart rate tracing. Heart block needs to be distinguished from bradycardia.

 For women with SLE, delivery at a facility equipped and staffed to provide maternal, fetal, and neonatal intensive care is recommended.

Postpartum Considerations
Maternal
- If maternal medication included steroids, the risk for infection (endometritis, surgical wound, urinary tract, etc) may be increased. Monitor closely and treat aggressively.
- SLE exacerbation can occur suddenly.
- Although rare, severe renal and/or cardiopulmonary complications can develop, especially for women with SLE who also have APLAs.

Neonatal
- Anticipate possible need for neonatal resuscitation.
- Occasionally, babies born to women with SLE will have "transient neonatal systemic lupus erythematosus," a benign and self-limited condition characterized by a rash and briefly elevated ANA levels, less often by transient hematologic abnormalities, hepatosplenomegaly, and pericarditis.
- Evaluate cardiac status. Monitor for arrhythmias, particularly heart block. Prognosis for babies with congenital heart block depends on several factors, including the degree of heart block. A pacemaker may be needed.
- Baby may be preterm and small for gestational age. Screen for corresponding risk factors. Provide care appropriate for size and gestational age (See Book I: Maternal and Fetal Evaluation and Immediate Newborn Care, Unit 6, Gestational Age and Size and Associated Risk Factors.)

E. Renal Disease

Women with renal disease are at increased risk for preterm labor, fetal growth restriction, in utero death, and preeclampsia. If the renal disease is uncomplicated by any other medical illness, the risk for development of these complications is relatively low.

Women with renal disease complicated by chronic hypertension or poor renal function, however, are at much higher risk for development of complications. Severe renal disease may be permanently worsened by pregnancy.

 Early detection of hypertension and/or deteriorating renal function is essential for optimal care of women with renal disease.

153

Prenatal Considerations
- Continue prepregnancy therapy during pregnancy.
- Evaluate renal function, particularly creatinine clearance (which is more reliable during pregnancy than blood urea nitrogen or serum creatinine), at the first prenatal visit and in each trimester.
- If renal function deteriorates, investigate other causes, such as urinary tract infection, dehydration, nephrotoxic drugs, and preeclampsia.
- Monitor for the development of preeclampsia. If renal function remains normal, follow management guidelines presented in Unit 1, Hypertension in Pregnancy, in this book.
- Begin the following at approximately 28 weeks' gestation:
  – Prenatal visits at least every 2 weeks
  – Daily fetal activity determinations
  – Antenatal testing of fetal well-being
  – Serial ultrasound evaluation of fetal growth

Note: *Renal transplant patients* usually tolerate pregnancy well if they enter pregnancy with normal renal function. If renal function begins to deteriorate, management can be very complex. Intrapartum management has no special requirements. Postpartum management depends on maternal immunosuppressive therapy. Cautions for newborn care relate only to breastfeeding, if the mother is taking specific immunosuppressive medications. Consult with maternal-fetal medicine specialists.

 Consultation with maternal-fetal medicine specialists is strongly recommended for the care of pregnant women with renal disease, especially if hypertension and/or declining renal function develop.

Intrapartum Considerations
- Placental function may be limited, especially if maternal hypertension is present.

Postpartum Considerations
Maternal
- Monitor renal function and blood pressure.

Neonatal
- Anticipate need for possible neonatal resuscitation.
- Feed early and screen for hypoglycemia (See Book I: Maternal and Fetal Evaluation and Immediate Newborn Care, Unit 8, Hypoglycemia.)
- If resuscitation is needed, monitor for post-resuscitation complications.

F. Neurologic Disease
1. **Seizure Disorders:** Consultation with a maternal-fetal medicine physician and a neurologist is recommended.

Prenatal Considerations
- Folate supplementation is recommended, beginning *before conception* or as early in pregnancy as possible. The neural tube, which develops into the brain and spinal cord, is formed during the first month of gestation. Many anticonvulsants interfere with folic acid metabolism, and folic acid deficiency has been associated with neural tube defects. Recommended folic acid dosage is 4.0 mg/day.

154

- Women with seizure disorders are at increased risk for delivering a baby with congenital anomalies. This is thought to be due to exposure to medications, rather than the seizure disorder alone.
- Phenytoin (Dilantin), phenobarbital, and carbamazepine (Tegretol) therapy increase the risk for congenital anomalies but, despite this, should be continued throughout pregnancy because seizures may result in severe maternal or fetal injury. If possible, however, anticonvulsant therapy with valproic acid should be avoided during pregnancy because of the greater risk for anomalies, such as a neural tube defect, in the fetus.
- Anticonvulsant levels tend to fall during pregnancy. Obtain serum levels every 2 to 4 weeks and readjust dosage as needed.
- Monitor closely for the development of pregnancy-specific hypertension. If preeclampsia develops, and seizures occur, consider that they may be due to eclampsia and not to the woman's seizure disorder. (See Unit 1, Hypertension in Pregnancy, in this book.)

Intrapartum Considerations
- If a woman's seizure disorder is under good control, with no recent symptoms, continue usual drug therapy during labor.
- If a woman has had recent symptoms, check blood level of anticonvulsant drug. Adjust medication dosage as needed.
- If seizures occur and are accompanied by hypertension and proteinuria, consider that they are due to eclampsia and treat accordingly to guidelines in Unit 1, Hypertension in Pregnancy, in this book.
- If uncontrollable seizures occur, which is rare, give oxygen and anticonvulsant medication.
  – Phenytoin (Dilantin) 10 to 15 mg/kg, intravenously
    ○ Give slowly so as not to exceed 50 mg/minute infusion rate.
    ○ Provide continuous cardiac monitoring.

OR
  – Diazepam (Valium) 10 mg intravenously
- Consider consultation with a maternal-fetal medicine specialist, a neurologist, and an anesthesiologist (for airway management).

Postpartum Considerations
Maternal
- Reevaluate anticonvulsant medication dosage and adjust as necessary.
- All anticonvulsant medications enter breast milk in small amounts. If the mother wishes to breastfeed, consider the following:
  – Phenobarbital may (rarely) make the baby drowsy; blood levels can be checked in the baby.
  – Phenytoin (Dilantin) has very rare reported ill effects on the baby.
  – Carbamazepine (Tegretol) has no reported ill effects on the baby.
  – Valproic acid (Depakene or Depakote) has very rare reported ill effects on the baby.
  – Lamotrigine, gabapentin, topiramate, and other newer antiepileptic medications have limited data available at this time regarding breastfeeding. Consult with a maternal-fetal medicine specialist, or a resource such as *Medications and Mothers Milk*, by Dr Thomas Hale, or www.reprotox.org.

Neonatal

- Evaluate for congenital malformations, depending on the anticonvulsive agent used to treat the mother.
- Check clotting studies; consider giving additional vitamin K if the mother was taking phenytoin.

G. Respiratory Disease

1. **Asthma**

Prenatal Considerations

- Treat acute asthma attacks medically. Neither asthma nor its treatment compromise a pregnancy unless an attack is severe and prolonged.
- If an acute attack occurs, requiring hospitalization beyond 26 to 28 weeks' gestation, monitor fetal heart rate and maternal oxygenation continuously. Although rare, fetal death can occur if an attack is serious enough to reduce maternal oxygenation below 90% saturation and/or to require artificial ventilation of the woman.
- If maternal disease is severe and persistent, monitor for fetal growth restriction.

Intrapartum Considerations

- Plan to deliver vaginally. Use cesarean delivery only for obstetric indications. (If needed, be sure anesthesia staff is aware of the patient's asthma so bronchospasm-inducing agents can be avoided.)
- Avoid bronchospasm during labor. Treat with steroids and/or bronchodilators.
- Monitor fetal heart rate, because bronchodilators given to the mother may increase the fetal heart rate.

Postpartum Considerations
Maternal

- Be aware that asthma attacks can occur at any time.

Neonatal

- Check for hypothyroidism and goiter if the mother received iodine-containing drugs (including over-the-counter cough and cold remedies) during pregnancy.

Self-test

Now answer these questions to test yourself on the information in the last section.

B1. True False Because of the risk of causing congenital anomalies, women with seizure disorders should *not* take phenytoin (Dilantin) during pregnancy.

B2. True False Bronchodilators given to an asthmatic pregnant woman may increase the fetal heart rate.

B3. True False Limited placental function in a woman with renal disease may result in a growth-restricted fetus who tolerates labor poorly.

B4. True False In some cases of maternal immune thrombocytopenic purpura, fetal platelets can be destroyed, putting the fetus and newborn at risk for internal and intracranial bleeding.

B5. True False If hemorrhage occurs in a woman with severe anemia, it is more likely to be life-threatening than it would be in a non-anemic woman.

B6. True False A woman with systemic lupus erythematosus may be stable or may become seriously ill during pregnancy.

B7. True False Sickle cell disease may be life-threatening to a woman and her fetus during pregnancy.

B8. True False Asthma rarely increases the risk of a pregnancy, unless an attack is so severe that hospitalization of the pregnant woman is required.

B9. True False Women with seizure disorders treated with phenytoin (Dilantin) maintain stable serum levels throughout pregnancy, making periodic readjustment of the drug dosage unnecessary.

B10. True False Women with sickle cell trait may benefit from oxygen by mask throughout labor.

B11. True False Women with renal disease are at increased risk for developing preeclampsia.

B12. True False Cardiac arrhythmias occur in all babies born to women with systemic lupus erythematosus.

B13. True False The risk of blood clot formation is increased during pregnancy for women with antiphospholipid syndrome.

B14. True False The risk of recurrent spontaneous abortion is increased for women with antiphospholipid syndrome and for women with systemic lupus erythematosus.

B15. True False Regardless of maternal medical illness, worsening hypertension increases the risk of complications for a woman and her fetus.

Check your answers with the list that follows the Recommended Routines. Correct any incorrect answers and review the appropriate section in the unit.

2. What Other Factors Can Adversely Affect Pregnancy?

A. Maternal Age

   1. **15 Years or Younger**

     Prenatal Considerations

     • Pregnant teenagers are at increased risk for pregnancy-specific hypertension, poor nutrition, drug use, domestic violence, and sexually transmitted infections (STIs), and having an underdeveloped bony structure that increases the likelihood of feto-pelvic disproportion.

- Poverty, educational interruption, disruption of the teenager's own growth and development, and other adverse social or economic factors may be present. Provide social service consultation, psychological counseling, and family support services as appropriate to individual needs. Counseling for pregnancy termination and adoption may be appropriate.
- Pregnancy may be unplanned and may create additional stress and social upheaval. Provide emotional support, pregnancy and childbirth information, parenthood preparation discussions, and other teaching and/or resources as appropriate to individual needs.
- Teenagers may benefit from counseling and prenatal care geared specifically for them. Counseling, teaching, and discussions in peer groups, rather than one-on-one, may be valuable.
- The risk of preterm delivery is increased in teenagers aged 18 years or younger.
- Provide frequent prenatal visits, dietary and drug counseling, contraceptive information, and information about transmission, consequences, and prevention of STIs.

Intrapartum Considerations
- Support from family and friends takes on more than the usual importance.
- A combination of praise, patience, encouragement, and gentle guidance from health care providers is especially valuable.

Postpartum Considerations
Maternal
- Provide parenting information and support.
- Provide child development and care instruction.
- Review contraceptive options and information about STIs.
- Provide emotional support and praise; recognize stress of parenting before the mother has herself achieved adulthood.

Neonatal
- Consult with social service.
  - Establish a system of follow-up care.
  - Assess the need for a support network for the mother and/or to oversee the welfare of the baby.

2. 35 Years or Older

Prenatal Considerations
- Older women are more likely to develop placenta previa and gestational hypertension or preeclampsia; to have underlying medical conditions, such as diabetes mellitus, chronic hypertension, and obesity; and to deliver a baby with a chromosomal abnormality.
- The risk of a newborn delivered at term having a trisomy 21, or Down syndrome, is 1 in 570 for women aged 33 years, and increases progressively until it is 1 in 353 for women aged 35 years and 1 in 35 for women aged 45 years.* Offer genetic counseling, aneuploidy screening, and diagnostic testing, such as chorionic villus sampling or amniocentesis.
- The risk of preterm delivery is increased in older women.

---

*American College of Obstetricians and Gynecologists. Invasive Prenatal Testing for Aneuploidy. ACOG Practice Bulletin #88. December 2007.

- Consider screening early for abnormal glucose tolerance early in pregnancy and again at 24 to 28 weeks' gestation. (See Unit 5, Abnormal Glucose Tolerance, in this book.)
- Begin antenatal testing as indicated by clinical condition.

Intrapartum Considerations
- Be aware that abnormal labor patterns are more likely to occur in older women.
- Older women have a greater risk of cesarean delivery.

Postpartum Considerations
Maternal
- Postpartum hemorrhage is more likely to occur.

Neonatal
- Evaluate and monitor according to the mother's medical diseases, if any.
- Evaluate for congenital malformations.

B. Psychological Maladaption to Pregnancy

Unresolved conflicts in a woman's life may interfere with normal emotional adaptation to pregnancy and preparation for parenting. An unwanted pregnancy, even for a woman with no underlying psychological conflicts or psychiatric disease, can create extreme emotional turmoil. A woman already stressed from inadequate income, social support, nutrition, or housing or from health concerns and difficult access to health care, may become more stressed during pregnancy. Reactions can vary widely but may include denial, depression, anger, withdrawal, self-destructive or risk-taking behavior, and child abuse.

Note: Women who have difficulty adapting to pregnancy, and/or are under severe emotional or social stress, are *not* more likely to be psychotic. Women with diagnosed mental illness, however, also may become pregnant. Consult a psychiatrist, because women with major psychosis may need antipsychotic medication and intensive counseling during pregnancy and postpartum. In general, prepregnancy medication is continued during pregnancy. Lithium and other psychotropic drugs, however, may be relatively contraindicated. Review the patient's medication regimen and consult with maternal-fetal medicine experts.

Prenatal Considerations
- Screen *all* women for psychosocial problems. Screening once may not be sufficient, because issues in a woman's life can change as the pregnancy progresses. Women who are screened once each trimester are less likely to have preterm or low birth weight babies than women who do not receive this psychosocial screening. Screening tools are available.*
- Provide emotional support and an outlet for expression of feelings. Also, a woman who adapted well to a previous pregnancy(ies) may encounter extreme difficulties with the current pregnancy, due to the added stress of another child and/or changes in financial, emotional, family, employment, or social circumstances.
- Involve family members, as appropriate, in establishing a support network during pregnancy and during the woman's adaptation to parenting after delivery.

---

*American College of Obstetricians and Gynecologists. Psychosocial Risk Factors: Perinatal Screening and Intervention. Committee Opinion #343. August 2006.

- Provide social service and other consultation, if there are specific stress factors that can be eliminated or alleviated by financial assistance, child care arrangements, changes in work or living arrangements, etc.
- Taking medication appropriately and/or following other medical care plans may be especially difficult for women with psychiatric illness or extreme emotional stress.

Intrapartum Considerations
- Emotional support from family and friends is especially important.
- Support of the woman's self-esteem throughout labor and delivery by health care providers is also particularly important.

Postpartum Considerations
Maternal
- Continue to assess adaptation to parenting after delivery.
- Be aware that some women, *without* preexisting mental illness, may experience serious depression and, rarely, postpartum psychosis. Recognition and intervention are crucial.
- Review prenatal support plan and revise as necessary.

Neonatal
- Arrange for ongoing follow-up care. Be aware that child neglect and/or abuse is more likely to occur.
- Consult with social service and other agencies as appropriate.

C. Substance Use

 Anyone can be a substance user. Routine investigation of possible substance use should be part of prenatal care for ALL women.

Depending on the substance, users can consume drugs orally, by injection (intradermal, intramuscular, and/or IV route), or through inhalation. For a specific substance, the effects on the fetus can be the same, regardless of the route of administration. Quite often, however, substance users use more than one drug, which may compound the effects on the woman and the fetus. Inform *all* pregnant women that smoking, drinking alcohol, and using illicit drugs are harmful to themselves *and* to their babies.

Discuss with every pregnant woman

- All legal and nonlegal substances she is using
- Psychosocial factors that may have an impact on pregnancy

 Overdose from any substance, or combination of substances, is an emergency. Maternal (and fetal) mortality is high with acute intoxication.

1. **Drugs:** Users of illicit drugs, particularly individuals who use needles to self-administer the drug(s), are at high risk for hepatitis, human immunodeficiency virus (HIV), STIs (see Unit 3, Perinatal Infections, in this book), other medical illnesses, and poor nutrition.

Drug-addicted women may not seek prenatal care, or may seek care from a variety of providers, with little chance for thorough assessment of maternal and fetal status or for continuity of care. The first contact with the health care system may not occur until labor begins, and sometimes not until labor is well-advanced. On the other hand, some drug-addicted women may seek early and consistent prenatal care. Women in either group may be extremely skilled at hiding their substance use or addiction. Health care providers need to be alert to subtle cues and willing to believe that pregnant women, from all walks of life, can be users of illicit drugs or excessive alcohol. Gentle, nonjudgmental, but thorough, investigation of findings suggestive of substance use is as important as any other aspect of maternal and fetal care.

 Risks from drug use are generally the same for recreational and hard-core users.

In addition to evaluation and care of the woman, involve social service as early as possible so that appropriate assessment of the home situation for postnatal care of the baby can be undertaken.

Narcotics: Maternal use is associated with fetal growth restriction, in utero death, and prematurity, and may result in neonatal abstinence syndrome (neonatal withdrawal). Fetal effects result from narcotics crossing the placenta and directly affecting the fetus and from diminished placental function that may accompany maternal narcotic use.

Prenatal Considerations
- Attempt to enroll the pregnant woman in a substance use treatment program.
- Consider methadone or buprenorphine maintenance therapy, in an established program.
- Begin serial ultrasound evaluation of fetal growth and antenatal testing for fetal well-being at approximately 28 weeks' gestation.

Intrapartum Considerations
- Acute narcotic use, whether from prescribed pain-relief medication or from illicit drug use, can cause decreased fetal heart rate variability.
- Be aware that the need for frequent and/or large doses of narcotic analgesia may indicate addiction in the woman.
- Consider requesting a urine drug screen if use is suspected.

Postpartum Considerations
Maternal
- Consult social service and other agencies, as appropriate, to assist the woman with substance use treatment program, parenting education, parenting, etc.
- Breastfeeding is contraindicated with maternal heroin use. Breastfeeding is usually NOT contraindicated for women in methadone or buprenorphine maintenance programs.

Neonatal
- If the baby is depressed at birth, provide assisted ventilation as necessary.
  – Do *not* give naloxone if maternal narcotic addiction is suspected. Naloxone will cause acute withdrawal in the baby, which may induce seizures.
- Consider obtaining a urine drug screen on the baby.
- Observe for signs of neonatal abstinence syndrome.
- Involve social service in planning for the baby's care post-discharge.

Amphetamines: Maternal use has been reported to be associated with placental abruption, fetal growth restriction, and in utero demise. At this time there is no clear evidence of an association with a specific syndrome or spectrum of congenital malformations.

Prenatal Considerations
- Attempt to enroll the pregnant woman in a substance use treatment program.
- Conduct ultrasound examination at 20 weeks to look for congenital abnormalities.

Intrapartum Considerations
- Communication with the woman may be extremely difficult. She may not be rational or respond appropriately to verbal instructions or inquiries. She also may be physically combative, which may be aggravated by physical restraint.
- Fetal bradycardia or tachycardia may be seen, depending on amphetamine dose and concurrent use of other drugs.

Postpartum Considerations
Maternal
- Mother's emotional state may remain unpredictable and irrational.
- Breastfeeding is contraindicated with maternal use of amphetamines.
- Consult social service and other agencies, as appropriate, to assist the woman with substance use treatment program, parenting education, parenting, etc.

Neonatal
- Consider obtaining a urine drug screen.
- Involve social service in planning for the baby's care post-discharge.

Cocaine: Maternal use is associated with premature rupture of membranes, preterm labor, abruptio placentae, fetal growth restriction, and fetal death. Fetal effects may result from cocaine crossing the placenta and directly affecting the fetus, as well as from the tachycardia, hypertension, and vasoconstriction that accompany maternal use, which may decrease placental perfusion.

Prenatal Considerations
- Attempt to enroll the pregnant woman in a substance use treatment program.
- Monitor for possible increase in maternal blood pressure.
- Begin serial ultrasound evaluation of fetal growth and antenatal testing for fetal well-being at approximately 28 weeks' gestation.

Intrapartum Considerations
- Otherwise unexplained loss of fetal heart rate variability may be due to maternal cocaine use or to narcotics. Consider requesting a drug screen on the woman.
- Consider abruptio placentae may be present if a non-reassuring fetal heart rate pattern develops.

Postpartum Considerations
Maternal
- Mother may have an increased need for pain medication.
- Breastfeeding is contraindicated with maternal cocaine use.

Neonatal
- Consider obtaining a urine drug screen on the baby.
- Involve social service in planning for the baby's care post-discharge.

- Maternal lifestyle may be chaotic, with many substance users coming from impoverished circumstances. In this regard, to date, most outcome studies indicate that poverty has greater impact than does maternal cocaine use, with no clear evidence of adverse childhood effects related solely to gestational cocaine exposure.

2. **Alcohol:** Chronic alcohol ingestion of 2 or more drinks per day (wine, beer, or hard liquor) may result in fetal alcohol syndrome (FAS). Fetal alcohol syndrome is characterized by subtle facial and brain malformations, including shortened palpebral fissures, broad upper lip, flattened nasal bridge, small philtrum, small jaw, small eyes, fetal growth restriction, and mental retardation. Congenital cardiac or other organ defects may also occur with this syndrome. Behavioral and learning difficulties may be demonstrated during childhood.

   The effects on the fetus range from mild to severe and do not always correlate with the amount of alcohol ingested. In addition, some babies of women who drink heavily during pregnancy are apparently unaffected. Nevertheless, FAS is the most common *preventable* cause of mental retardation.

   Although the effects on the fetus are different from those of other drugs, women who chronically consume large quantities of alcohol need much the same care as women addicted to other drugs.

   Prenatal Considerations
   - If high alcohol intake occurs throughout the first trimester, discuss pregnancy termination.
   - Attempt to enroll the woman in an alcohol treatment program.
   - Encourage good maternal nutrition.
   - Consider serial ultrasound examinations if fetal growth restriction is suspected.

   Intrapartum Considerations: None specific to alcohol use

   Postpartum Considerations
   Maternal
   - If not enrolled earlier, attempt to enroll the woman in an alcohol treatment program.
   - Monitor for signs and symptoms of withdrawal.

   Neonatal
   - Examine baby for evidence of FAS. Findings in the neonatal period, however, may be very nonspecific.
   - In nearly all cases, acute maternal intake of alcohol will be eliminated from the baby by the time delivery occurs. In rare cases, a woman with a high blood alcohol level will deliver an intoxicated newborn. Provide resuscitation, as necessary; give supportive care; and monitor the baby until symptoms disappear.
   - Involve social service in planning for the baby's care post-discharge.

3. **Smoking:** Smoking tobacco increases the risk of fetal growth restriction and abruptio placentae. Fetal effects result, at least in part, from uterine vasoconstriction caused by nicotine and from diminished oxygen delivery to the placenta caused by carbon monoxide inhaled with cigarette smoke. In addition, the incidence of sudden infant death syndrome (SIDS) is significantly increased in babies born to women who smoked during pregnancy.

Controversy exists over whether smoking marijuana has similar detrimental effects on the fetus. Breastfeeding, however, is contraindicated with maternal marijuana use.

Prenatal Considerations
• Encourage the woman to stop or decrease smoking during pregnancy.

Intrapartum Considerations: None specific to smoking

Postpartum Considerations
Maternal
• If the mother continues to smoke, encourage her to stop or decrease smoking.
• Nicotine is present in breast milk in concentrations between 1.5 and 3.0 times the simultaneous maternal plasma concentrations.
• If either or both parents smoke, encourage them to avoid smoking near the baby.

Neonatal
• Increased risk for pneumonia, bronchiolitis and, perhaps, SIDS in the presence of secondhand smoke.

D. Adverse Social and/or Economic Factors
Each of the following factors is associated with increased perinatal morbidity and mortality. These adverse socioeconomic factors increase the risk for preterm labor, fetal growth restriction, medical illness in the pregnant woman, and/or difficulty in recovering from surgery (if an operative delivery is required).

• Minimal or absent prenatal care
• Low income, poor housing
• Nutritional deficiency, obesity, low prepregnancy weight, or inadequate weight gain
• Heavy manual labor or hazardous work environment

These factors may occur together, or one may contribute to another. For example, poverty may be one cause for poor dietary intake, which may result in maternal iron deficiency anemia and suboptimal fetal growth. Compliance with medical regimens may be hampered by emotional stress, physically and/or psychologically abusive domestic situation, low income, difficult work schedule, or child care and family demands.

Investigate what a woman sees as adverse circumstances for herself, provide information about her pregnancy and risk factors she can address, and consult with social service and/or other agencies. Alleviating any risk factor may help to improve the outcome of a pregnancy.

 Investigate the possibility of domestic violence with EVERY pregnant woman. Battering can include physical, psychological, and/or sexual abuse.

Be aware that domestic violence
• Affects approximately 10% of all pregnancies (reported range is 4% to 20%), making it one of the most common complications of pregnancy
• Is more likely to start, or increase, when a woman is pregnant
• Affects women of every income level and educational background
• Has an impact on all members of a victim's family

Self-test

Now answer these questions to test yourself on the information in the last section.

C1. What level of alcohol intake is considered dangerous to the fetus?

_____

C2. List at least 3 socioeconomic factors that may adversely affect pregnancy outcome.

_____

_____

_____

C3.	**True**	**False**	Maternal cocaine use is associated with the occurrence of fetal cardiac defects.
C4.	**True**	**False**	Maternal use of illicit drugs may affect the fetus by interfering with placental function and/or directly by crossing the placenta.
C5.	**True**	**False**	Minimal or absent prenatal care increases the risk of pregnancy complications, regardless of a woman's economic status.
C6.	**True**	**False**	Maternal smoking increases the risk for fetal growth restriction.
C7.	**True**	**False**	Cocaine use during pregnancy is associated with placental abruption.
C8.	**True**	**False**	Women with low-risk pregnancies may have significant emotional difficulties adapting to parenthood and child care.
C9.	**True**	**False**	A woman older than 35 years is less likely to deliver a baby with Down syndrome.
C10.	**True**	**False**	Acute narcotic use may cause increased beat-to-beat variability.
C11.	**True**	**False**	Excessive need for pain medication during labor may indicate maternal narcotic addiction.
C12.	**True**	**False**	Women who have difficulty adapting to pregnancy are much more likely to commit suicide than women who do not have difficulty adapting to pregnancy.
C13.	**True**	**False**	Occasional recreational drug use is not as harmful to the fetus as chronic maternal addiction.

C14. Which of the following risks are increased for women who inject illicit drugs?

Yes	**No**	
____	____	Becoming infected with human immunodeficiency virus
____	____	Developing diabetes mellitus
____	____	Causing permanent fetal damage
____	____	Becoming infected with hepatitis B virus

Check your answers with the list that follows the Recommended Routines. Correct any incorrect answers and review the appropriate section in the unit.

165

Obstetric Risk Factors and Their Implications

1. What Are Obstetric Risk Factors?

A. Obstetric History

B. Current Pregnancy

1. What Are Obstetric Risk Factors?

A. Obstetric History

Repeated pregnancy losses, endocrine diseases, uterine abnormality, and certain medical illnesses may pose obstacles to conception and/or to carrying a fetus to term. Some conditions experienced in one pregnancy have an increased risk of recurring in subsequent pregnancies.

Not all risk factors are presented in the following text. Only risk factors not covered in other units (such as obstetric hemorrhage, preterm labor, etc) are discussed here.

It is important to obtain a thorough, detailed history during the first prenatal visit. Attempt to obtain complete copies of a woman's earlier reproductive health care records, including records of care delivered elsewhere. If fetal death or neonatal death occurred, those records, including autopsy findings, can be extremely valuable in counseling the parents and in providing future care.

1. **Previous Uterine Surgery:** Surgery that entered the uterine cavity carries increased risk. No additional risk is associated with surgical procedures that did not cut through the full thickness of the myometrium.

   Prenatal Considerations

   - Previous surgery may increase the risk of uterine rupture during labor.
   - Consider cesarean delivery before the onset of labor and discuss the risks and benefits of this plan with the pregnant woman.

   Intrapartum Considerations

   - Risk for uterine rupture during labor is increased. See Section 6, Intrapartum Considerations, Signs of Uterine Rupture.

   Postpartum Considerations

   Maternal: None specific to previous uterine surgery

   Neonatal: None specific to previous uterine surgery

2. **Previous Macrosomic Newborn** (>4,000 g [8 lb, 13 oz] birth weight)

   Prenatal Considerations

   - Many babies of excessive size are born to women without any medical complications. Abnormal maternal glucose tolerance and diabetes mellitus, however, are associated with fetal macrosomia. Evaluate the woman for glucose intolerance. (See Unit 5, Abnormal Glucose Tolerance, in this book.)
   - Counsel the woman to avoid excessive weight gain, as appropriate for her prepregnancy BMI.
   - Estimate fetal weight by clinical and/or ultrasound examination near term. If an earlier delivery was complicated by shoulder dystocia with sequelae, consider cesarean delivery if the fetus is comparable in size to the previous baby.
   - Vaginal delivery of a macrosomic fetus may be accompanied by shoulder dystocia, brachial plexus injury in the newborn, and vaginal lacerations in the mother. Shoulder dystocia is a life-threatening and unpredictable complication.
     - Shoulder dystocia (encountered with 10% to 15% of babies >4,000 g)
     - Brachial plexus injury (Approximately 1 in 1,000 babies with shoulder dystocia will have *permanent* nerve damage, commonly called Erb palsy.)

- Planned induction of labor for suspected macrosomia does *not* decrease the risks associated with delivery of a big baby, increases the risk of cesarean delivery, and may result in unintended preterm delivery.
- Together with the patient, a decision about delivery route should be made based on history, current pregnancy, and clinical judgment.

Intrapartum Considerations
- Reevaluate fetal size and review delivery plans with the parents.
- If vaginal delivery is the route planned, reevaluate the plan frequently based on labor progress.

Postpartum Considerations
Maternal
- If vaginal delivery, check for cervical, vaginal, and perineal lacerations.

Neonatal
- If baby is large, screen for hypoglycemia (Book I: Maternal and Fetal Evaluation and Immediate Newborn Care, Unit 8, Hypoglycemia) and check for brachial plexus injury (Erb palsy) and other palsies.

3. **Previous Perinatal Death, Including Stillborn Baby**

Prenatal Considerations
- Review previous maternal and fetal records (including autopsy report and karyo-type, whenever possible) to provide the parents with the most accurate and complete information regarding the risks in the current pregnancy.
- Evaluate the woman for syphilis, diabetes mellitus, thyroid malfunction, isoimmunization to rare blood types, and immunologic diseases (SLE and APS) because all are associated with an increased risk for fetal demise.
- Begin daily fetal activity determinations at approximately 28 weeks.
- At a time prior to when the previous loss occurred, begin weekly
  - Antenatal testing of fetal well-being and growth
  - Prenatal visits

Intrapartum Considerations
- Use fetal heart rate monitoring as early as possible.

Postpartum Considerations
Maternal
- Mother and/or father may continue to need support and counseling regarding loss of previous baby.

Neonatal
- Evaluation of this baby depends on the cause of the previous perinatal death, as well as problems, if any, experienced during this pregnancy, labor, and delivery.

4. **Previous Congenital Malformation(s) or Hereditary Disease**

Prenatal Considerations
- Some malformations and diseases have a predictable pattern of inheritance, but many do not. Parents need to know the cause, treatment, prognosis, and risk of recurrence. Arrange for genetic counseling before pregnancy or as early in pregnancy as possible. Discuss possible prenatal diagnosis of the fetus. Consultation with a maternal-fetal medicine specialist or geneticist is recommended.

- If the previous disorder was, or can be, clearly identified, use diagnostic tests specific for that malformation. Specific tests are not available for all malformations.
- The risk of neural tube defects (eg, anencephaly, meningomyelocele) has been shown to be reduced with folic acid supplementation. Folate (4.0 mg/day) is recommended for all women, beginning before conception or as early in pregnancy as possible.

5. **High Parity (several previous births)** (Note: Traditionally, the definition of *grand multiparity* is ≥5 previous births [a woman in her sixth pregnancy]). Currently, *women of high parity* is used to indicate women at risk for certain complications because of numerous previous pregnancies and deliveries.

Prenatal Considerations
- Observe closely for signs of hypertension and placenta previa.
- Risk for abruptio placentae is also increased, particularly if the woman smokes or has hypertension.

Intrapartum Considerations
- There is an increased risk for rapid labor and for uterine rupture.

Postpartum Considerations

Maternal
- Women of high parity are at increased risk for postpartum hemorrhage.

Neonatal: None specific to high maternal parity

6. **Previous Cesarean Section**

Repeat cesarean section
- If a repeat cesarean delivery is planned for a time prior to the onset of spontaneous labor, fetal maturity criteria outlined in Book I: Maternal and Fetal Evaluation and Immediate Newborn Care, Unit 2, Fetal Age, Growth, and Maturity, should be fulfilled.
- The date of a planned cesarean delivery may not need to be scheduled. Another approach that should be considered is to wait for the spontaneous onset of labor. This may be especially important if there is a question about a woman's due date.

Vaginal birth after cesarean (VBAC): Repeat cesarean deliveries account for approximately one-third of all cesarean deliveries. The overall success rate for VBAC is 60% to 80%, but is generally higher for women who have had a previous vaginal birth and lower for women whose previous cesarean delivery was due to dystocia. Although they occur infrequently, serious risks are associated with VBAC, including

- Uterine rupture, which can be life-threatening for the woman and the fetus
- Non-reassuring fetal status

Contraindications to VBAC
- Previous vertical uterine incision
- Contracted pelvis
- Non-reassuring fetal status
- Lack of obstetrical physician and anesthesia staff immediately available to provide emergency care*

---

*American College of Obstetricians and Gynecologists. Vaginal Birth After Previous Cesarean Delivery. ACOG Practice Bulletin #115. August 2010.

Prenatal Considerations

Consider a trial of labor if all the following conditions exist:

- One previous cesarean delivery with low transverse incision confined entirely to the non-contractile lower uterine segment; no other uterine scars

  Note: A trial of labor may be considered in women with 2 prior low transverse cesarean deliveries. The risk of uterine rupture may be as high as double the rate for women with one prior cesarean delivery. A history of prior vaginal birth and 2 prior cesarean deliveries is associated with higher success than women without a history of vaginal birth.

- Clinically adequate maternal pelvis
- Vertex presentation (some experts use VBAC selectively with breech presentation, twins, and other high-risk situations)
- No fetal contraindications to vaginal delivery
- Indication for the previous cesarean section is not recurrent
- Availability of continuous fetal and uterine monitoring
- Capability for immediate cesarean delivery and hysterectomy, if necessary
- Woman who is well-informed and well-prepared

 A trial of labor may not be appropriate for all women with a prior cesarean delivery, even if they meet all the conditions. Individual history must be carefully considered.

Intrapartum Considerations

- Misoprostol should not be used for third trimester cervical ripening or labor induction in patients who have had a cesarean delivery or major uterine surgery. Induction of labor for maternal or fetal indications remains an option for women undergoing trial of labor after cesarean delivery.
- Epidural anesthesia and oxytocin infusion may be used judiciously.
  - Epidural anesthesia does not seem to affect the success rate for VBAC, and its use rarely hides the signs of uterine rupture (if one occurs).
  - No relationship between the use of oxytocin and uterine rupture has been found, although some studies have suggested a relationship between high-dose oxytocin and uterine rupture.
- *Signs of uterine rupture:* Sudden cessation of labor, variable fetal heart rate decelerations that progress to late decelerations and bradycardia, uterine or abdominal pain, or fetal position that regresses from the station that had been achieved are the hallmarks of uterine rupture. Vaginal bleeding may not be present. If present, low blood pressure and signs of shock also may appear.

Postpartum Considerations

Maternal

- There seems to be little need for routine exploration of the uterus following a successful vaginal delivery. Asymptomatic separation of an old scar generally heals well without surgical repair. There is no indication that surgical repair of an asymptomatic scar rupture improves future pregnancy outcome.
- If uterine rupture occurred during this pregnancy, cesarean delivery should be planned for all future pregnancies.

Neonatal: None specific to VBAC

7. **Previous Blood Group Incompatibility (Rh or other isoimmune disease)**

Prenatal Considerations

- Women with known Rh sensitization require careful, frequent, and complex prenatal assessment of fetal well-being. Fetal therapy may include intrauterine fetal blood sampling and/or transfusion(s).
- The severity of isoimmunization can vary and determination of how seriously the fetus may be affected is complex, requiring testing of the mother and father, ultrasound evaluation of fetal middle cerebral artery with Doppler velocimetry, and amniocentesis for amniotic fluid analysis for bilirubin and of fetal cell DNA to determine the fetal Rh status.
- Timing of delivery requires a balance between fetal status and fetal gestational age.
- Risk of pregnancy-specific hypertension is increased if fetal hydrops is present.
- If fetal hydrops is found before the onset of labor, transfer of the woman for delivery at a regional perinatal center is strongly recommended. Fetuses with hydrops fetalis generally do not tolerate labor well, will require neonatal intensive care, and have a high mortality rate.

 Because of the high risk of fetal death or serious neonatal illness associated with Rh disease, comanagement with and/or referral to maternal-fetal medicine specialists is strongly recommended for all Rh-sensitized women.

Intrapartum Considerations

- If hydrops is found during labor, and transfer of the woman is unwise at that time, it is usually an indication for a cesarean delivery because fetuses with hydrops usually tolerate labor poorly.
- If you plan to deliver a woman with Rh sensitization electively in your hospital,
  - If hydrops is not present, monitor carefully and deliver vaginally, unless there are obstetric indications for cesarean delivery.
  - Plan to have blood ready in the delivery room for emergency transfusion if a seriously anemic newborn is anticipated. The blood volume of babies with Rh disease is often normal, or even high. If transfusion is needed for anemia, it must be given cautiously, and perhaps as an exchange transfusion. Blood that may be used includes

    ○ O, Rh-negative red blood cells, *crossmatched against the mother's blood*
    OR

    ○ Type-specific blood (same as fetal blood type)
    OR

    ○ Maternal washed, packed red blood cells, donated and prepared in advance of delivery (preferable, but requires specialized preparation techniques)
- Anticipate and plan for neonatal care the baby may need. (See the following text.)

Postpartum Considerations
Maternal

- Provide counseling regarding future pregnancies.

Neonatal

- Consult with pediatric specialists and your hospital's blood bank.
- Be prepared to resuscitate the baby and/or provide continued respiratory support if hydrops is present.

- Check blood pressure, hematocrit, bilirubin, reticulocytes, peripheral smear, and Coombs test.
- Be prepared to start intensive phototherapy treatment for hyperbilirubinemia soon after delivery.
- Anticipate need for exchange transfusion(s), as well as thoracentesis and/or paracentesis if the baby has hydrops.

Self-test

Now answer these questions to test yourself on the information in the last section.

D1. Match each condition in the left column with the most closely associated condition on the right.

____ Shoulder dystocia	a. Cesarean delivery
____ Brachial plexus injury	b. Macrosomic newborn
____ Neonatal hypoglycemia	
____ Previous uterine surgery	
____ Abnormal maternal glucose tolerance	

D2. The risk of uterine rupture during labor is increased when previous uterine surgery entered the

_____.

D3. Soon after delivery, women who give birth vaginally to large babies should be checked for

_____.

D4. True   False   The presence of hydrops fetalis suggests that the fetus will tolerate labor poorly and the baby will need intensive care.

D5. True   False   Vaginal birth is successful for 60% to 80% of women with a previous cesarean section.

D6. True   False   When Rh disease is present, the baby may require a transfusion in the delivery room for severe anemia.

D7. True   False   All congenital malformations have a predictable pattern of inheritance.

D8. True   False   Vaginal birth after cesarean is contraindicated when a previous classical (vertical) cesarean section was done.

D9. True   False   Autopsy reports of a previous fetal or neonatal death are rarely useful in providing information to parents about future pregnancies.

D10. True   False   Evaluation of fetal death may include testing of the woman for various medical illnesses.

D11. Large babies, especially those over 4,000 g birth weight, should be screened for _____ whether or not their mothers were known to have abnormal glucose intolerance during pregnancy.

D12. A 27-year-old woman who has had 6 previous deliveries is at risk for which of the following?

Yes	No	
____	____	Post-term pregnancy
____	____	Uterine rupture
____	____	Postpartum hemorrhage
____	____	Abruptio placentae
____	____	Rapid labor
____	____	Fetal chromosomal abnormality

Check your answers with the list that follows the Recommended Routines. Correct any incorrect answers and review the appropriate section in the unit.

B. Current Pregnancy

A woman's current pregnancy may experience problems in 4 ways:

- A woman who has had one or more uncomplicated pregnancies may develop significant problems, for the first time, during the current pregnancy.
- Certain high-risk or emergent situations may develop during labor or delivery, without warning or history of previous risk factors.
- Some women with known high-risk factors may develop complications during labor or delivery, unrelated to the previously identified risk factors.
- Screening tests may indicate an abnormality in the fetus.

1. **Early Antenatal Testing***: Women with either low-risk or high-risk pregnancies may have a fetus with an abnormality. Screening tests are designed to identify the pregnancies most likely to be affected by any of a variety of abnormalities. These tests should be offered to *all* pregnant women.

While the risk of a chromosomal abnormality is higher in women aged 35 years and older, there are fewer births among this age group. Most babies, and thus most babies with chromosomal abnormalities, are born to women younger than 35 years. It is also important to remember that there are more babies born with birth defects with normal chromosomes, than babies born with chromosome abnormalities.

- Early pregnancy dating is essential. For many screening tests, accurate determination of gestational age is necessary for interpretation of test results. Test values change with gestational age. Results considered high or low may be normal if a fetus is older or younger than first thought.
- Depending on test results, discuss the options available to the family during pregnancy, including diagnostic testing, such as amniocentesis or CVS. Depending on the results of diagnostic testing pregnancy options, such as termination, placement of baby for adoption, or pediatric care after delivery, should be discussed. Consultation with experts is recommended.
- If a fetal abnormality is present, it may influence the route and location of delivery.

Screening Tests: Negative (normal) screening results do not guarantee that a fetus is normal. Certain risk factors (eg, family history or advanced maternal age) may indicate the need for other diagnostic tests, even if initial screening results are normal. Positive (abnormal) screening results do not guarantee a fetus is abnormal. False positive results or incorrect gestational age of the fetus used in calculating test results are common reasons for abnormal results.

- *Maternal serum alpha fetoprotein (MSAFP)* can be used at 15 to 20 weeks' gestation (most accurate at 16 to 18 weeks), as a screening tool for open neural tube defects (will detect about 85% of neural tube defects), ventral wall defects (gastroschisis, omphalocele), and a variety of other chromosomal or congenital abnormalities in the fetus. Most babies with neural tube defects (90% to 95%) are born to families with no risk factors. All pregnant women should be informed of the availability of the test, and its limitations. When abnormal MSAFP values (either high or low) are found, additional testing is recommended.

---

*American College of Obstetricians and Gynecologists. Screening for fetal chromosomal abnormalities. Practice Bulletin #77. January 2007 (reaffirmed 2008).

- *Multiple markers*: When interpreted in relation to maternal age, MSAFP, unconjugated estriol (uE_3), inhibin-A and human chorionic gonadotropin can be used in combination to identify approximately 80% of fetuses with trisomy 21 (Down syndrome), and a smaller proportion of fetuses with other chromosome abnormalities.

 Screening tests cannot diagnose, or completely rule out, a problem. In general, positive results identify patients who need to be offered additional diagnostic testing.

Diagnostic Tests

- *Comprehensive ultrasound* can be used as early as 18 to 20 weeks' gestation to detect fetal structural abnormalities.
- *Analysis of amniotic fluid* obtained by amniocentesis, usually at 15 to 20 weeks' gestation, can detect fetal chromosomal, biochemical, and enzymatic abnormalities.
- *CVS* and *PUBS* (also called cordocentesis) are generally available only at highly specialized perinatal centers, and may be used to assess certain fetal abnormalities or illnesses.
  - Optimal timing for a CVS procedure is 10 to 12 weeks. Cervical infections with gonorrhea, *Chlamydia*, or herpes are contraindications to CVS.
  - PUBS can be done from 18 weeks' gestation to term.

2. **Multifetal Gestation:** Complications of twin gestation include preterm delivery, twin-twin transfusion, discordant growth and/or intrauterine growth restriction, placenta previa, abruptio placentae, abnormal presentation, non-reassuring fetal status, in utero death, and umbilical cord prolapse. Both fetuses, or sometimes just one fetus, may be affected by certain risk factors. Each additional fetus further increases the risk of complications, the possibility of preterm labor, and the likelihood of fetal malformations.

 It is recommended that women pregnant with triplets, or any higher-order multiple gestation, be referred to regional center specialists for prenatal care, delivery, and neonatal care. The risk for fetal complications, extremely preterm birth, and neonatal illness is very high. Bed rest or decreased activity, intensive fetal surveillance, and careful planning for delivery and neonatal care are generally required for optimal outcome.

Prenatal Considerations

- Preterm birth is the most common threat to twins and all other multifetal gestations. Institute preterm labor precautions given in Unit 7, Preterm Labor, in this book. While aggressive management of preterm labor may be able to prolong gestation, the likelihood of delivery before term is still very high. It is recommended that this be discussed with the woman and plans made in advance for delivery at a hospital staffed and equipped to care for preterm newborns.
- Maternal risk for anemia is increased. Give extra folic acid and iron supplementation.
- Maternal risk for abnormal glucose tolerance is increased. Consider early glucose screening.
- Risk for development of pregnancy-specific hypertension is increased.

- Schedule frequent prenatal visits (at least every 2 weeks during the second trimester and every week during the third trimester).
- Use serial ultrasound examinations to
  - *Evaluate each fetus for growth restriction.*
  - *Estimate the volume of amniotic fluid in each sac.* If there is marked discrepancy between the sacs, consultation with a maternal-fetal medicine specialist is recommended.
  - *Identify a single sac.* Absence of a membrane separating twins indicates monoamniotic twins, which is an unusual occurrence that allows twins to move about each other in the same sac. This carries a high risk of in utero or intrapartum death from intertwining umbilical cords. Cesarean delivery is recommended if one or both of the twins is alive at the start of labor.
  - *Identify conjoined twins.*
- Begin NST or BPP at approximately 32 weeks' gestation or earlier if ultrasound examination shows abnormal fetal growth. Antepartum testing in multifetal gestations has not been shown to be clearly beneficial because intervention on behalf of one fetus may be to the detriment of the other fetus.
- Near term, use ultrasound to determine
  - Fetal presentation.
  - Placental location. (Increased size of a fused placenta or 2 single placentas increases the likelihood of placenta previa.)

Intrapartum Considerations
- When the woman presents in labor, use ultrasound to document the fetal presentations. Delivery route is usually determined by fetal presentation, gestational age, and provider skill (Table 4.1).
- Even when a vaginal delivery is expected, anesthesia personnel and facilities should be *immediately* available throughout the second stage of labor, in case an emergency delivery becomes necessary. If anesthesia personnel and facilities cannot be present during the second stage of labor, a cesarean delivery early in labor should be considered regardless of fetal presentation.

Table 4.1. Delivery of Twins		
Fetal Presentation*	**Gestational Age**	**Recommended Route of Delivery**
(first twin-second twin)		
Vertex-vertex	Term or preterm	Vaginal delivery[†]
Vertex-nonvertex	Term	Vaginal delivery[†]
Vertex-nonvertex	Preterm	Cesarean or vaginal delivery[†]
Nonvertex-vertex	Term or preterm	Cesarean delivery
Nonvertex-nonvertex	Term or preterm	Cesarean delivery

*If monoamniotic twins are suspected, cesarean section is the recommended route of delivery, regardless of fetal presentation.

[†]Acute fetal heart rate abnormalities and malpresentation of the second twin, requiring intrauterine fetal manipulation, occurs quite often. Use vaginal route only if the physician is experienced and skilled in delivery of abnormal presentation. If physician expertise for breech extraction is lacking, plan for cesarean delivery.

- If vaginal delivery is planned, fetal monitoring of *both* fetuses throughout labor is essential. Monitoring of the second twin should continue during and after delivery of the first twin because there is an increased likelihood of cord prolapse, placental separation, and cessation of uterine contractions during this time.
- Labor may stop following delivery of the first twin. Oxytocin augmentation may be used.
- Anticipate likelihood of postpartum hemorrhage with either vaginal or cesarean delivery. Insert a large-bore IV line for rapid-fluid infusion and consider having blood crossmatched for the woman, in case transfusion/volume expansion is needed.
- Plan to have a neonatal team for each baby attend delivery.

Postpartum Considerations
Maternal
- Risk of postpartum hemorrhage is increased. Check blood pressure and heart rate. Monitor for excessive bleeding.

Neonatal
- Be prepared with a delivery room team for *each* baby.
- Check blood pressure and hematocrit.

3. **Abnormal Volume of Amniotic Fluid:** There are several methods to define hydramnios and oligohydramnios, but all use ultrasound measurement to estimate amniotic fluid volume. AFI is one system of measuring amniotic fluid.

The procedure used to obtain AFI measurements is as follows:
- Position the pregnant woman supine.
- Identify 4 equal quadrants of the uterus by using the umbilicus to divide the uterus into upper and lower halves and into left and right halves (Figure 4.1).
- Hold the ultrasound transducer perpendicular to the flat surface on which the woman is supine and align it longitudinally with her spine.
- Measure, in centimeters or millimeters, the vertical size of the largest clear amniotic fluid pocket in each of the 4 quadrants.
- Add the 4 measurements together to obtain the AFI.

Amniotic fluid volume varies significantly with gestational age. It increases from 16 weeks until it peaks at approximately 27 weeks, stays stable until approximately 33 weeks, then decreases steadily through 42 weeks. The AFI for any patient can be compared to the chart of normal values, for each week of gestation from 16 to 42 weeks, as shown in Table 4.2.

Hydramnios (abnormally large amount of amniotic fluid; formerly termed polyhydramnios)
Common definitions include
- A vertical pocket of amniotic fluid of 8 cm or larger
OR
- Free-floating fetus, not touching any uterine surface
OR
- AFI of 25 cm or more, regardless of gestational age
OR
- AFI greater than the 95th percentile for the specific gestational age of the fetus

Most cases of hydramnios have no identifiable cause. In more than half the cases, the fetus is normal. Nevertheless, hydramnios may be associated with

- Multifetal gestation
- Placental abnormalities
- Rh and other isoimmune diseases
- Non-immune hydrops
- Maternal diabetes mellitus
- Fetal abnormalities, including
  - Anencephaly
  - Gastrointestinal tract abnormality
  - Chromosomal defect, in particular Down syndrome and Turner syndrome, or other genetic defect

Prenatal Considerations
- If fundal height is more than 3 to 4 cm *higher* than expected, or if palpation of the uterus suggests excessive fluid, obtain an ultrasound examination to assess amniotic fluid volume.
- If hydramnios is found, evaluate the woman and fetus for the conditions listed above.

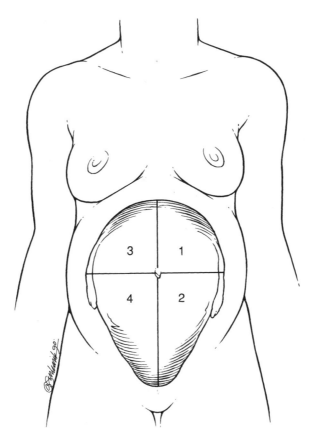

Figure 4.1. Uterine Quadrants for Amniotic Fluid Measurements.
Reproduced with permission from Gabbe SG, Niebyl JR, Simpson JL, eds. *Obstetrics: Normal and Problem Pregnancies.* 3rd ed. Churchill Livingstone: New York, NY; 1996:288.

Table 4.2. Amniotic Fluid Index in Normal Pregnancy* (in millimeters)			
Week of Gestation	5th Percentile (oligohydramnios)	50th Percentile	95th Percentile (hydramnios)
16	79	121	185
17	83	127	194
18	87	133	202
19	90	137	207
20	93	141	212
21	95	143	214
22	97	145	216
23	98	146	218
24	98	147	219
25	97	147	221
26	97	147	223
27	95	146	226
28	94	146	228
29	92	145	231
30	90	145	234
31	88	144	238
32	86	144	242
33	83	143	245
34	81	142	248
35	79	140	249
36	77	138	249
37	75	135	244
38	73	132	239
39	72	127	226
40	71	123	214
41	70	116	194
42	69	110	175

*Adapted with permission from Moore TR, Cayle JE. The amniotic fluid index in normal human pregnancy. *Am J Obstet Gynecol.* 1990;162:1172.

- Women with hydramnios, regardless of the cause, are at increased risk for development of premature rupture of membranes and preterm labor and delivery.
- Discuss findings, particularly those that might influence the route of delivery or plans for neonatal care, with pediatric practitioners.
- Perform serial ultrasound examinations to assess change in amniotic fluid volume.
- If maternal respiratory compromise develops (from pressure on the diaphragm), amniocentesis to remove excess fluid may be helpful. Repeated amniocenteses may be needed because fluid usually re-accumulates in a few days. Preterm labor, premature rupture of membranes, or placental abruption may occur with this degree of hydramnios, and repeated amniocenteses carry an increased risk for infection.

Intrapartum Considerations
- When membranes rupture with hydramnios present, there may be a sudden loss of a large amount of fluid and corresponding rapid decrease in intrauterine volume. Immediately check the following:
  - *Vaginal examination*: A rush of excess fluid increases the risk for umbilical cord prolapse when the presenting part is unengaged.
  - *Fetal heart rate and maternal blood pressure*: Sudden decompression of an over-distended uterus may lead to placental abruption.
  - *Uterine tone*: Tense, "board-like" consistency suggests a partial abruption with blood collection between the placenta and uterine wall.
- An over-distended uterus generally does not contract well during labor or after delivery. Consider the use of an internal uterine contraction monitor to assess the strength of contractions; be prepared for the possibility of a postpartum hemorrhage. If contractions are poor, oxytocin augmentation of labor may be needed. (See Unit 8, Inducing and Augmenting Labor, and Unit 9, Abnormal Labor and Difficult Deliveries, in this book.)

Postpartum Considerations
Maternal
- Check blood pressure and monitor for excessive bleeding. Women with hydramnios often have poor progress during labor and are at increased risk for postpartum hemorrhage due to uterine atony.

Neonatal
- Evaluate for abnormality of swallowing (ie, gastrointestinal obstruction or neurologic malfunction).
- Consider evaluation for neurologic, genetic, and/or chromosomal abnormality.

Oligohydramnios (abnormally small amount of amniotic fluid)

Common definitions include
- Largest vertical pocket of amniotic fluid is less than or equal to 2 cm

OR
- AFI of less than or equal to 5 cm, regardless of gestational age

OR
- AFI less than the 5th percentile for the specific gestational age of the fetus

Errors in obtaining an AFI are more common when there is little amniotic fluid. When an AFI of less than 10 cm (100 mm) is obtained, it is recommended that 2 additional AFI measurements be taken and the 3 averaged together.

Oligohydramnios may be associated with
- Postmaturity
- Fetal growth restriction
- Fetal abnormalities, including
  - Pulmonary hypoplasia
  - Certain chromosomal defects
  - Congenital infection
  - Genitourinary tract abnormalities
- Fetal death
- Unrecognized rupture of membranes
- Reduced fetal urine output due to chronic utero-placental insufficiency

Prenatal Considerations
- If fundal height is more than 3 to 4 cm *lower* than expected or if palpation of the uterus suggests meager fluid, obtain an ultrasound examination to assess amniotic fluid volume.
- If oligohydramnios is found, take the following actions:
  – Attempt to rule out rupture of membranes.
  – Reassess pregnancy dates as the volume of amniotic fluid declines in post-term pregnancies.
  – Perform comprehensive ultrasound examination to evaluate for genitourinary tract abnormalities or fetal growth restriction.
  – Obtain NST, BPP, or Doppler study of umbilical arterial blood flow.
  – Consider fetal chromosomal analysis.
- Consultation with maternal-fetal medicine specialists is recommended to identify additional tests that may be indicated, as well as the place and timing of delivery. Certain genitourinary tract abnormalities require prompt neonatal surgery.

Intrapartum Considerations
- Anticipate the likelihood of umbilical cord compression during labor.
- Because of the increased risk for abnormal fetal heart rate patterns, an emergency cesarean delivery may be needed.
- If non-reassuring fetal heart rate patterns develop and are thought to be due to cord compression (without prolapse) after membranes rupture, the fetus may respond well to amnioinfusion. Amnioinfusion is the infusion of fluid into the uterus. There are several appropriate protocols; one is the following:
  – Insert a Foley or amnioinfusion catheter into the uterus, beyond the fetal head (it may not be necessary to inflate the bulb), and connect to a bag or bottle of sterile saline or Ringer's solution.
  – Infuse 300 to 600 mL initially over 1 hour, followed by continuous infusion of 60 to 180 mL/hour for as long as fluid continues to come out of the uterus. (Fluid leak may stop as the fetus descends in the birth canal.)

Note: *Avoid over-distending the uterus with infused fluid.*

Postpartum Considerations

Maternal: None specific to oligohydramnios

Neonatal
- Be prepared for possibility of a newborn with severe respiratory distress due to underdeveloped lungs (pulmonary hypoplasia) if oligohydramnios has been present since the early second trimester.
- Evaluate the baby for urinary tract obstruction or absent kidneys (fetal urine is a major source of amniotic fluid).
- Evaluate for positional deformities, which may occur as a result of uterine pressure on the fetus without the cushion of amniotic fluid.
- Evaluate for congenital infection and/or genetic defect.

Self-test

Now answer these questions to test yourself on the information in the last section.

E1. **True** **False** Maternal serum alpha fetoprotein testing is used as a screening tool for the detection of a neural tube defect in the fetus.

E2. **True** **False** Antenatal testing has become so precise that every fetal defect can be identified early in pregnancy.

E3. **True** **False** Gastrointestinal obstruction in the fetus is associated with hydramnios.

E4. **True** **False** Intrauterine growth restriction can affect one twin but not the other.

E5. **True** **False** Oligohydramnios is associated with an increased risk for umbilical cord compression and non-reassuring fetal heart rate status during labor.

E6. **True** **False** Fetal genitourinary tract abnormality is associated with oligohydramnios.

E7. What is the single biggest threat to multifetal gestation? _____

E8. What are 3 identifiable causes for hydramnios?

_____

_____

_____

E9. Multifetal gestation increases the risk for

Yes	No	
____	____	Preterm delivery
____	____	Pregnancy-specific hypertension
____	____	Intrauterine growth restriction
____	____	Placenta previa
____	____	Abnormal presentation
____	____	Fetal death
____	____	Umbilical cord prolapse
____	____	Postpartum hemorrhage

E10. When hydramnios is present and membranes rupture, what 2 things may happen?

_____

_____

E11. **True** **False** Twins in nonvertex-vertex position is an indication for cesarean delivery.

E12. **True** **False** When longstanding oligohydramnios is present, you should be prepared for the possibility of a newborn with severe respiratory distress.

E13. **True** **False** The second twin should be monitored during and following delivery of the first twin.

E14. **True** **False** Most fetuses with hydramnios have a congenital malformation or chromosomal defect.

E15. **True** **False** Oligohydramnios indicates the need for thorough evaluation of fetal well-being.

E16. Which of the following risks are increased after delivery of the first twin?

Yes	No	
____	____	Umbilical cord prolapse
____	____	Arrest of labor
____	____	Placental abruption

E17. Which of the following risks are increased with hydramnios?

Yes	No	
____	____	Postpartum hemorrhage
____	____	Pregnancy-specific hypertension
____	____	Hypotonic uterus
____	____	Fetal positional deformities
____	____	Preterm labor

E18. Which of the following tests are used to screen for or detect chromosomal abnormalities in a fetus?

Yes	No	
____	____	Multiple markers: combination of maternal age, maternal serum alpha fetoprotein, estriol, and hCG
____	____	Fetal activity determinations
____	____	Analysis of amniotic fluid
____	____	Maternal serum alpha fetoprotein
____	____	Biophysical profile

Check your answers with the list that follows the Recommended Routines. Correct any incorrect answers and review the appropriate section in the unit.

---

4. **Growth-Restricted Fetus:** Intrauterine growth restriction (IUGR) may be difficult to determine antenatally and *diagnosis requires accurate pregnancy dating*. The causes of IUGR vary widely and cannot always be clearly identified.

Intrauterine growth restriction may be suspected if repeated measurements of fundal height are lower than expected for gestational age. Diagnosis is confirmed when serial ultrasound examinations show an estimated fetal weight that is less than 10% of the expected weight for the weeks of gestation examined. The more severe the growth restriction, the greater the risk of fetal and neonatal complications and death.

Symmetric growth restriction: Head circumference, body length, and weight are equally affected. Causes for symmetric growth restriction include congenital infection, genetic defect, chromosomal defect, or very early onset utero-placental insufficiency.

Asymmetric growth restriction: Head circumference, body length, and weight are not equally affected. Generally, body weight will be affected first. Then, with increasing severity of factors limiting growth, abdominal circumference, body length, and finally, but rarely, head growth will be affected. Asymmetric growth restriction may be associated with utero-placental insufficiency resulting from maternal hypertension or other medical illnesses, or from smoking, or with severe maternal malnutrition.

Regardless of the type of growth restriction, take the following actions:

Prenatal Considerations
- Obtain ultrasound examination.
  - Check for fetal anomalies (if found, consult with specialists).
  - Obtain AFI (oligohydramnios is often found with growth restriction).
- Treat underlying maternal condition(s). Consider obtaining titers for the TORCHS infections, to identify possible infection and provide antimicrobial therapy (available for some TORCHS infections). Consult with maternal-fetal and infectious disease experts.
- Consider amniocentesis or PUBS for chromosomal analysis, if no other reason for severe growth restriction can be found or if fetal anomalies are seen on ultrasound examination. Consult with maternal-fetal medicine specialists.
- Conduct antenatal testing for fetal well-being 1 or 2 times per week, starting as soon as growth restriction is identified. Growth-restricted fetuses have an increased risk for in utero death. Doppler umbilical artery blood flow studies may be useful in the evaluation of fetal status.

- Deliver the fetus as soon as pulmonary maturity is documented and/or there is evidence of deteriorating fetal condition.
- If growth restriction is severe, consider referral for delivery at a regional center because likelihood of serious neonatal illness is high.

Intrapartum Considerations
- Placental function may be limited, increasing the risk for fetal heart rate abnormalities during labor. Look specifically for late decelerations and minimal variability.
- Check for meconium-stained amniotic fluid when membranes rupture.
- Plan for vaginal delivery, but likelihood of fetal intolerance of labor is high, so be prepared for possible emergency delivery by cesarean section or forceps/vacuum extraction, depending on fetal condition and station. Anticipate possible need for neonatal resuscitation.

Postpartum Considerations
Maternal
- Review risk factors associated with growth restriction, especially smoking, substance use, maternal medical disease, etc.

Neonatal
- If resuscitation is needed, monitor for possible post-resuscitation complications.
- Screen for hypoglycemia (make first check within 30 minutes of birth). Begin early feedings and/or IV fluids. (See Book I: Maternal and Fetal Evaluation and Immediate Newborn Care, Unit 8, Hypoglycemia.)
- Check hematocrit (polycythemia is common).
- Evaluate for congenital malformation, infection, and/or chromosomal abnormality.

5. **Post-term Fetus** (beyond the first day of the 42nd week of gestation): Nutritional support for the growing fetus wanes as the placenta ages beyond the end of the 41st week, which may lead to fetal weight loss, loss of subcutaneous fat, and skin peeling. While weight loss occurs in some post-term fetuses, about one-fourth of these babies continue to gain weight and become macrosomic. Amniotic fluid decreases in prolonged gestation. The likelihood of diminished placental function and umbilical cord compression increases the risk of fetal intolerance of labor.

 The risk of fetal death dramatically increases in gestations that go beyond 41 weeks. There is little evidence of any increase in risk, however, during the 2 weeks between the beginning of 40 weeks and the end of 41 weeks of gestation.

Prenatal Considerations
- If spontaneous labor does not occur by 41 weeks, discuss the risks and benefits of induction, and the risks associated with a pregnancy lasting longer than 41 weeks.

 While it may be prudent to recheck how pregnancy dates were calculated, do NOT change a reasonably established due date based on one ultrasound examination obtained in late pregnancy, when the margin of error can be as much as 3 weeks.

183

- Consider comprehensive ultrasound investigation to check for
  - Anencephaly (associated with post-term fetus)
  - Fetal size
  - Amniotic fluid volume
- Establish a management plan.
  - *Induce labor* during the 41st week of gestation. Induction of labor is associated with less risk and greater likelihood of success when the woman is multiparous and when the cervix is ripe.

    OR
  - *Follow the pregnancy* beyond the end of 41 weeks' gestation with intensive testing of fetal well-being, consisting of daily fetal activity determinations and either
- Amniotic fluid volume determination once a week and NST twice a week

or

- Biophysical profile at least once per week

Allow the spontaneous onset of labor, unless an abnormality of antenatal testing indicates the need for earlier delivery. Consider consultation with a maternal-fetal medicine specialist.

Intrapartum Considerations

- Plan for vaginal delivery, but be prepared for possible emergency delivery.
- If the fetus seems to be macrosomic (estimated fetal weight >4,000 g), discuss with the patient the risk of shoulder dystocia, birth trauma, brachial plexus injury (Erb palsy) and other palsies, and maternal birth canal lacerations.
- If meconium is seen in the amniotic fluid, a period of fetal stress *may* have occurred. Fetal stress can cause the rectal sphincter to relax and result in meconium passage. Functional maturation in a post-term fetus can also cause the fetus to pass meconium in utero, without any evidence of stress (natural emptying of a full rectum).
- If the amniotic fluid is meconium-stained, be prepared for management of meconium for the baby, as well as possible need for neonatal resuscitation. (See Book I: Maternal and Fetal Evaluation and Immediate Newborn Care, Unit 5, Resuscitating the Newborn.)

Postpartum Considerations

Maternal: None specific to post-term pregnancy

Neonatal

- Anticipate possible need for neonatal resuscitation.
- If meconium is present, follow the guidelines in Book I: Maternal and Fetal Evaluation and Immediate Newborn Care, Unit 5, Resuscitating the Newborn, and manage according to the baby's condition (vigorous or not).
- If resuscitation is needed, monitor for possible post-resuscitation complications.
- If the baby is large, examine for signs of birth trauma.
- Begin early feedings and screen for hypoglycemia. (See Book I: Maternal and Fetal Evaluation and Immediate Newborn Care, Unit 8, Hypoglycemia.)

Self-test

Now answer these questions to test yourself on the information in the last section.

F1. True False Uteroplacental insufficiency is rarely a cause of fetal growth restriction.

F2. True False When a fetus is suspected of being post-term, it is valuable to obtain ultrasound measurement of the amniotic fluid volume.

F3. True False The likelihood of fetal distress during labor is increased in post-term pregnancies.

F4. True False Intrauterine viral infection is one cause of symmetric fetal growth restriction.

F5. True False A baby born post-term is at increased risk for neonatal hypoglycemia.

F6. True False Because of their small size, babies with intrauterine growth restriction rarely develop hypoglycemia.

F7. True False A growth-restricted fetus at term is at increased risk for fetal distress during labor.

F8. True False Serial ultrasound measurements of fetal size are usually needed to identify intrauterine growth restriction.

F9. True False Meconium in the amniotic fluid is always an indication of fetal stress.

F10. What are 2 identifiable causes for asymmetric growth restriction?

_____   _____

F11. With an uncomplicated, low-risk pregnancy, a clearly increased risk of fetal death begins at
  A. 38 weeks' gestation
  B. 40 weeks' gestation
  C. 42 weeks' gestation

F12. Post-term newborns are at increased risk for all of the following, *except:*
  A. Anemia
  B. Macrosomia
  C. Meconium-stained amniotic fluid
  D. Hypoglycemia

F13. Two recommended approaches to the management of post-term pregnancy are
  1. Induce labor during _____ week.

  OR
  2. Follow the pregnancy beyond _____ weeks, with _____.

F14. Match each condition on the left with the best choice from the right.
  _____ Positional deformities in the fetus a. Hydramnios
  _____ Placental abruption b. Oligohydramnios
  _____ Postpartum hemorrhage c. Intrauterine growth restriction
  _____ Pulmonary hypoplasia
  _____ Chronic maternal medical illness
  _____ Neonatal hypoglycemia

Check your answers with the list that follows the Recommended Routines. Correct any incorrect answers and review the appropriate section in the unit.

Various High-Risk Conditions

Recommended Routines

All the routines listed below are based on the principles of perinatal care presented in the unit you have just finished. They are recommended as part of routine perinatal care.

Read each routine carefully and decide whether it is standard operating procedure in your hospital. Check the appropriate blank next to each routine.

Procedure Standard in My Hospital   **Needs Discussion by Our Staff**

_____   _____   1. Establish a system of prenatal consultation and referral, as appropriate, for the
   • Evaluation and care of high-risk pregnant women
   • Evaluation and care of at-risk or sick fetuses
   • Anticipated care of at-risk or sick newborns

_____   _____   2. Attempt vaginal birth after cesarean labor only when physician(s), anesthesia staff, and neonatal staff are immediately available to provide emergency care, possible hysterectomy, and neonatal resuscitation.

Self-test Answers

These are the answers to the self-test questions. Please check them with the answers you gave and review the information in the unit wherever necessary.

A1. False. The reverse is accurate. Oral anticoagulants are harmful to the fetus and should be replaced with heparin therapy during pregnancy.

A2. True

A3. False. A woman with that degree of heart disease is likely to develop complications, especially congestive heart failure, during labor or postpartum.

A4. False. Thyroid storm is a possible complication of *hyper*thyroidism.

A5. False. For most women with heart disease, anesthesia and surgery pose a greater risk than labor.

A6. False. Antibiotics are recommended only for women who have a fever.

A7. True

A8. True

A9.
Yes	No	
	X	Plan to deliver by cesarean section.
X		Evaluate frequently for evidence of congestive heart failure.
X		Keep intravenous fluids during labor to a minimum amount.

A10.
Yes	No	
	X	Heart rate of 60 beats per minute
X		Sweating
X		Shortness of breath
X		Fever
	X	Dry skin
	X	Deep, labored breathing
X		Heart rate of 150 beats per minute

B1. False. While phenytoin therapy during pregnancy carries increased risk for congenital anomalies, the risk to the woman for serious injury is greater if anticonvulsant medication is stopped and seizures occur.

B2. True

B3. True

B4. True

B5. True

B6. True

B7. True

B8. True

B9. False. Anticonvulsant levels tend to fall during pregnancy and should be checked every 2 to 4 weeks, with dosage readjusted as necessary to maintain therapeutic levels in the woman.

B10. True

B11. True

B12. False. Cardiac arrhythmias (most often heart block) occur only in a very small number of babies born to women with systemic lupus erythematosus.

B13. True

B14. True

B15. True

C1. Frequent intake of 2 or more drinks per day of beer, wine, or hard liquor

C2. Any 3 of the following: minimal or absent prenatal care, low income, poor housing, nutritional deficiency, obesity, inadequate weight gain, heavy manual labor, hazardous work, domestic violence

C3. False. Maternal *amphetamine* use is associated with the occurrence of fetal cardiac defects.

C4. True

C5. True

C6. True

C7. True

C8. True

C9. False. Women older than 35 years (advanced age) are *more* likely to deliver a baby with Down syndrome.

C10. False. Acute narcotic use (pain medication or illicit use) is likely to *decrease* beat-to-beat variability.

C11. True

C12. False. Women who have difficulty adapting to pregnancy are *not* more likely to commit suicide. Ongoing emotional stress is associated with a variety of problems during pregnancy (greater risk for pregnancy-specific hypertension, preterm labor, etc) and postpartum (depression, difficulty with parenting, etc), but the risk for suicide is *not* increased.

C13. False. The fetal effects of maternal drug use, especially cocaine, are unpredictable. Infrequent use has been associated with serious problems in the fetus while, conversely, chronic use does not always cause injury to the fetus. That is the basis for "any use is abuse," particularly during pregnancy.

C14. Yes   No

  X   Becoming infected with human immunodeficiency virus

        X   Developing diabetes mellitus

  X   Causing permanent fetal damage

  X   Becoming infected with hepatitis B virus

D1. b Shoulder dystocia   a. Cesarean delivery

    b Brachial plexus injury   b. Macrosomic newborn

    b Neonatal hypoglycemia

    a Previous uterine surgery

    b Maternal glucose intolerance

D2. Contractile upper uterine segment

D3. Lacerations of the birth canal

D4. True

D5. True

D6. True

D7. False. Many congenital malformations are not related to a genetic disease or chromosomal defect. Sometimes fetal deformities develop with no identifiable cause. Sometimes they result from adverse fetal environment during embryogenesis. For example, high maternal blood glucose (and, therefore, high fetal blood glucose, because glucose easily crosses the placenta) early in pregnancy is associated with congenital malformations. Maternal ingestion of some drugs considered *un*safe for the fetus can also result in deformities.

D8. True

D9. False. Autopsy reports of a previous fetal or neonatal death can be *extremely useful* in providing information to parents about future pregnancies. The cause of the previous death may indicate therapy or surveillance measures that can be instituted to avoid another tragedy.

D10. True

D11. Hypoglycemia

D12.

Yes	No	
____	_X_	Post-term pregnancy
_X_	____	Uterine rupture
_X_	____	Postpartum hemorrhage
_X_	____	Abruptio placentae
_X_	____	Rapid labor
____	_X_	Fetal chromosomal abnormality

E1. True

E2. False. Antenatal testing can provide a tremendous amount of detailed and useful information, but cannot be counted on to identify 100% of fetal defects.

E3. True

E4. True

E5. True

E6. True

E7. Preterm birth

E8. Any 3 of the following: multifetal gestation, Rh isoimmune disease, maternal diabetes mellitus, fetal gastrointestinal abnormality, anencephaly, Down and Turner syndromes, placental abnormalities

E9.

Yes	No	
_X_	____	Preterm delivery
_X_	____	Pregnancy-specific hypertension
_X_	____	Intrauterine growth restriction
_X_	____	Placenta previa
_X_	____	Abnormal presentation
_X_	____	Fetal death
_X_	____	Umbilical cord prolapse
_X_	____	Postpartum hemorrhage

E10. Possible umbilical cord prolapse with rush of excess fluid.
Possible placental abruption with sudden uterine decompression.

E11. True

E12. True

E13. True

E14. False. While some fetuses with hydramnios have a congenital malformation or chromosomal defect, most fetuses with hydramnios are normal.

E15. True

E16.

Yes	No	
_X_	____	Umbilical cord prolapse
_X_	____	Arrest of labor
_X_	____	Placental abruption

E17.

Yes	No	
_X_	____	Postpartum hemorrhage
_X_	____	Pregnancy-specific hypertension
_X_	____	Hypotonic uterus
____	_X_	Fetal positional deformities
_X_	____	Preterm labor

E18.

	Yes	No	
	X	___	Multiple markers: combination of maternal age, maternal serum alpha fetoprotein, estriol, and hCG
	___	X	Fetal activity determinations
	X	___	Analysis of amniotic fluid
	X	___	Maternal serum alpha fetoprotein
	___	X	Biophysical profile

F1. False. The reverse is accurate. Utero-placental insufficiency is often a cause of fetal growth restriction.

F2. True

F3. True

F4. True

F5. True

F6. False. Babies with intrauterine growth restriction have decreased stores of glycogen and fat to metabolize after delivery and, therefore, are at increased risk for developing hypoglycemia after birth.

F7. True

F8. True

F9. False. Meconium in the amniotic fluid may or may not be an indication of fetal distress. In mature fetuses, the rectum may simply empty when it is full. If a fetus is in distress, the rectal sphincter also may relax and release meconium into the amniotic fluid.

F10. Any 2 of the following:
Maternal hypertension, renal disease, or other medical illnesses, smoking, severe maternal malnutrition

F11. C

F12. A

F13. 1. Induce labor during 41st week.
2. Follow the pregnancy beyond 41 weeks, with intensive testing of fetal well-being.

F14.
b	Positional deformities in the fetus	a. Hydramnios
a	Placental abruption	b. Oligohydramnios
a	Postpartum hemorrhage	c. Intrauterine growth restriction
b	Pulmonary hypoplasia	
c	Chronic maternal medical illness	
c	Neonatal hypoglycemia	

Unit 4 Posttest

If you are applying for continuing education credits, a posttest for this unit is available online. Completion of unit posttests and the book evaluation form are required to achieve continuing education credit. For more details, visit www.cmevillage.com.

Unit 5: Abnormal Glucose Tolerance

Objectives

In this unit you will learn

A. How gestational diabetes mellitus is defined and diagnosed

B. Which pregnant women should be screened for abnormal glucose tolerance

C. Why it is important to identify women with abnormal glucose tolerance

D. How screening is done for gestational diabetes mellitus

E. How gestational diabetes mellitus is managed during pregnancy

F. How the fetus is monitored during pregnancy complicated by gestational diabetes mellitus

G. How gestational diabetes mellitus is managed during labor

H. What postpartum follow-up should be provided to women with gestational diabetes mellitus

Unit 5 Pretest

Before reading the unit, please answer the following questions. Select the *one best* answer to each question (unless otherwise instructed). Record your answers on the test and check them against the answers at the end of the book.

1. **True** **False** After diagnosis is confirmed, gestational diabetes mellitus should be treated with insulin therapy.

2. **True** **False** Because the hormonal changes of pregnancy make a woman more resistant to the insulin her body produces, gestational diabetes mellitus is extremely common.

3. **True** **False** Pregnant teenagers are at increased risk for gestational diabetes mellitus.

4. **True** **False** It is desirable to keep maternal fasting blood glucose above 120 mg/dL throughout pregnancy.

5. **True** **False** African American women are at increased risk for gestational diabetes mellitus.

6. **True** **False** Pregnant women with an early pregnancy screening blood glucose level above 130 to 140 mg/dL should have a standard 3-hour glucose tolerance test.

7. **True** **False** Women with preconception diabetes mellitus and women with gestational diabetes mellitus have the same risk of having a baby with congenital malformation(s).

8. **True** **False** Nearly all women with gestational diabetes mellitus will develop diabetes mellitus later in life.

9. **True** **False** Women with abnormal glucose tolerance are at increased risk for developing preeclampsia.

10. **True** **False** For gestational diabetes mellitus to be diagnosed, results from 2 or more testing periods (fasting, 1 hour, 2 hours, or 3 hours after drinking glucose syrup) must be abnormal.

11. **True** **False** Generally, a planned delivery at 36 to 37 weeks' gestation is recommended when gestational diabetes mellitus is diagnosed.

12. **True** **False** Insulin therapy may be needed during labor for women with gestational diabetes mellitus, even if insulin was not needed earlier in pregnancy.

13. During the peripartum period, women with gestational diabetes should routinely have all of the following, *except:*
    A. Postpartum glucose tolerance test
    B. Oral medications to control blood glucose
    C. Dietary intake of 60 to 65 g of protein each day
    D. Capillary blood glucose home monitoring

14. Increased neonatal risks from maternal gestational diabetes mellitus include

Yes	No	
____	____	Neonatal hypoglycemia
____	____	Birth trauma
____	____	Neonatal diabetes mellitus
____	____	Neonatal hyperbilirubinemia

15. Which of the following indicate that a woman might be at increased risk for the development of gestational diabetes mellitus?

Yes	No	
____	____	Pre-pregnancy weight of 200 lb or more
____	____	Eastern European heritage
____	____	Gestational diabetes mellitus in a previous pregnancy
____	____	Maternal age of 35 years or older

16. Which of the following are recommended for pregnant women with gestational diabetes mellitus?

Yes	No	
____	____	Begin testing for fetal well-being at approximately 28 weeks.
____	____	Consider use of insulin if blood glucose is consistently 80 to 100 mg/dL.
____	____	Plan to deliver at 36 to 37 weeks' gestation unless tests of fetal well-being indicate a need for earlier delivery.
____	____	Estimate fetal weight prior to undertaking vaginal delivery.

1. Is Management of Pregestational Diabetes Mellitus in Pregnancy Included in This Unit?

No. Management of abnormal glucose tolerance, or *gestational* diabetes mellitus, which develops during pregnancy in some women, is the subject of this unit.

Normal changes in metabolism that come with pregnancy and fetal growth make management of insulin-dependent diabetes mellitus during pregnancy, labor, and delivery exceedingly complex. Meticulous, individualized evaluation and ongoing monitoring of maternal renal function, retinal vascularity, chronic infection(s), cardiac function, and fetal growth and well-being are required for optimal pregnancy outcome.

Diabetes mellitus poses significant risks to maternal and fetal well-being.

Prenatal care and delivery at a regional center, by specialists trained and experienced in the management of insulin-dependent diabetes mellitus during pregnancy, is recommended.

2. Why Do Some Pregnant Women Develop Abnormal Glucose Tolerance?

The normal hormonal changes of pregnancy make pregnant women more resistant to insulin. For diabetic women, these changes usually require a woman to increase her daily dose of insulin to maintain the same degree of control over her blood glucose that she had before pregnancy.

Nondiabetic pregnant women produce more insulin every day to maintain normal blood glucose levels. Some nondiabetic women cannot produce sufficient insulin during pregnancy, which results in their blood glucose level rising higher than normal after meals. This condition is called abnormal glucose tolerance. This may be just a temporary effect of pregnancy, with a natural return to normal glucose control after the pregnancy ends.

For some nondiabetic women, however, the pregnancy changes may lead to the earliest stage of diabetes mellitus. After delivery, these women may continue to have elevated blood glucose levels after meals. Some may require ongoing insulin therapy.

During pregnancy, it is not possible to know whether a woman with abnormal glucose tolerance has developed true diabetes mellitus or simply has temporary glucose intolerance due to pregnancy. Without preexisting diabetes mellitus, abnormal glucose tolerance during pregnancy is described as gestational diabetes mellitus (GDM).

Gestational diabetes mellitus is estimated to occur in 1% to 14% of nondiabetic pregnant women. The prevalence of GDM varies by ethnic group, personal and family history, and body mass index (BMI).

3. Why Is It Important to Identify Women With Gestational Diabetes Mellitus?

A. Maternal Risks From GDM

Continuous exposure to elevated blood glucose in women with GDM may lead to all the metabolic problems that can develop with non—pregnancy-related diabetes mellitus. In this way, maternal health may be compromised by uncontrolled or poorly controlled blood glucose.

In addition, women with GDM are more likely to develop preeclampsia and to need a cesarean delivery than women without GDM.

197

B. Fetal and Neonatal Risks From Maternal GDM

Alterations of maternal glucose metabolism may lead to fetal hyperglycemia (high blood glucose) because maternal blood glucose readily crosses the placenta. Fetal hyperglycemia may result in excessive fetal growth. The fetus is not diabetic and responds to the maternal hyperglycemia with hypersecretion of insulin.

After birth, the baby is cut off from high maternal glucose levels but still has increased insulin production, causing a drop in newborn blood glucose levels. For this reason, babies born to women with GDM are at risk for neonatal hypoglycemia (Book I: Maternal and Fetal Evaluation and Immediate Newborn Care, Unit 8, Hypoglycemia). Fetal and neonatal risks from maternal GDM include

- Macrosomia
- Operative delivery
- Shoulder dystocia, and subsequent adverse neonatal outcomes, such as brachial plexus injury or clavicular fracture
- Neonatal hypoglycemia
- Neonatal hyperbilirubinemia

C. Fetal and Neonatal Risks From Preexisting Diabetes Mellitus

Babies born to women with pre-pregnancy diabetes mellitus (type 1 or type 2) are also at risk for fetal macrosomia and related problems, neonatal hypoglycemia, and neonatal hyperbilirubinemia. In addition, they are at increased risk for the following problems:

- Congenital malformations during certain stages of embryo development, early in the first trimester
- Second trimester miscarriage; intrauterine fetal death
- Polycythemia
- Hypocalcemia
- Increased risk of respiratory distress syndrome (Regardless of gestational age, babies born to diabetic women have delayed ability to produce surfactants.)

4. Which Women Should Be Screened for Abnormal Glucose Tolerance?

Through *either* history (family, medical, obstetrical) and identification of risk factors *or* laboratory determination of blood glucose levels, the American College of Obstetricians and Gynecologists recommends universal screening of all pregnant women.[*]

Women at increased risk for GDM include those with

- Gestational diabetes mellitus in a previous pregnancy (as many as one-half of women with GDM in one pregnancy will have a recurrence in a subsequent pregnancy)
- Pre-pregnancy (or early pregnancy) BMI greater than 25 kg/m²
- Family history of a first-degree relative with diabetes mellitus
- Previous large-for-gestational-age baby, or baby with birth weight of 4,000 g (8 lb, 13 oz) or more
- African American, Hispanic, Native American, South or East Asian, or Pacific Islander heritage
- Maternal age 35 years or older
- Previous newborn with nonchromosomal congenital anomalies
- History of unexplained stillbirths or miscarriages beyond the first trimester

---

[*]American College of Obstetricians and Gynecologists, Practice Bulletin, *Gestational Diabetes*. September 2010.

5. How Is Blood Glucose Screening Done During Pregnancy?

Women at increased risk for GDM should have laboratory screening as soon as the elevated risk is identified. Women with abnormal glucose tolerance during the first half of pregnancy are more likely to demonstrate severe hyperglycemia later in pregnancy.

Women at increased risk should be screened *again* at 24 to 28 weeks, even if the earlier results showed normal blood glucose.

This glucose screening does not require a period of fasting. A solution containing 50 g of glucose is given orally. A blood glucose level is drawn 1 hour later.

Women with an elevated screening blood glucose level should have a standard 3-hour glucose tolerance test (GTT). Different thresholds for defining an abnormal screening test have been proposed, and range from 130 to 140 mg/dL. Know what threshold your institution uses.

6. How Is Gestational Diabetes Mellitus Diagnosed?

A standard 3-hour GTT is used. For at least 3 days before the test, the woman should follow an unrestricted diet, consuming at least 150 g of carbohydrates per day. The woman should not eat anything and should drink only water for 8 to 14 hours overnight before the GTT. The next morning, her fasting blood glucose level is drawn.

She should sit during the test and not smoke immediately before or during the test. After the fasting blood glucose is drawn, the woman drinks a 100-g portion of glucose solution. Blood glucose levels are drawn hourly for the next 3 hours (Table 5.1).

When results from any 2 sampling periods reach or exceed the upper limit of normal, the GTT is abnormal and the woman is considered to have gestational diabetes mellitus.

Example: If a woman's results are 165 mg/dL 2 hours and 150 mg/dL 3 hours after drinking the glucose solution, she has gestational diabetes, even if her fasting and 1-hour glucose levels are within normal limits.

7. How Do You Care for Women With Gestational Diabetes Mellitus?

The principal goal for women with abnormal glucose tolerance is to achieve normal blood glucose levels throughout the remainder of their pregnancy. When normal blood glucose is maintained, the complications and risks of gestational diabetes are reduced for the woman, fetus, and newborn. Care is based on diet, exercise, and monitoring blood levels.

  A. Diet

      The goal of diet therapy for a woman with GDM is to achieve normal blood glucose levels, provide adequate nutrition for normal weight gain, and avoid ketosis.

Table 5.1. Upper Limits of Normal Plasma Glucose for Glucose Tolerance Test*	
• Fasting evening to morning (8-14 hours)	95 mg/dL
• 1 hour after glucose syrup	180 mg/dL
• 2 hours after glucose syrup	155 mg/dL
• 3 hours after glucose syrup	140 mg/dL

*From American Diabetes Association. Diagnosis and classification of diabetes mellitus. *Diabetes Care.* 2005;28:S37-S42.

For healthy pregnant women of normal weight for height, without diabetes mellitus or abnormal glucose tolerance, the recommended diet contains 30 kcal per kilogram of nonpregnant body weight per day (kcal/kg/day). Similarly, underweight women should consume roughly an additional 200 calories/day.

Example: For a woman with normal weight for her height (ie, a BMI of 19 to 24, and a pre-pregnancy weight of 120 lb [54.5 kg]), the recommended caloric intake is approximately 1,635 calories/day (54.5 × 30).

Another woman, also weighing 120 lb, but significantly underweight for her height (ie, BMI ≤18), should have an intake of approximately 1,835 calories/day.

Obese women (BMI ≥30) should restrict their intake slightly, to 25 kcal/kg/day of ideal nonpregnant weight. This caloric restriction has been associated with improved pregnancy outcome regarding the incidence of macrosomia, but also carries the possibility of starvation ketosis. There is limited evidence that a build-up of ketones in maternal blood (subsequently in urine) during the second and third trimesters is inversely related to impaired psychomotor and cognitive development in their babies, through 9 years of age. In general, the less ketosis, the better the baby's outcome. Although the data are limited, it is recommended that ketosis be avoided during pregnancy, and that weekly checks be made for the possible onset of ketonuria.

Amounts of fat and carbohydrate in the diet may be varied to taste, as long as a pregnant woman obtains 60 to 65 g of protein each day.

These recommendations are also appropriate for women with GDM, with the following suggestions:
- *Avoid concentrated sweets,* such as candy, refined sugars, soft drinks (soda pop), etc.
- *Spread out meals to 4 to 6 smaller meals each day.* This is done by splitting breakfast and eating part of it in mid-morning, eating part of the noon meal in mid-afternoon, and part of the evening meal later in the evening. These recommendations may be adjusted to individual dietary habits to foster compliance.

B. Exercise

Regular exercise uses glucose in the blood, thus helping the body reduce the need for insulin production. Diet and exercise together have been shown to improve both fasting blood glucose levels and response to a 50-g glucose challenge in women with GDM. Recommended minimum amount of exercise is 20 to 30 minutes, 3 or 4 times per week.

Exercise should not cause pain or significant impact. Walking, stretching, yoga, gardening, and swimming are examples of appropriate exercise during pregnancy.

C. Blood Tests

1. *Home Blood Glucose Monitoring*

Teaching should be provided regarding diet and exercise, and the woman should be allowed a few days to adjust to her new regimen. After a few days, capillary blood glucose monitoring is recommended to establish the normal variations of blood glucose during the woman's typical diet, work, and exercise. After a few days of monitoring capillary blood glucose 1 to 2 hours after meals, it will become clear whether normal blood glucose can be maintained with diet and exercise (Table 5.2).

The optimal glucose testing regimen has not been determined. It has been shown, however, that more intensively monitored women with GDM have fewer primary cesarean deliveries, fewer macrosomic babies, and fewer babies who develop newborn hypoglycemia.

Table 5.2. Recommended Capillary Blood Glucose Levels During Pregnancy	
• Fasting evening to morning	60-90 mg/dL
• 1 hour after a meal	<140 mg/dL
• 2 hours after a meal	<120 mg/dL

The preferred timing of glucose testing also has not been determined. It is believed, however, that the fetus may be most sensitive to high maternal blood glucose. Post-meal monitoring, therefore, is recommended, although it has not been determined whether 1-hour or 2-hour post-meal monitoring is superior.

 Most women with GDM can achieve and maintain normal blood glucose with diet and exercise.

8. Are Oral Antidiabetic Medications Useful With Gestational Diabetes Mellitus?

Glyburide, a second-generation sulfonylurea, when compared to insulin, has been shown to provide similar glucose control, as well as pregnancy outcomes, including rates of cesarean delivery, preeclampsia, macrosomia (>4 kg), and neonatal hypoglycemia. Cord serum analyses showed no detectable glyburide in the babies. Due to these results, as well as increased patient satisfaction, many obstetricians are using glyburide as a first choice for medical management of gestational diabetes. Approximately 20% of women will not achieve ideal glycemic control with glyburide within 1 to 2 weeks of starting therapy, and will need to be switched to insulin therapy.

9. How Do You Know When Insulin Therapy Is Needed?

Persistent failure to maintain normal blood glucose with diet and exercise may require insulin therapy to provide control of blood glucose. Table 5.3 indicates blood levels that should prompt consideration of insulin therapy.

Women with gestational diabetes mellitus who require insulin therapy to maintain normal blood glucose or who have complications, such as hypertension, should be managed in the same way as women with pre-pregnancy insulin-dependent diabetes mellitus. Risks to maternal and fetal health increase dramatically whenever complications develop or glucose intolerance becomes severe enough to require insulin for blood glucose control.

 Referral to care by experts is strongly recommended if a woman with gestational diabetes mellitus develops a complication(s) or need for insulin therapy.

Table 5.3. Blood Test Results That Indicate Insulin Therapy May Be Needed	
Blood Glucose	
• Fasting evening to morning (8-14 hours)	>95 mg/dL
• 1 hour after a meal	>140 mg/dL
• 2 hours after a meal	>120 mg/dL

Self-test

Now answer these questions to test yourself on the information in the last section.

A1. **True** **False** Women at high risk for gestational diabetes mellitus should be screened as soon as their risk status is identified, and again at 24 to 28 weeks' gestation.

A2. **True** **False** Healthy pregnant women produce more insulin to maintain normal blood glucose.

A3. **True** **False** Fasting blood glucose levels that remain above 105 mg/dL, despite diet and exercise, are likely to require insulin therapy during pregnancy.

A4. **True** **False** Pregnant women with early pregnancy screening blood glucose levels above 130 to 140 mg/dL should have a standard 3-hour glucose tolerance test.

A5. **True** **False** Babies born to women with gestational diabetes mellitus diagnosed in the second trimester are more likely to have congenital malformation(s) than if diabetes is diagnosed before pregnancy.

A6. List at least 3 factors that suggest a woman may be at increased risk for gestational diabetes mellitus.

_____
_____
_____

A7. What are the 3 main components of gestational diabetes mellitus management?

_____
_____

A8. What are 2 fetal or neonatal risks due to maternal gestational diabetes mellitus?

_____
_____

Check your answers with the list that follows the Recommended Routines. Correct any incorrect answers and review the appropriate section in the unit.

10. How Do You Monitor the Fetus?

A. Fetal Well-being

The risk of fetal death in utero is increased with insulin-dependent maternal diabetes mellitus. The risk is significantly lower in women with controlled GDM who do not require insulin therapy. Nevertheless, it is generally believed that increased fetal surveillance should be conducted for both of these pregnancies.

Recommendations for antenatal testing include

- Daily fetal activity determinations beginning at 28 weeks' gestation.
- Testing twice weekly with either non-stress test, biophysical profile, or modified biophysical profile starting at 32 weeks' gestation, or earlier if there are additional risk factors.
- Women whose GDM is uncontrolled, who require insulin, who are diagnosed early in pregnancy or have other risk factors, such as hypertension or adverse obstetric history, should be managed the same as individuals with preexisting diabetes mellitus.

B. Fetal Size

Because macrosomia is of concern in pregnancies complicated by GDM, serial ultrasound measurements may be useful in revealing the rate of fetal growth, and hence the likelihood of a large fetus. Ultrasonography, however, has *not* been shown to be more accurate than clinical measures in estimating actual fetal weight during labor.

Early delivery to avoid the development of macrosomia and the possibility of associated shoulder dystocia is *not* recommended. *Cesarean delivery, at term* and before the onset of labor, is recommended by some experts if the fetal weight is estimated to be such that shoulder dystocia becomes a significant concern.

11. What Care Should You Provide During Labor?

During labor, maternal blood glucose should be monitored hourly and kept between 80 and 120 mg/dL. Insulin therapy may become necessary if the blood glucose cannot be kept in this range.

If volume expansion is needed (for hydration, preload before epidural anesthesia, or any reason), *avoid* use of glucose-containing solutions. If maternal blood glucose levels are high during labor, hyperglycemia, followed by rebound hypoglycemia, may occur in the newborn (Book I: Maternal and Fetal Evaluation and Immediate Newborn Care, Unit 8, Hypoglycemia).

12. What Postpartum Follow-up Is Needed?

Approximately 10% of women with gestational diabetes will continue to have fasting hyperglycemia after delivery. A random blood glucose should be obtained in the immediate postpartum period. Any value less than 200 mg/dL is within the normal range. It is also recommended that women with GDM have a 2-hour, 75-g GTT in the postpartum period.

Evaluation of glucose tolerance in a woman who delivered a large-for-gestational-age baby should be considered. She may have had unrecognized GDM.

Because delivery of the placenta removes the hormones that induce insulin resistance, a larger dose (75 g) of glucose is given orally for the postpartum GTT. The test may be done at the time of the 6-week postpartum visit or after cessation of breastfeeding, whichever comes later.

Women who had gestational diabetes and have abnormal GTT postpartum may have early diabetes mellitus and should be evaluated for insulin or oral hypoglycemic drug therapy.

Counsel women with abnormal glucose tolerance regarding future pregnancies, and the particular importance of glucose control before conception and during early pregnancy. Hyperglycemia very early in gestation, during the formation of fetal organs, is thought to be responsible for the higher incidence of congenital malformations in babies of diabetic women.

13. What Long-term Care and Advice Should You Give a Woman With Gestational Diabetes?

Up to one-half of women with gestational diabetes go on to develop insulin-dependent diabetes mellitus within 20 years of the pregnancy in which GDM was discovered, even if their initial postpartum GTT was normal. Teach women about the increased likelihood of developing

Table 5.4. Postpartum Evaluation of Women With Gestational Diabetes Mellitus*			
	Plasma Glucose Levels		
	Normal	Prediabetes[†]	Diabetes Mellitus
Fasting	<110 mg/dL	110-125 mg/dL	126 mg/dL
2 hour	<140 mg/dL	140-199 mg/dL	200 mg/dL

*Table created from content from American Diabetes Association. Diagnosis and classification of diabetes mellitus, *Diabetes Care.* 2005;28:S37-S42.
[†]High risk for future development of diabetes mellitus.

diabetes mellitus and what signs and symptoms to report, including increased thirst, increased urination, and unexplained weight loss.

Advice regarding weight control, regular exercise, and diet may be helpful in delaying the onset of diabetes mellitus, if it is going to develop. Refer your patient to a registered dietitian/diabetes educator for individualized help with meal planning, exercise, and blood glucose management. Annual examination of fasting blood glucose is recommended (Table 5.4).

Self-test

Now answer these questions to test yourself on the information in the last section.

B1. **True** **False** Women with gestational diabetes mellitus should have their blood glucose monitored throughout labor and maintained between 80 to 120 mg/dL.

B2. **True** **False** A woman who delivered a very large newborn should be evaluated for abnormal glucose tolerance.

B3. **True** **False** Women with gestational diabetes mellitus will develop diabetes mellitus in the immediate postpartum period.

B4. **True** **False** Women with gestational diabetes mellitus should have a glucose tolerance test done in the postpartum period.

B5. **True** **False** Up to one-half of women with gestational diabetes go on to develop insulin-dependent diabetes within 20 years of the pregnancy in which gestational diabetes occurred.

B6. If volume expansion is needed during labor for a woman with gestational diabetes mellitus, what type of fluids should be used?

_____

B7. Which of the following are recommended for pregnant women with gestational diabetes?

Yes	No	
____	____	Begin testing of fetal well-being at approximately 28 weeks.
____	____	Consider use of insulin if blood glucose is consistently over 80 mg/dL.
____	____	Plan to deliver at 35 to 36 weeks unless tests of fetal well-being indicate need for earlier delivery.
____	____	Estimate fetal weight prior to undertaking vaginal delivery.

Check your answers with the list that follows the Recommended Routines. Correct any incorrect answers and review the appropriate section in the unit.

Abnormal Glucose Tolerance

Recommended Routines

All the routines listed below are based on the principles of perinatal care presented in the unit you have just finished. They are recommended as part of routine perinatal care.

Read each routine carefully and decide whether it is standard operating procedure in your hospital. Check the appropriate blank next to each routine.

Procedure Standard in My Hospital　　**Needs Discussion by Our Staff**

_____　_____　1. Establish a protocol to screen all women for abnormal glucose tolerance through
  • History and identification of risk factors and/or
  • Laboratory determination of blood glucose levels, as early in pregnancy as possible

_____　_____　2. Establish a protocol of laboratory screening of women at high risk for abnormal glucose tolerance early in pregnancy, and again at 24 to 28 weeks, even if their earlier results were within normal limits.

_____　_____　3. Establish a protocol for estimation of fetal weight on admission to the labor unit for women with gestational diabetes mellitus.

_____　_____　4. Establish a protocol for management of gestational diabetes mellitus during labor.

Self-test Answers

These are the answers to the self-test questions. Please check them with the answers you gave and review the information in the unit wherever necessary.

A1. True

A2. True

A3. True

A4. True

A5. False. Women with diabetes mellitus pre-pregnancy are at increased risk of having a baby with a congenital malformation, especially if blood glucose is uncontrolled at conception and shortly thereafter, during fetal organ formation. Hyperglycemia later in pregnancy does not carry the same risk.

A6. Any 3 of the following:
- Gestational diabetes mellitus in a previous pregnancy
- Pre-pregnancy or early pregnancy weight greater than 90 kg (200 lb)
- Family history of diabetes mellitus
- Previous large-for-gestational-age baby, or baby with birth weight of 4,000 g (8 lb, 13 oz) or more
- African American, Hispanic, Native American, South or East Asian, or Pacific Islander heritage
- Maternal age 35 years or older
- Previous babies with nonchromosomal congenital anomalies
- History of unexplained stillbirths or miscarriages beyond the first trimester

A7. Diet, exercise, capillary glucose monitoring

A8. Any 2 of the following:
- Macrosomia
- Cesarean delivery
- Shoulder dystocia, birth trauma
- Neonatal hypoglycemia
- Neonatal hyperbilirubinemia

B1. True

B2. True

B3. False. About 10% of women with gestational diabetes mellitus continue to have fasting hyperglycemia postpartum. As many as one-half of women with gestational diabetes mellitus will develop diabetes mellitus within 20 years of the pregnancy in which gestational diabetes mellitus occurred, even when their initial postpartum glucose tolerance test was normal.

B4. True

B5. True

B6. Fluids that do not contain glucose

B7.

	Yes	No	
	X	____	Begin testing of fetal well-being at approximately 28 weeks.
	____	X	Consider use of insulin if blood glucose is consistently over 80 mg/dL.
	____	X	Plan to deliver at 35 to 36 weeks unless tests of fetal well-being indicate need for earlier delivery.
	X	____	Estimate fetal weight prior to undertaking vaginal delivery.

Unit 5 Posttest

If you are applying for continuing education credits, a posttest for this unit is available online. Completion of unit posttests and the book evaluation form are required to achieve continuing education credit. For more details, visit www.cmevillage.com.

Unit 6: Premature Rupture and/or Infection of the Amniotic Membranes

Objectives

In this unit you will learn

A. What maternal, fetal, and neonatal risks are associated with

- Premature rupture of membranes
- Chorioamnionitis
- Prolonged rupture of membranes

B. How to determine whether the amniotic membranes are ruptured

C. What signs and symptoms indicate chorioamnionitis

D. How to treat chorioamnionitis

E. How to manage premature rupture of membranes when there are no signs of infection

- Term fetus
- Preterm fetus

F. What post-delivery maternal and neonatal care to provide for patients with a history of premature rupture and/or infection of the amniotic membranes

Unit 6 Pretest

Before reading the unit, please answer the following questions. Select the *one best* answer to each question (unless otherwise instructed). Record your answers on the test and check them against the answers at the end of the book.

1. Which of the following are associated with premature rupture of membranes?

Yes	No	
____	____	Amniotic fluid embolism
____	____	Umbilical cord compression
____	____	Neonatal sepsis
____	____	Abruptio placentae

2. True   False If the amniotic fluid is foul smelling and maternal fever is present, you should begin treatment for intra-amniotic infection.

3. True   False Rupture of membranes for 18 hours or longer increases the risk of neonatal infection for preterm babies, but not for term babies.

4. True   False Chorioamnionitis can occur only after the membranes have ruptured.

5. True   False When chorioamnionitis develops in a preterm gestation, early use of intravenous antibiotics usually allows the pregnancy to continue for at least another 1 to 2 weeks.

6. True   False Chorioamnionitis increases the risk for postpartum endometritis.

7. Premature rupture of membranes has occurred at 32 weeks' gestation. There are no signs or symptoms of labor or infection, and fetal heart tones are reassuring. For which of the following reasons should a sterile speculum examination be performed?

Yes	No	
____	____	Assess cervical dilatation and effacement.
____	____	Obtain samples for group B beta-hemolytic streptococcus, *Chlamydia,* and gonorrhea testing.
____	____	Collect amniotic fluid from the vaginal pool to test for phosphatidyl glycerol.
____	____	Place internal fetal heart rate and uterine contraction monitoring devices.

8. A woman has chorioamnionitis at 38 weeks' gestation, with foul-smelling amniotic fluid, maternal fever of 38.6°C (101.6°F), tender uterus, and fetal tachycardia. There is no other evidence of fetal distress; presentation is vertex. You should begin intravenous antibiotics and

A. Induce labor.

B. Perform a cesarean delivery.

C. Wait for spontaneous onset of labor.

D. Perform an amnioinfusion.

9. Which of the following are appropriate for the management of preterm, premature rupture of membranes at 30 weeks' gestation, when a woman is not in labor and there are no signs of infection?

Yes	No	
____	____	Start antibiotics.
____	____	Use sterile speculum examination to check for prolapsed umbilical cord.
____	____	Obtain urine for analysis and culture.
____	____	Periodically palpate the uterus.
____	____	Give corticosteroids.
____	____	Perform digital cervical examination to assess cervical dilatation.

10. True   False   When a woman is treated during labor for chorioamnionitis, intravenous antibiotic therapy should be continued for 10 to 14 days after she becomes afebrile.

11. True   False   In the presence of asymptomatic maternal colonization with group B beta-hemolytic streptococcus, there is no reason to use prophylactic antibiotics during labor.

12. True   False   Neonatal sepsis can follow premature rupture of membranes, even if the woman showed no sign of illness.

1. What Is Premature Rupture of Membranes?

The amniotic (fetal) membranes may rupture before, coincident with, or after the onset of labor. Rupture of fetal membranes before the onset of labor is abnormal and is termed **premature** rupture of membranes, with "premature" referring to the timing of membrane rupture (before labor) and not to fetal gestational age.

To eliminate possible confusion and misuse of the acronym PROM, some prefer to abbreviate rupture of membranes as ROM and then specify whether there is premature ROM or preterm, premature ROM.

2. What Are the Causes of Premature Rupture of Membranes?

The cause of premature ROM is not entirely understood. Infection, however, is strongly associated with premature ROM. While premature ROM can occur without infection known to be present, the risk is particularly increased when genital tract infection or colonization with group B beta-hemolytic streptococcus (GBS) is present. Urinary tract infection (UTI) is also associated with premature ROM. In some cases, premature ROM and/or preterm labor may be an early sign of chorioamnionitis.

In most cases of premature ROM, there is no identifiable risk factor. The risk for premature ROM is increased, however, with each of the following risk factors:

- *Prior preterm delivery,* especially if associated with preterm, premature ROM
- *Uterine over-distension* (hydramnios, multifetal gestation)
- *Maternal genital tract infection,* especially *Trichomonas,* gonorrhea, *Chlamydia,* or bacterial vaginosis
- *Vaginal bleeding after 14 weeks' gestation*
- *Bacteriuria,* with or without symptoms of UTI
- *Maternal smoking*
- *Lower socioeconomic status*
- *Incompetent cervix and/or procedures involving the cervix,* including cerclage and conization
- *Amniocentesis* (<1% risk that premature ROM will occur because of the procedure; if it does, fluid leakage almost always stops spontaneously)

3. What Are the Risks of Premature Rupture of Membranes?

A. Maternal and/or Neonatal Infection

While infection may be a *cause* of premature ROM, infection also can be a *result* of premature ROM, even if no preexisting infection can be identified. Ascending infection, in the absence of recognized maternal infection, can still result in chorioamnionitis and/or fetal infection. Ascending infection (vertical pathway from vagina to uterus) can be caused by normal vaginal flora or by pathogenic organisms.

The membranes that surround the amniotic fluid and fetus, and the thick cervical mucus, normally provide a barrier to ascending infection. When the membranes rupture, this protective barrier is broken, creating a portal of entry for organisms. This puts the woman at risk for chorioamnionitis, sepsis, and/or postpartum endometritis and the fetus at risk for in utero infection, preterm birth, and/or neonatal sepsis. The risk of maternal and/or fetal infection increases with decreasing gestational age at the time of membrane rupture and, the longer pregnancy continues after membrane rupture, the greater the risk of infection.

Note: Although uncommon, intrauterine infection and/or fetal infection also can occur with intact membranes.

The degree of maternal illness may not correlate with the degree of neonatal illness. In some cases, fatal neonatal sepsis will follow premature ROM, with little or no evidence of maternal infection.

B. Preterm Birth

Preterm labor often follows preterm, premature ROM. In the absence of infection (which does not always develop), prematurity poses the greatest risk to the baby. If infection is also present, the threat of neonatal illness or death is significantly increased.

C. Umbilical Cord Consequences

1. *Compression:* Leakage of amniotic fluid can result in oligohydramnios. Without the cushion of amniotic fluid, the umbilical cord can become compressed between the fetus and the uterine wall, whether or not labor is present.

2. *Prolapse:* Premature ROM increases the risk for umbilical cord prolapse, especially if the fetus is breech and/or the presenting part is not engaged.

D. Oligohydramnios Complications

Prolonged oligohydramnios, particularly if ROM occurs during the second trimester, can result in pulmonary hypoplasia. The absence of fluid limits the growth and development of the terminal airways and alveoli that normally occurs with fetal respiratory movements of a fluid-filled lung. Deformation of the fetus, with abnormal facies and limb positioning deformations, also may occur because of restriction of fetal growth and movement. These complications do not always develop, even at the youngest gestational ages, and rarely develop when ROM occurs after 26 weeks' gestation.

E. Abruptio Placentae

For reasons that are not clearly identified, premature ROM is associated with an increased risk for placental abruption. If blood (even a small amount) is passed vaginally, or if there are any other signs of an abruption, check maternal blood pressure, begin fetal monitoring, and investigate the cause of the bleeding.

F. Fetal Death

The risk of in utero death is increased in all cases of premature ROM. The risk increases with decreasing gestational age and is highest for fetuses less than 26 weeks' gestation. The cause is unclear but is probably related to cord compression with fetal hypoxia and/or to infection.

4. How Do You Determine Whether the Membranes Have Ruptured?

A. History

A woman usually will note a gush of fluid from her vagina. Less often, she may be aware of smaller amounts of watery discharge. In more than 90% of cases, maternal history is correct. In some cases, however, membrane rupture may be confused with leakage of urine. In addition, painless cervical dilatation of an incompetent cervix is sometimes accompanied by a watery discharge, without ROM. Lastly, normal vaginal discharge of pregnancy or discharge associated with bacterial vaginosis may be mistaken by the woman for fluid leakage.

If the history includes a description of foul-smelling and/or cloudy amniotic fluid, clinical suspicion for chorioamnionitis should be very high.

B. Examination

1. *Sterile Speculum Examination* (see also the skill units that follow this unit)

To decrease the risk of introducing infectious organisms, digital pelvic examinations should not be done unless a decision has been made to proceed promptly with delivery.

Perform a sterile speculum examination to
- Look for a prolapsed umbilical cord.
- Assess cervical dilatation and effacement by visual inspection.
- Look for leakage of fluid through the cervix; if fluid is leaking, a pool may form in the posterior fornix.
- Note color, consistency, and odor of the fluid.
  — Nitrazine paper test to determine pH (see Skill Unit: Tests With Suspected or Proven Rupture of Membranes)
  — Phosphatidyl glycerol (PG) determination to assess fetal pulmonary maturity (if the estimated gestational age is between 34 and 36 weeks)

Note: Amniotic fluid obtained from a vaginal pool will give accurate results for PG, but not for lecithin-sphingomyelin ratio and certain other tests of fetal pulmonary maturity.
- Obtain cultures.
  — Cervical culture or DNA probe test for gonorrhea and *Chlamydia*
  — Vaginal and rectal cultures for GBS

2. *Placental Alpha Microglobulin-1 (PAMG-1) Assay*
   - This is a commercially available product (AmniSure)* that detects PAMG-1 protein marker in the amniotic fluid.
   - It can be used in place of or in addition to a sterile speculum examination to test for ROM.
   - Follow manufacturer's instructions for use.

3. *Ultrasound Examination*

   If premature ROM is suspected, but not confirmed, an abdominal ultrasound examination may be able to identify a decrease in the volume of amniotic fluid. Ultrasound also may be useful in assessing fetal size, well-being, and presentation.

   Fetal malpresentation is increased with preterm, premature ROM.

4. *Amniocentesis*

   When the diagnosis of premature ROM cannot be made with sterile speculum and abdominal ultrasound examination(s), and the diagnosis is critical to management decisions (such as when ROM before 34 weeks' gestation is suspected), consider amniocentesis and dye test.

 Amniocentesis in this situation (possible ROM with decreased fluid volume) requires special expertise. Consultation with maternal-fetal medicine specialists is strongly recommended.

---

*info@amnisure.com; 617/234-4441.

If amniocentesis is appropriate,

a. *Withdraw fluid for analysis.* If analysis of amniotic fluid would be useful, fluid must be withdrawn *before* dye is injected.

Useful amniotic fluid analyses include
- Tests of fetal pulmonary maturity
- Culture
- Gram stain (for leukocytes or bacteria)
- Leukocyte (white blood cell [WBC]) count
- Glucose concentration (low concentration suggests glucose is being consumed by bacteria)

b. *Instill dye into the amniotic space* after withdrawal of fluid sample. Use indigo carmine (1 mL of dye diluted with 9 mL sterile normal saline).

Note: Methylene blue dye should NEVER be used for this test, because it can bind to fetal hemoglobin and cause methemoglobinemia.

c. *Observe for leakage of the dye.* Place a sterile gauze high in the woman's vagina. If possible, have the woman walk or sit for 20 to 30 minutes, then retrieve the gauze. Dye on the gauze indicates rupture of membranes.

Note: Indigo carmine dye will be absorbed systemically within a short period and then be excreted in the urine, making the urine blue. Gauze placed in the vagina, rather than a pad on the perineum, will make certain that any dye on the gauze is due to amniotic fluid leakage, rather than urine leakage.

Once the diagnosis of premature ROM is made, admit the woman to a hospital. In most cases, further care will require continued hospitalization until delivery.

Self-test

Now answer these questions to test yourself on the information in the last section.

A1. **True** **False** The risk of premature rupture of membranes is increased when gonorrhea or *Chlamydia* infection is present.

A2. **True** **False** Ultrasound examination may be able to identify a decrease in amniotic fluid, which may help to confirm suspected rupture of membranes.

A3. **True** **False** Although rare, chorioamnionitis can occur with intact membranes.

A4. **True** **False** Life-threatening neonatal illness can develop following premature rupture of membranes, even when there is no evidence of chorioamnionitis.

A5. **True** **False** Digital pelvic examinations should not be done when preterm premature rupture of membranes occurs and labor does not begin.

A6. **True** **False** Umbilical cord compression and cord prolapse are possible complications of premature rupture of membranes.

A7. **True** **False** Urinary tract infection increases the risk for premature rupture of membranes.

A8. **True** **False** Following rupture of membranes, amniotic fluid obtained from a vaginal pool can be used for a lecithin-sphingomyelin ratio.

A9. List at least 3 complications associated with premature rupture of membranes.

_____

_____

_____

A10. The main risk associated with premature rupture of membranes is maternal and/or neonatal

_____ .

A11. Following amniocentesis and a dye test for rupture of membranes, a sterile gauze should be placed

_____ .

Check your answers with the list that follows the Recommended Routines. Correct any incorrect answers and review the appropriate section in the unit.

5. How Should You Respond to Premature Rupture of Membranes?

In the absence of infection, approximately 75% of all women with premature ROM will deliver within 7 days. However, the more preterm the pregnancy, the longer the length of time will be between ROM and spontaneous onset of labor.

Treatment is dictated primarily by 2 factors.

1. Fetal gestational age
2. Whether infection is present

   A. Evaluate Fetal Status

     Establish or confirm fetal gestational age. Evaluate fetal well-being with fetal heart rate monitoring and/or biophysical profile (BPP). If not done earlier (see Section 4B3), use abdominal ultrasound examination to assess amniotic fluid volume, fetal size, and fetal presentation.

   B. Evaluate for Evidence of Infection

     Obtain maternal vital signs, complete blood count with differential, and perform physical examination. Obtain urine for analysis and culture. If not done earlier (see Section 4), obtain a vaginal/rectal culture for GBS and appropriate specimens to test for gonorrhea and *Chlamydia*.

The diagnosis of intra-amniotic infection is made when temperature of 38°C (100.4°F) or higher plus 2 of the following additional findings are present:

- Uterine tenderness
- Cloudy and/or foul-smelling amniotic fluid
- Fetal tachycardia (baseline heart rate >160 beats per minute)
- Maternal tachycardia

 In women with premature ROM, development of any of these signs indicates chorioamnionitis, whether or not amniotic fluid cultures are positive.

Less frequent findings in chorioamnionitis include the following:

- Low BPP score (≤6).
- Maternal malaise ("I just don't feel well").
- Elevated maternal leukocyte (WBC) count. (Without other signs of infection, this may *not* be helpful, especially if antenatal corticosteroids have been used.)

If none of these clinical signs and symptoms clearly indicate infection, but you still suspect chorioamnionitis, amniocentesis is sometimes used to aid in the diagnosis. The following findings in amniotic fluid (obtained by amniocentesis) suggest infection:

- Amniotic fluid glucose concentration less than 15 mg/dL
- Positive Gram stain (for leukocytes or bacteria)

Note: By itself, positive Gram stain is a better test than low glucose but, together, these tests provide stronger evidence for infection than either test alone.

- Amniotic fluid white cell count greater than 100/mm³
- Positive amniotic fluid culture

6. What Should You Do if There Is Evidence of Infection?

When there is evidence of intrauterine infection, the woman and the fetus may develop serious complications. The fetus must be delivered, regardless of fetal gestational age. Antibiotic therapy should be started promptly, but antibiotics cannot cure chorioamnionitis without delivery.

 If chorioamnionitis develops, the specific infectious organism and the length of time until delivery are key factors in determining the severity of maternal illness.

The longer the fetus and placenta remain in the uterus, the more serious the intrauterine infection is likely to become.

A. Begin Antibiotic Therapy
Promptly begin intravenous administration of broad-spectrum antibiotics, either a second- or third-generation cephalosporin or the combination of a penicillin and gentamicin. The following combination of antibiotics gives excellent coverage for GBS and *Escherichia coli*, 2 major causes of neonatal sepsis:

- Penicillin G, 5 million units initially, intravenously, then 2.5 million units intravenously every 4 hours until delivery

OR

- Ampicillin, 2 g first dose, intravenously, then 1 g intravenously every 4 hours until delivery

AND

- Gentamicin, 1.5 mg/kg, intravenously, every 8 hours

If cesarean delivery becomes necessary, the risk of postpartum endometritis is significantly increased. If drug therapy with ampicillin or penicillin and gentamicin is used, add antibiotic coverage for anaerobic organisms immediately *after* the cord is clamped. Recommendations include

• Clindamycin, 900 mg, intravenously, every 8 hours

OR

• Metronidazole, 500 mg, intravenously, every 12 hours

Alternatively, if an extended-spectrum cephalosporin was used for intrapartum antibiotic therapy and cesarean delivery becomes necessary, cephalosporin treatment should be continued postpartum.

Adding an additional antibiotic for improved anaerobic coverage may be indicated. Adjust antibiotic choices when culture and sensitivity reports are known. Consider consultation with an infectious disease specialist.

B. Deliver the Fetus

Provide continuous fetal heart rate and uterine contraction monitoring. If labor does not start spontaneously, or progress is inadequate, augment uterine contractions with oxytocin as clinically indicated. Use internal monitoring as clinically indicated. Minimize digital pelvic examinations, but examine frequently enough to know that labor is progressing. Dysfunctional labor is more common in the presence of chorioamnionitis, and the likelihood that cesarean delivery is necessary will be increased.

In addition, due to ineffective uterine contraction, postpartum hemorrhage is more likely. Have an increased index of suspicion for this obstetric emergency and make appropriate preparations.

 Chorioamnionitis is life-threatening for a woman and her fetus. Delivery needs to occur.

Corticosteroids are recommended for women with preterm premature ROM between 24 and 34 weeks' gestation to help mature fetal lungs, because these women are at increased risk for preterm delivery. Corticosteroids should be administered even if labor has begun, because they many provide benefit before delivery occurs. At present, there is insufficient evidence regarding the administration of corticosteroids in the setting of overt intra-amniotic infection. Consultation with maternal-fetal medicine specialists is strongly recommended.

7. What Should You Do if There Is *No* Evidence of Infection?

A. Term Fetus

1. *Term Gestation, Woman **in Labor,** No Evidence of Infection*
   • Assess the degree of risk for early-onset neonatal GBS sepsis. (See also Unit 3, Perinatal Infections, in this book.)
     – Maternal recto-vaginal or urine culture positive for GBS: initiate prophylaxis
     – Maternal recto-vaginal or urine culture negative for GBS: prophylaxis not indicated

- Maternal GBS status unknown: prophylaxis indicated if any of the following conditions are met:
  - o Prior child with early onset GBS sepsis
  - o Gestational age less than 37 weeks
  - o Maternal intrapartum fever (>100.4°F)
  - o Prolonged rupture of membranes (>18 hours)
- Use internal fetal heart rate and uterine contraction monitoring only when clinically indicated and not as a matter of routine.
- Keep the number of digital pelvic examinations to the minimum necessary to ensure normal progress of labor.
- Evaluate the woman and fetus for evidence of chorioamnionitis.
- Consider amnioinfusion, if persistent variable decelerations occur. Amnioinfusion may provide a sufficient cushion of fluid to relieve cord compression. If variable decelerations cannot be corrected, cesarean delivery may become necessary.

  Note: Amnioinfusion is described in the oligohydramnios section of Unit 4, Various High-Risk Conditions, in this book.

2. *Term Gestation, Mother* **Not** *in Labor, No Evidence of Infection*

More than 90% of pregnancies greater than 37 weeks will enter labor spontaneously and deliver within 24 hours of ROM.

Discuss management options with the patient and her family. There are 2 commonly followed approaches—either immediate induction of labor or a period of observation while awaiting spontaneous onset of labor.

a. *Immediate induction of labor* carries higher risks for failed induction (which might then require cesarean delivery) and for operative vaginal delivery, but is associated with a lower risk for infection.

b. *Observation until spontaneous labor begins* carries a higher risk for infection but is associated with a lower risk for operative delivery. Generally, it is not advisable to wait longer than 24 to 72 hours for spontaneous labor to begin. If labor does not begin spontaneously within this observation period, consider labor induction. This approach is associated with an increased rate of infections in women who are carriers of GBS.

Either management plan requires continued surveillance for infection. If evidence of infection develops, labor should be induced. Digital cervical examinations should be avoided.

Continuous external fetal heart rate monitoring is recommended. Decreased amniotic fluid increases the risk for cord compression by the body of the fetus, even if labor is not present.

B. Preterm Fetus

 Consultation with maternal-fetal medicine specialists is recommended, especially when the pregnancy is extremely preterm.

1. *Preterm Gestation, Mother* **in Labor,** *No Evidence of Infection*
   a. *Give antibiotics:* Review the GBS section in Unit 3, Perinatal Infections, in this book, and treat accordingly.
   b. *Consider tocolysis* (see Unit 7, Preterm Labor, in this book): Tocolysis may not stop labor entirely, but it may be useful in gaining time for the administration of antibiotics and corticosteroids.

c. *Give corticosteroids* (see Unit 7, Preterm Labor, in this book): When there is premature ROM but no evidence of chorioamnionitis, antenatal corticosteroid therapy is recommended for patients between 24 and 34 weeks' gestation. The corticosteroid benefits include reducing the neonatal risks of respiratory distress syndrome, intraventricular hemorrhage, necrotizing enterocolitis, and death.

2. *Preterm Gestation, Mother* **Not** *in Labor, No Evidence of Infection*

a. *Give antibiotics*: Even in the absence of labor or clinical evidence of infection, antibiotics given prophylactically have demonstrated several benefits when used for patients with premature ROM before 35 weeks' gestation. These benefits include
- Significantly prolonging pregnancy
- Reducing the incidence of
  - Maternal infection (chorioamnionitis and postpartum endometritis)
  - Neonatal sepsis
  - Neonatal intraventricular hemorrhage

Several antibiotic regimens are acceptable. One effective one is
- Ampicillin 2 g and erythromycin 250 mg intravenously every 6 hours for 48 hours

then
- Amoxicillin 250 mg and erythromycin 333 mg orally every 8 hours for an additional 5 days

If the course of prophylactic antibiotic therapy is completed before the onset of labor, the need for intrapartum antibiotic therapy (for prevention of neonatal GBS disease) should be reassessed when labor begins.

b. *Give corticosteroids* (see Section 7B1c and Unit 7, Preterm Labor, in this book).

c. *Consider management options*: Three options may be available. Discuss these, and their respective risks and benefits, with the pregnant woman and her family.
- *Labor induction*: Labor induction may be appropriate if the pregnancy is 32 to 36 weeks and pulmonary maturity can be documented.
- *Prolonged hospitalization*: If the pregnancy is significantly preterm, hospitalization with bed rest and frequent reassessment of maternal and fetal condition may be required for weeks or months.
- While most studies have used a daily nonstress test and/or daily BPP testing to assess cord compression and fetal well-being, the optimal testing scheme and frequency of testing is not known. Any abnormal test results, however, should prompt further investigation.
- Consultation with maternal-fetal medicine specialists for the care of the woman and the fetus is strongly recommended, particularly if the fetus is extremely preterm. The onset of labor may occur at any time, and is likely to progress rapidly, so transfer for continued in-patient observation and delivery at a regional center also should be considered.

Note: Optimal management of preterm, premature ROM when *cervical cerclage* is in place has not yet been established. Consult with and/or refer to maternal-fetal medicine specialists.

8. What Post-delivery Care Should You Provide?

A. Maternal Care

1. *Premature ROM, Without Clear Evidence of Intrauterine Infection*
   Continue to observe for evidence of infection. Endometritis, if untreated, can progress to life-threatening maternal sepsis. (See the puerperal endometritis section in Unit 3, Perinatal Infections, in this book).

   If antibiotics were started during labor, but there is no evidence of infection, antibiotic therapy may be stopped at or shortly after delivery.

2. *Strongly Suspected or Proven Chorioamnionitis*
   Current post-delivery recommendations for women with chorioamnionitis are to administer the next scheduled dose of antibiotics after the baby is delivered, and to add clindamycin 900 mg at the time of cord clamping for women undergoing cesarean delivery. Continued antibiotic therapy beyond this point should be individualized based on ongoing maternal fever or other objective evidence of infection.

B. Neonatal Care
   Prolonged ROM is defined as ROM for 18 hours or longer. Prolonged ROM can occur with or without premature ROM. Sometimes membranes rupture after the start of labor, but a lengthy labor then creates the situation of prolonged rupture by the time the baby is born.

   Either premature or prolonged ROM increases the risk for neonatal sepsis. Although many babies do not become sick, some can become infected and gravely ill, even when there is no evidence of maternal infection. Even if a woman does not appear to be ill, a complete obstetric history should be conveyed promptly to neonatal care providers.

   Neonatal management following premature or prolonged ROM requires consideration of several factors, including obstetric history, gestational age, the woman's intrapartum treatment and current clinical condition, and the baby's clinical condition. This issue is addressed in Book III: Neonatal Care, Unit 8, Infections.

Self-test

Now answer these questions to test yourself on the information in the last section.

B1. Rupture of membranes occurs in a pregnancy at 29 weeks' gestation. There is no evidence of infection or preterm labor. Which of the following should be done?

Yes	No	
____	____	Check urinalysis.
____	____	Check maternal vital signs.
____	____	Give corticosteroids.
____	____	Consider transfer to regional center.
____	____	Begin antibiotics.

B2. A 28-year-old woman pregnant with her third baby presents with premature rupture of membranes and a temperature of 39°C (102.2°F) at 36 weeks' gestation. Her uterus is very tender, but labor has not started and there have been no other pregnancy complications. What should you do?

Yes	No	
____	____	Obtain specimens for GBS, gonorrhea, and *Chlamydia*.
____	____	Begin broad-spectrum antibiotics intravenously.
____	____	Obtain complete blood count with differential.
____	____	Notify pediatrics of maternal condition.
____	____	Perform cesarean delivery.
____	____	Begin oxytocin induction of labor.

B3. List at least 4 signs of chorioamnionitis.

_____

_____

_____

_____

B4. In which of the following situations might it be appropriate to use amniocentesis with instillation of dye into the amniotic cavity to confirm suspected rupture of membranes?

Yes	No	
____	____	32 weeks' gestation with no evidence of infection
____	____	40 weeks' gestation with maternal fever and fetal tachycardia
____	____	30 weeks' gestation with uterine tenderness and fetal biophysical score of 4
____	____	38 weeks' gestation with maternal hypertension

B5. Premature rupture of membranes occurred in a pregnancy at 39 weeks' gestation. There is no evidence of infection. Membranes ruptured 8 hours earlier, but labor has not yet started. The fetus is in cephalic presentation. Which of the following are appropriate actions?

Yes	No	
____	____	Begin induction of labor.
____	____	Observe. Begin induction if labor does not start spontaneously in 24 to 72 hours.
____	____	Deliver by cesarean section.

B6. **True** **False** With chorioamnionitis, the specific infectious organism and length of time until delivery are the key factors in determining the severity of maternal illness.

Check your answers with the list that follows the Recommended Routines. Correct any incorrect answers and review the appropriate section in the unit.

223

Premature Rupture and/or Infection of the Amniotic Membranes

Recommended Routines

All the routines listed below are based on the principles of perinatal care presented in the unit you have just finished. They are recommended as part of routine perinatal care.

Read each routine carefully and decide whether it is standard operating procedure in your hospital. Check the appropriate blank next to each routine.

Procedure Standard in My Hospital	Needs Discussion by Our Staff	
_____	_____	1. Establish a system for consultation and referral for women with preterm, premature rupture of membranes.
_____	_____	2. Establish a system to notify nursery personnel of women whose babies are at risk for infection, including women • With evidence of chorioamnionitis • Who received antibiotics during labor, and the indication for their treatment • With premature rupture of membranes • With prolonged rupture of membranes

_____	_____	3. Establish a protocol for the care of all women with premature rupture of membranes that includes
		• Evaluation for umbilical cord prolapse and compression
		• Evaluation for infection
		• Minimization of digital cervical examinations
		   – None for women not in labor or not expected to have immediate induction of labor
		   – As few as necessary for women in labor and, as appropriate, administration of
		     o Antibiotics
		     o Corticosteroids

225

Self-test Answers

These are the answers to the self-test questions. Please check them with the answers you gave and review the information in the unit wherever necessary.

A1. True

A2. True

A3. True

A4. True

A5. True

A6. True

A7. True

A8. False.   Fluid from a vaginal pool following rupture of membranes can be used to test for phosphatidyl glycerol, but not for lecithin-sphingomyelin ratio, or certain other tests of fetal lung maturity.

A9. Any 3 of the following: infection (chorioamnionitis, maternal sepsis, puerperal endometritis, fetal and/or neonatal sepsis), preterm birth, prolapsed umbilical cord, umbilical cord compression, complications of oligohydramnios, abruptio placentae, fetal death

A10. Infection

A11. High in the vagina

B1.
Yes	No	
X	___	Check urinalysis.
X	___	Check maternal vital signs.
X	___	Give corticosteroids.
X	___	Consider transfer to regional center.
X	___	Begin antibiotics.

B2.
Yes	No	
X	___	Obtain specimens for testing for group B beta-hemolytic streptococcus, gonorrhea, and *Chlamydia*.
X	___	Begin broad-spectrum antibiotics intravenously.
X	___	Obtain complete blood count with differential.
X	___	Notify pediatrics of maternal condition.
___	X	Perform cesarean delivery.
X	___	Begin oxytocin induction of labor.

B3. Any 4 of the following: maternal fever 38°C (100.4°F) or higher, elevated white blood cell count, uterine tenderness, cloudy or foul-smelling amniotic fluid, maternal malaise, fetal tachycardia, biophysical profile score of 6 or lower

B4. Yes   No

     X   ____   32 weeks' gestation with no evidence of infection. (If all other means to determine whether the membranes are ruptured are inconclusive, and knowing that is essential to clinical decision making, an amniocentesis and dye test is likely to be helpful to determine whether membranes are ruptured and to reveal presence or absence of bacteria in the amniotic fluid. Consultation with and/or referral to a regional center is recommended.)

    ____   X   40 weeks' gestation with maternal fever and fetal tachycardia. (Term newborn with findings suggestive of infection; induction of labor is indicated; dye test unlikely to add useful information because the baby needs to be delivered; assess fetal well-being and consider consultation with a regional center.)

    ____   X   30 weeks' gestation with uterine tenderness and fetal biophysical score of 4. (Evidence of an ill fetus and infection; delivery is needed; amniocentesis with dye test is an invasive procedure unlikely to add useful information in this situation; consultation with and/or referral to a regional center is recommended.)

    ____   X   38 weeks' gestation with maternal hypertension. (Term fetus; dye test is unlikely to add useful information in this situation; assess fetal well-being and consider consultation with a regional center.) (If adequate amniotic fluid cannot be obtained with a sterile speculum examination, amniocentesis may be appropriate to collect fluid for culture and sensitivities and Gram stain.)

B5. Yes   No

     X   ____   Begin induction of labor.

     X   ____   Observe. Begin induction if labor does not start spontaneously in 24 to 72 hours.

    ____   X   Deliver by cesarean section.

B6. True

227

Unit 6 Posttest

If you are applying for continuing education credits, a posttest for this unit is available online. Completion of unit posttests and the book evaluation form are required to achieve continuing education credit. For more details, visit www.cmevillage.com.

SKILL UNIT

Sterile Speculum Examination

This skill unit will teach you how to perform a sterile speculum examination. *Not everyone* will be required to learn and practice this skill. *Everyone,* however, should read this unit and attend a skill session to learn the equipment needed and the sequence of steps to be able to assist with a sterile speculum examination.

Study this skill unit, then attend a skill demonstration and practice session. To master the skill, you will need to demonstrate correctly each of the steps listed below. You may be asked to demonstrate your proficiency with either a manikin and/or a patient (who requires the procedure).

1. Explain the procedure and be able to answer questions a pregnant woman might ask about the examination (in particular why it is needed, what is involved, and how she can help during the examination).
2. Collect and prepare the equipment, including supplies for anticipated tests.
3. Position the woman for the examination.
4. Insert a sterile speculum.
5. Position the speculum so the cervix is clearly visible.
6. Withdraw the speculum and complete the examination.
7. Describe your findings accurately and completely regarding color, consistency, and odor of fluid; leakage of fluid; cervical dilatation and effacement; and any other pertinent findings.

Note: Illustrations in this skill unit are reproduced with permission from Martin EJ, ed. *Intrapartum Management Modules: A Perinatal Education Program.* 3rd ed. Philadelphia, PA: Lippincott Williams & Wilkins; 2002:85-86.

PERINATAL PERFORMANCE GUIDE

Sterile Speculum Examination

ACTIONS	REMARKS

Deciding When to Use a Sterile Speculum Examination

1. What are the indications for an examination?
   - Is there doubt as to whether the membranes are ruptured?
   - Do cervical/vaginal cultures need to be obtained (whether or not the membranes are ruptured)?
   - If the membranes are ruptured, would it be helpful to clinical care to know if phosphatidyl glycerol (PG) is present in the amniotic fluid without doing an amniocentesis?
   - Is visual inspection for a prolapsed umbilical cord and/or cervical dilatation and effacement needed?

   Yes: Perform a sterile speculum examination if the answer is "yes" to any of these questions.

   No: A sterile speculum examination may not be needed.

These are the common indications for a sterile speculum examination. A sterile speculum examination may be indicated for other reasons in individual clinical situations.

A sterile speculum examination, rather than a digital examination, is preferable whenever there is an increased risk of intrauterine infection. If labor is not present, *only* sterile speculum examination(s) should be used until a decision about whether to proceed with delivery has been made.

Preparing the Woman for the Examination

2. Talk to the woman about the examination.
   - Explain the procedure.
     - Why it is needed
     - What is involved
     - What she can do to help during the examination
   - Ask the woman to empty her bladder.

This is an intrusive procedure.
Understanding the purpose of the examination and how it will be carried out may help a woman to relax and cooperate more fully during the procedure.

The examination is easier to perform and more comfortable when the woman's bladder is empty.

Collecting and Preparing the Equipment

3. Collect the necessary equipment.
   - Sterile speculum
   - Sterile gloves
   - Moveable, adjustable lamp
   - Stool for the examiner to sit on

Select the size and type of speculum according to the woman's history. A Pedersen speculum (flatter and more narrow blades) may be more comfortable for primigravidas and very tense women than the more common Graves speculum, which has wider blades and comes in 2 sizes (standard and large).

ACTIONS	REMARKS

Collecting and Preparing the Equipment (continued)

• Equipment for anticipated tests (gonorrhea, *Chlamydia,* and group B beta-hemolytic streptococcus); Nitrazine paper; containers for specimens to test for PG, immunochromatographic assay for ruptured membranes (AmniSure), as appropriate.	Check to be sure you know the specific specimen containers needed for these tests in your hospital.
4. Set up a sterile tray. Open the packages of sterile supplies onto the tray.	Take care to maintain strict aseptic technique.
5. Position the tray so that it is within easy reach of where the examiner will be sitting on the stool at the end of the examining table.	Be sure the tray and equipment are protected from contamination while you position the woman.

Positioning the Woman

6. Ask the woman to remove the clothes below her waist and then to lie on the examining table with • A pillow under head • Her legs in stirrups • Her arms at her sides or across her abdomen or chest	Be sure that she is as comfortable as possible before you begin the examination. Abdominal muscles are more likely to be tense when a woman puts her arms and hands above or behind her head.
7. Drape the woman's legs with a sheet so her knees are covered but the pubic area is exposed.	Be sure that you will be able to see her face when you are seated on the stool.
8. Position the lamp so the perineum and the anticipated visual field, once the speculum is positioned properly, will be well-lighted.	Be sure the light does not shine directly in the woman's eyes when she is looking toward you at the end of the table.
9. Position the stool so you will be comfortable performing the examination.	
10. If the woman is tense, encourage her to use relaxation breathing techniques or slow, deep breathing.	Relaxed abdominal and perineal muscles make insertion of the speculum easier and more comfortable.

Inserting and Positioning a Sterile Speculum

11. Wash your hands and put on the sterile gloves.	Talk with the woman and help her relax.
12. Sit comfortably on the stool and ask the woman to open her legs.	*Cleansing the perineum is not necessary, and antiseptics such as povidone-iodine can interfere with test results.*

ACTIONS	REMARKS

Inserting and Positioning a Sterile Speculum (continued)

13. Touch the inside of the woman's leg with the *back* of the hand *not* holding the speculum, before you touch the perineum.

    This helps to avoid startling the woman when you touch the more sensitive perineum.

14. With this same hand, place your index and middle finger on either side of the vaginal opening. Exert gentle downward pressure with your fingers and spread the opening slightly.

15. With the other hand (hand holding the speculum), tip the speculum slightly to one side and keep the blades closed as you pass them over your spread fingers and into the vagina.

    Avoid use of lubricants. Antiseptics and lubricants can cause test results to be inaccurate. In addition, a lubricant is usually not needed because vaginal secretions and/or amniotic fluid provide adequate moisture.

    If a patient is very dry and a lubricant seems essential, use only sterile water. When the amount of amniotic fluid is small, however, even water may dilute it enough to give misleading results.

    Turning the speculum blades 45° off midline avoids the urethra getting pinched.

    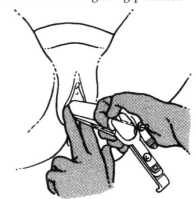

16. Maintain a slight downward pressure until the blades are fully inserted into the vagina.

    Take care to ensure that no tissue is caught between the blades as they are being inserted.

    Downward pressure will avoid pressing on the sensitive urethra.

    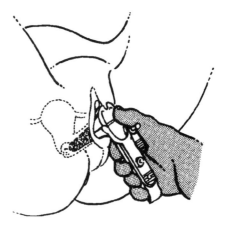

17. After the blades are fully inserted, remove your fingers from the vaginal opening, rotate the handle so it is vertical, and lift the tip of the blades to a more horizontal position.

    Let the woman know what you are doing and that she may feel some pressure.

ACTIONS   **REMARKS**

Inserting and Positioning a Sterile Speculum (continued)

18. Use the thumb piece on the speculum to open the blades and look for the cervix.

    BEWARE: Premature rupture of membranes (ROM), especially preterm, premature ROM, carries an increased risk for umbilical cord prolapse. If the cord is seen, withdraw the speculum carefully and proceed to management of a prolapsed cord.

    If you cannot see the cervix, reposition the speculum more anteriorly, posteriorly, or laterally until the cervix is completely in view.

Tell the woman she may feel more pressure as the blades are opened and positioned.

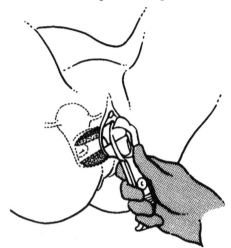

19. Once the cervix is clearly in view, tighten the thumbscrew to hold the blades open to that position.

When the speculum is properly positioned, the cervix will be between the upper and lower blades.

Obtaining Information From the Examination

20. Look at the cervix and determine if any fluid is leaking through it. If fluid is leaking, assess its color, consistency, and odor.
    • Is the fluid clear or very pale yellow?

    • Is the fluid dark yellow?

    • Is the fluid dark greenish brown and thick?
    • Is the fluid bloody? If it is bloody, is the blood bright red or dark red? What is the volume of blood?

    • Is there a foul odor?

Second trimester amniotic fluid is pale yellow, similar to the color of dilute urine. Near term, the fluid becomes less yellow and has vernix floating in it.
This indicates passage of meconium sometime in the past.
This indicates recent passage of meconium.

A small amount of blood might be from normal bloody show late in labor. It also might be due to one of the causes of obstetric hemorrhage. There is an increased risk of abruptio placentae with premature ROM.
Normal amniotic fluid has an odor but it is not unpleasant. A foul odor suggests infection.

21. Look at the cervix and determine if there is any evidence of dilatation or effacement.

ACTIONS   **REMARKS**

Obtaining Information From the Examination (continued)

22. Obtain specimens for testing. (See Skill Unit: Tests With Suspected or Proven Rupture of Membranes.)

23. When you have completed visual inspection of the cervix and collection of test samples, begin to withdraw the speculum.
    - Release the thumbscrew, but continue to hold the blades open.
    - Hold the blades open until the cervix is no longer visible between the upper and lower blades.
    - Allow the blades to close as the speculum is being withdrawn, so that they close completely just before reaching the vaginal opening.

    An assistant will make specimen collection and proper handling of the specimens easier.

24. If appropriate, obtain additional specimens from the lower blade. (See Skill Unit: Tests With Suspected or Proven Rupture of Membranes.)

Removing the Speculum and Completing the Examination

25. Remember that, once the sterile speculum has been inserted, it is contaminated by body fluids and should be handled accordingly.

26. Wipe any fluid from the perineum and help the woman assume a more comfortable position.

27. Finish preparation of the collected specimens. (See Skill Unit: Tests With Suspected or Proven Rupture of Membranes.)

28. Record
    - Observations made
      - Absence or presence (and degree) of cervical dilatation and effacement
      - Absence or presence of leakage of fluid
      - If leakage present, note color, consistency, and odor of fluid
    - Specimens obtained
      - Those sent for laboratory analysis
      - Those with results available at bedside

    Proceed to additional evaluation of maternal condition and/or fetal well-being, as warranted by your findings.

234

SKILL UNIT

Tests With Suspected or Proven Rupture of Membranes

This skill unit will teach you how to obtain test specimens during a sterile speculum examination. *Not everyone* will be required to learn and practice this skill. *Everyone,* however, should read this unit and attend a skill session to learn the equipment needed for each test and the sequence of steps to be able to assist with collection and correct handling of the specimens.

Study this skill unit, then attend a skill demonstration and practice session. To master the skills, you will need to demonstrate correctly each of the steps listed below. You may be asked to demonstrate your proficiency with either a manikin and/or a patient (who requires the test[s]), at the same time that you perform a sterile speculum examination.

pH Test (also known as Phenapthazine paper or nitrazine test)

1. Moisten the test device with fluid in the vagina.
2. Interpret the results.
3. Identify possible causes for inaccurate results.

Immunochromatographic assay for Placental alpha microglobulin-1 (info@amnisure.com; 617/234-4441)

A commercially available test for ruptured membranes is now available in many hospitals. This test detects the presence of placental alpha microglobulin-1. The procedure for performing the test is described in the package insert, but does not require a speculum examination. This test is reported to be highly sensitive and specific for ruptured membranes.

Tests for Gonorrhea, Chlamydia, and Group B Beta-Hemolytic Streptococcus

Analysis for Phosphatidyl Glycerol

1. Collect correct specimen containers.
2. Obtain specimens.
3. Prepare specimens for laboratory analysis.

Note: Illustration in this skill unit is reproduced with permission from Martin EJ, ed.
     Intrapartum Management Modules: A Perinatal Education Program. 3rd ed.
     Philadelphia, PA: Lippincott Williams & Wilkins; 2002:86.

PERINATAL PERFORMANCE GUIDE

Nitrazine Paper Test

ACTIONS   **REMARKS**

Deciding When to Obtain a Nitrazine Paper Test

1. Is rupture of membranes (ROM) suspected but not confirmed?

When moistened with a fluid, Nitrazine paper changes color in response to the fluid pH. Different colors indicate different pH values.

   Yes: Nitrazine paper test can help confirm or rule out ROM, but cannot provide a definitive diagnosis.

   No: There is no reason to obtain a Nitrazine paper test.

Results are unreliable when blood, mucus, semen, and certain vaginal infections are present, which have pH values close to that of amniotic fluid. Contamination with urine also may result in inaccurate results.

2. Is it appropriate to perform a sterile speculum or digital pelvic examination?

   Yes: Obtain a Nitrazine paper test.

   No: Wait to obtain the test until an examination is done.

Nitrazine paper can be tested during either a sterile speculum examination or a digital examination, although there is a greater risk of contamination and false values when it is tested as part of a digital examination.

Performing the Test During a Sterile Speculum Examination

3. Collect the equipment and prepare the patient for a sterile speculum examination.

In addition to the equipment needed for a sterile speculum examination, you will need a piece of Nitrazine paper.

4. During a sterile speculum examination, fluid may be applied to Nitrazine test paper.

 • Grip a piece of test paper with sterile forceps, then dip the paper in fluid that has collected in the posterior fornix.

OR

 • Moisten Nitrazine paper with fluid collected in the hollow area of the lower speculum blade, immediately after the speculum is withdrawn.

OR

 • Place a sterile cotton-tipped swab deep in the vagina and moisten it with fluid collected there. Then touch the swab to a piece of Nitrazine paper, making sure the paper is wet thoroughly.

If an assistant is not available, tear a piece from the spool of test paper when you prepare for the examination. The paper is not sterile, so it should not be put on the sterile tray, but it can be placed in a convenient spot where you can reach it with sterile forceps that have been placed on the sterile tray.

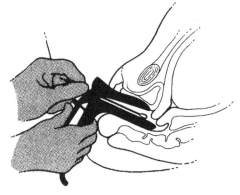

Performing the Test During a Digital Examination

5. Grip a 2- to 3-inch piece of Nitrazine paper between your index and middle finger. Insert your fingers with the paper into the vagina.

If you withdraw and then reinsert your hand into the woman's vagina more than once during an examination, put on a new sterile glove each time.

Interpreting the Test Results

6. Compare the color of the moistened section of Nitrazine paper with the color chart on the Nitrazine paper box.

   The membranes are *probably intact* if the test paper is
   • Yellow   pH = 5.0
   • Olive yellow   pH = 5.5
   • Olive green   pH = 6.0

   The membranes are *probably ruptured* if the test paper is
   • Blue-green   pH = 6.5
   • Blue-gray   pH = 7.0
   • Deep blue   pH = 7.5

7. Record your findings.

Be sure to note if you suspect that
   • There was an inadequate amount of amniotic fluid for accurate results.
   and/or
   • Contamination with other fluids may have occurred.

What Can Go Wrong?

1. The test paper may be contaminated
   • With other body fluids (blood, mucus, semen, etc)
   • From lubricants or antiseptics used previously

Results may be falsely positive or falsely negative, depending on the source of the contamination.

2. There may be too little amniotic fluid to obtain an accurate result.

If you think membranes are ruptured, but fluid is not apparent during a sterile speculum examination, ask the woman to cough or bear down. This action usually causes fluid to leak through the cervix if the membranes are ruptured.

3. The Nitrazine paper may be outdated.

Periodically check the expiration dates on the boxes and discard any that have expired. Make it a habit to check the date again before each time you use Nitrazine paper.

4. The Nitrazine paper may have been stored improperly.

Exposure to light for long periods or to moisture can interfere with the accuracy of the paper.

237

PERINATAL PERFORMANCE GUIDE

Collecting Specimens for

• Tests for Gonorrhea, Chlamydia, and Group B Streptococcus
• Analysis for Phosphatidyl Glycerol

ACTIONS	REMARKS
Deciding When to Obtain These Tests	

1. Consider the following:

    • Should cultures for group B streptococcus (GBS) and tests for gonorrhea and chlamydia be obtained?

    • Are the membranes ruptured and, if so, is there a need to estimate fetal lung maturity? (See Book I: Maternal and Fetal Evaluation and Immediate Newborn Care, Unit 2, Fetal Age, Growth, and Maturity.)

Consider cultures for GBS and testing for gonorrhea and chlamydia in all women with premature ROM.

If clinical decisions might be influenced by the pulmonary maturity of the fetus, a sample of amniotic fluid should be collected to determine if phosphatidyl glycerol (PG) is present.

If the delivery must occur, regardless of fetal maturity, the value of the information in planning care for the baby should be weighed against the cost of the test.

Collecting the Equipment

2. Collect the necessary equipment.

    • *Culture:* one sterile culture tube with swab for GBS culture
    • Gonorrhea and chlamydia: collect specimen container specific to the test used in your hospital
    • *PG:* 10-mL syringe and 5F feeding tube or flexible intravenous catheter

Transport media and protocols for specimens vary. Check the requirements of the laboratory in your hospital.

Various tests can be used to detect gonorrhea and chlamydia. Learn which one is used in your hospital.

Collecting the Specimens

3. GBS

    Use the sterile swab to sample the lower vagina and then the rectum, then place the swab into the transport medium.

The area sampled is important to the accurate determination of the presence or absence of GBS.

Clinical management is the same regardless of the reservoir of GBS, so only one swab is needed.

238

ACTIONS	REMARKS

Collecting the Specimens (continued)

4. Gonorrhea and chlamydia
   - Use a sterile swab to swab the endocervix, then place the swab in the appropriate transport container or medium.

5. *PG:* Aspirate the pool of fluid in the posterior vagina with a 5F catheter or flexible intravenous catheter attached to the syringe.

Place into the proper transport medium. Many laboratories require 2.0 mL for PG analysis. Check with your laboratory for the amount needed.

6. Label the specimens and send to the appropriate laboratories for culture and analysis.

Unit 7: Preterm Labor

Objectives

In this unit you will learn

A. The definition of preterm labor

B. The impact preterm birth has on neonatal morbidity and mortality

C. What factors increase the risks for preterm labor

D. What you can do to avoid preterm labor and delivery

E. How to evaluate preterm labor

F. How to treat preterm labor

G. How to manage a preterm delivery

H. What you should anticipate for the care of a preterm baby

Unit 7 Pretest

Before reading the unit, please answer the following questions. Select the *one best* answer to each question (unless otherwise instructed). Record your answers on the test and check them against the answers at the end of the book.

1. **True   False**   Fluid restriction may stop preterm uterine contractions if true labor has not developed.

2. **True   False**   Maternal hyperglycemia (high blood glucose) is a possible side effect of magnesium sulfate.

3. **True   False**   Cervical cerclage at 12 to 14 weeks is recommended for women who are known to have cervical insufficiency.

4. **True   False**   The risk of preterm delivery is increased with multifetal gestation.

5. **True   False**   Tocolysis may be appropriate for a woman with intact membranes and preterm labor, even when the cervix is dilated 4 cm or more.

6. **True   False**   Optimal benefits from antenatal steroid administration are achieved when treatment is given 24 to 48 hours before delivery.

7. Corticosteroids are given to a pregnant woman to help
   A. Prevent preterm labor.
   B. Mature the fetus's lungs when preterm delivery is unavoidable.
   C. Treat genital herpes infection.
   D. Ripen the cervix when induction of labor is planned.

8. In which of the following situations is tocolysis *most* appropriate?
   A. Preterm labor at 32 weeks with worsening maternal preeclampsia
   B. Preterm labor at 36 weeks with premature rupture of membranes
   C. Preterm labor at 34 weeks with uterine tenderness and maternal fever
   D. Preterm labor at 32 weeks with 2-cm cervical dilatation and 80% effacement

9. Which of the following conditions increase the risk for preterm labor and delivery?

Yes	No	
____	____	Hypertension
____	____	Urinary tract infection
____	____	Cigarette smoking
____	____	Previous cesarean delivery
____	____	Maternal cocaine use
____	____	Uterine malformation

10. All of the following may indicate the onset of preterm labor *except*
    A. Decreased fetal movement
    B. "Ballooning" of the lower uterine segment
    C. Pelvic pressure
    D. Softened, anterior position of the cervix

11. **True   False**   When beta-mimetic tocolytic medications are used, maternal heart rate should be maintained above 140 beats per minute.

12. **True   False**   One reason tocolysis is used is to allow time for administration of corticosteroids.

13. True   False   A negative fetal fibronectin test indicates delivery is unlikely to occur within the next 2 weeks.

14. True   False   Asymptomatic bacteriuria during pregnancy is common and rarely requires treatment.

15. True   False   Administration of corticosteroids should be considered only when the membranes are intact.

16. True   False   Vaginal delivery of a 2,000-g preterm fetus in breech presentation carries the same degree of risk to the fetus as a cesarean delivery.

Preterm labor does not necessarily have to result in preterm delivery. With early recognition, prompt intervention, and aggressive management, it may be possible to stop preterm labor and prolong a pregnancy.

1. What Are the Risks of Preterm Labor?

Preterm labor is defined as labor occurring prior to the completion of 37 weeks of gestation (before the start of the 38th week). Approximately 10% of babies born in the United States are born preterm.

The most serious threat from preterm labor is the risk of preterm birth. Prematurity is, over-whelmingly, the most common cause of neonatal morbidity and mortality. It accounts for approximately 75% of neonatal deaths that are not due to congenital malformations. Although *most* preterm babies who survive *do not* develop physical or mental impairment, preterm babies are much more likely to have some degree of impairment than are babies born at term. The lower the gestational age at birth, the greater the risk of death or long-term problems.

If a likely explanation for preterm labor can be identified, that factor (maternal medical illness, infection, multifetal gestation, etc) may pose additional maternal, fetal, and/or neonatal risks. The specific risks posed by those illnesses or conditions are described in other units within this book.

2. What Are the Causes of Preterm Labor?

In most cases, a cause cannot be clearly identified. There are many factors, however, that are known to increase the risk of preterm labor. These factors have an additive effect. The more risk factors a woman has, the greater her risk is for preterm labor. Intervention to reduce or eliminate any risk factor may help improve the outcome of a pregnancy.

    A. Maternal Medical Conditions

        Any serious medical disease increases the risk for preterm delivery, either because the risk of spontaneous preterm labor is increased or because preterm delivery may become necessary to preserve maternal and/or fetal health. The following conditions are especially likely to be associated with early birth:

- Hypertension, either chronic or pregnancy-related
- Diabetes mellitus
- Severe anemia
- Hemoglobinopathy
- Systemic lupus erythematosus
- Intra-amniotic infection
- Upper urinary tract infection, either symptomatic or asymptomatic
- Substance use (especially cocaine use)

    B. Adverse Socioeconomic and Lifestyle Conditions

        All of the following conditions are associated with an increased risk for preterm labor:

- Maternal age of 18 years or younger or 40 years or older
- Little or no prenatal care
- Inadequate nutrition, poor weight gain, and/or low pre-pregnancy weight
- Poverty, poor housing
- Heavy manual labor and/or very long work hours with extreme fatigue
- Severe emotional stress
- Trauma (due to a fall, traffic accident, domestic violence, etc)
- Maternal smoking

C. Obstetric Conditions

Risk factors may be related to obstetric history and/or to the current pregnancy. Some factors may recur from pregnancy to pregnancy, while others are a threat only in the present pregnancy.

1. *Obstetric History*
   - Cervical insufficiency
   - Uterine malformations, such as unicornuate or bicornuate uterus
   - Uterine fibroids
   - Spontaneous *second* trimester abortion(s)
   - Multiple first trimester dilatation and curettage procedures
   - **Previous preterm delivery***: The risk of preterm labor is *significantly* increased for women who have experienced a previous preterm delivery. The risk increases with the number of previous preterm births and decreases with the number of term births.

2. *Current Pregnancy*
   - Uterine overdistension
     - Hydramnios
     - **Multifetal gestation***: Multifetal gestation occurs in about 1% of all pregnancies, but accounts for 10% of all preterm births.
   - Antepartum obstetric bleeding
   - Chorioamnionitis
   - **Preterm premature rupture of membranes***

 Because prediction of preterm labor is very difficult, care aimed at early recognition of preterm labor and prevention of preterm delivery should be routinely provided to all women.

3. What Can You Do to Avoid Preterm Delivery?

A. Educate All Patients

All pregnant women should be taught the signs and symptoms of preterm labor. Women often think that only painful contractions indicate labor. Cervical dilatation can occur, however, even with relatively painless contractions.

The presence of any one of the following findings may indicate preterm labor:
- Abdominal cramping (may feel like gas pains or menstrual cramps)
- Increase in vaginal discharge, onset of watery or mucoid discharge
- Low backache, intermittent or constant
- Pelvic pressure, sense of heaviness in the vagina

The earlier intervention to stop preterm labor is started, the more likely it is to be successful. Any indication of preterm labor should be reported as soon as a woman becomes aware of it. Provide information about how to contact care providers and report symptoms, 24 hours a day, 7 days a week.

---

*Factors identified with an asterisk (*) put a pregnancy at particularly high risk for preterm labor. However, only about 20% to 30% of women with any risk factor(s) for preterm labor will actually experience preterm labor. Preterm labor occurs in many pregnancies that have no recognizable risk factors. Some risk factors are present only because of events that occurred in a previous pregnancy and, therefore, cannot be identified during a first pregnancy.

Instruct all pregnant women in the signs and symptoms of preterm labor.

B. Recognize and Address Risk Factors

Obtain a thorough history at the first prenatal visit. Be sure it includes a comprehensive review of maternal medical conditions; social, economic, and lifestyle risk factors; obstetric history and, for multigravidas, any changes since the previous pregnancy.

1. *Medical Conditions*

Assess maternal condition and current treatment, and determine if treatment needs to be modified. Establish a plan to monitor maternal and fetal health. Consult with and/or refer the woman for care by specialists, as appropriate.

Be sure to investigate substance use with *all* patients. Drug use crosses all socioeconomic boundaries. This includes cigarette smoking and alcohol intake, in addition to the use of illicit or prescription drugs. Enlist the help of social service resources if substance use counseling or treatment is indicated.

2. *Socioeconomic and Lifestyle Factors*

These factors, like substance use, can be extremely difficult to change. Alleviating any one factor, however, may improve pregnancy outcome. Consider what actions you, the woman, and/or an outside agency might be able to take to

- **Help ensure compliance with prenatal visit schedule.** Consider assistance with transportation or child care, scheduling to see the same care provider with each visit, and/or other intervention.
- **Improve nutritional status.** Consider dietary education, information about normal weight gain and body changes during pregnancy, meal preparation instruction, financial assistance, and/or other intervention.
- **Improve living conditions.** Consider assistance in locating adequate housing or in dealing with landlord of present housing, financial assistance, and/or other intervention.
- **Reduce demanding physical labor or extreme fatigue.** Consider modification of employment or living conditions.
- **Modify an abusive situation.** Consider support person or group, safe haven, legal aid, and/or other assistance or intervention.
- **Relieve extreme emotional stress.** Consider intervention to alleviate the most pressing social, economic, or other problem.

Keep in mind, what you see as a problem may not be what the patient sees as a problem, and what she sees as a problem may go unrecognized by you. Make every effort to involve the woman in decisions affecting her care and the care of her fetus. Involvement of the woman in identifying adverse conditions and in planning for change, including what she can do without outside assistance and what outside help she would accept, is essential for change to occur. Involve social service, counseling, education, and other resources, as appropriate, as early as possible in addressing these issues that can adversely affect the health of a pregnant woman.

3. *Obstetric Factors*

    a. *History of a prior preterm birth* is the most reliable predictor of risk of preterm birth in the current pregnancy. Weekly administration of 17 α-hydroxyprogesterone (250-mg intramuscular injection), beginning between 16 and 20 weeks' estimated gestational age, has been shown to reduce the recurrence risk of preterm birth. This treatment should be offered to all women who have had a prior delivery at less than 37 weeks due to spontaneous preterm labor or preterm premature rupture of membranes.

    Progesterone supplementation for asymptomatic women with an incidentally identified short cervical length (<15 mm) may be considered; however, routine cervical length screening is not recommended.

    b. *Establish pregnancy dates*: Determine the dates of every pregnancy, even low-risk, uncomplicated pregnancies, as early and as accurately as possible. If problems develop later in a pregnancy, this information can be invaluable in deciding an appropriate course of action.

    c. *Treat all infections*

    Routinely screen all women at the first prenatal visit for asymptomatic bacteriuria, vaginal infections, and sexually transmitted infections (STIs). Treat, retest, and re-treat as necessary.

    Urinary tract infections (including asymptomatic bacteriuria), symptomatic vaginal infections, and STIs are associated with the occurrence of preterm labor, and should be treated.

    d. *Reassess risk throughout pregnancy*

    Risk factors can change. Risk factors may stay the same but care needs to change as gestation progresses. New risk factors can develop.

Self-test

Now answer these questions to test yourself on the information in the last section.

A1. Preterm labor is defined as labor occurring before the *start* of the _____th week of gestation (or before the *end* of the _____th week).

A2. Prematurity accounts for approximately _____% of neonatal deaths that are not due to congenital malformations.

A3. Approximately _____% of babies born in the United States are born preterm.

A4. **True** **False** Preterm labor rarely occurs in women who do not have at least one risk factor.

A5. **True** **False** Routine screening for and treatment of asymptomatic bacteriuria may help prevent preterm labor.

A6. **True** **False** The earlier intervention to stop preterm labor is started, the more likely it is to be successful.

A7. What symptoms of preterm labor would you tell a pregnant woman to report?

_____

_____

A8. Which of the following conditions increase the risk for preterm labor and delivery?

Yes	No	
____	____	Chorioamnionitis
____	____	Severe anemia
____	____	Gonorrhea
____	____	Maternal age 18 years or younger
____	____	Cocaine use
____	____	Cervical insufficiency
____	____	Absence of prenatal care
____	____	Preterm premature rupture of membranes

A9. List at least 3 conditions that put a pregnancy at *particularly* high risk for preterm labor.

_____

_____

_____

Check your answers with the list that follows the Recommended Routines. Correct any incorrect answers and review the appropriate section in the unit.

4. What Should You Do for Women Known to Be At Risk for Preterm Labor?

A. Treat Conditions That Can Be Treated

1. *Cervical Insufficiency*

The cause of cervical insufficiency is often unknown, but may result from trauma resulting from obstetric or gynecologic procedures in the past or from in utero exposure to diethylstilbestrol. Diethylstilbestrol was in use from 1940 to 1971. It is estimated that 1 to 1.5 million women were exposed in utero to this medication. As a result, those women have a dramatically increased risk for spontaneous abortion and preterm birth because of maldevelopment of their uterus and cervix.

If a woman is known to have cervical insufficiency, cerclage is often effective when done early, before cervical dilatation. An ultrasound examination should be done to confirm fetal heart beat and to rule out gross anomalies. If there are no fetal contraindications, prophylactic cerclage is generally performed at 12 to 14 weeks. Vaginal

249

examinations are done every 1 to 2 weeks until 24 weeks' gestation, to assess the sutures that comprise the cerclage to be sure there is no erosion of the cervix. If this problem has not developed by 24 weeks, it is unlikely it will until near term. In rare instances, replacement of the cerclage may be indicated.

The cerclage remains in place until 36 to 37 weeks is reached or labor begins. Labor can result in uterine rupture if the cerclage is not removed.

2. *Suspected Cervical Insufficiency*
Cervical insufficiency may be suspected from a previous pregnancy that ended spontaneously between 12 and 20 weeks. If cervical insufficiency is suspected, but the condition is not clear enough to warrant cerclage, weekly vaginal examinations should begin at 10 to 14 weeks to assess for cervical dilatation and effacement. If cervical changes are found, consider hospitalization for monitoring to determine if uterine contractions are present. If no contractions are found, cervical cerclage may be appropriate.

Ultrasound examination also may be started at completion of the first trimester to assess the length of the cervix and presence or absence of "funneling" of the cervix. A short cervix and/or the appearance of funneling, but without the presence of cervical dilatation, may be an early sign of cervical insufficiency. These ultrasound findings also may be an early indication of the onset of labor. For this reason, it is difficult to know if cervical cerclage or treatment for preterm labor is the better course of action. Consultation with maternal-fetal medicine specialists is recommended.

3. *Urinary Tract Infections* (See Unit 3, Perinatal Infections, in this book.)
Preterm labor may be associated with the presence of a urinary tract infection, whether or not the infection is symptomatic. The risk is particularly increased with pyelonephritis. The apparent mechanism for this is the release of toxins from the infecting organism into the bloodstream. *Escherichia coli,* in particular, releases a toxin that has an oxytocin-like effect.

Routinely screen *all* pregnant women for bacteriuria at the first prenatal visit. Confirm a positive screening test result with a urine culture. Whether symptomatic or asymptomatic, treat bacteriuria promptly and aggressively. Recommended antibiotics, until sensitivities are known, include trimethoprim/sulfamethoxazole, nitrofurantoin, and cephalexin. Obtain follow-up urine culture 10 to 14 days after completion of antibiotic therapy. For women treated for bacteriuria, symptomatic or otherwise, periodically rescreen during pregnancy. If it recurs, suppressive antibiotic therapy for the remainder of the pregnancy is usually recommended.

B. Provide Increased Surveillance
If a woman had a previous preterm labor or is at high risk for preterm labor, institute preterm labor precautions.

1. *Increase the Frequency of Prenatal Visits*
Women at high risk for preterm delivery should be seen every 1 to 2 weeks, beginning at approximately 20 weeks.

2. *Inspect the Cervix*
Examine the cervix at 18 to 24 weeks to determine its condition and to establish its baseline status, by which to compare future changes. As with measurements of fundal height, accuracy is improved when the same examiner performs all subsequent examinations.

Check the cervix every 1 to 2 weeks from 20 weeks' to 34 weeks' gestation. Check for cervical changes, including

- Effacement
- Dilatation
- Softening
- Anterior position
- "Ballooning" of the lower uterine segment so the anterior vaginal wall appears to bulge into the vagina

Instruct the woman and her partner to abstain from sexual intercourse if cervical changes have occurred.

3. *Provide Patient Education*
   Review the symptoms of preterm labor and the importance of seeking prompt medical care if any symptoms occur.

5. How Do You Evaluate Preterm Labor?

Investigate, as quickly as possible, *any* evidence of preterm labor. You will need to decide if true labor is present and, if it is present, whether an attempt should be made to stop it.

The following things need to be accomplished:

- Provide intravenous (IV) hydration and rest.
- Evaluate maternal health.
- Evaluate fetal health, size, and gestational age.
- Determine whether true labor is present.
- Make a plan of care.

   A. Assess the Condition of the Woman and Her Fetus
   With the woman resting in bed, monitor and evaluate the woman and the fetus.
   Outpatient evaluation in an antenatal testing or labor area is recommended because some women will not be in labor and can safely go home after observation and assessment. For those patients who require further treatment, formal hospital admission can be arranged after this period of evaluation.

 The onset of labor before term has a cause, although the cause may not be obvious. Look for a cause, and evaluate maternal and fetal well-being. Try to determine whether continuation of the pregnancy would jeopardize the health of the woman or the fetus.

   1. *Examine the Woman*
      Perform a physical examination and check the woman's vital signs. Look for evidence of intra-amniotic infection (chorioamnionitis) (see Unit 6, Abnormal Rupture and/or Infection of the Amniotic Membranes, in this book). Obtain a medical and obstetric history, if that is not already known.

   2. *Hydrate the Patient and Institute Bed Rest*
      Start an IV and give an initial bolus of 500 mL of an isotonic crystalloid solution. Dehydration can initiate contractions. Rehydration and complete rest usually inhibits contractions that are due to dehydration and not accompanied by cervical changes.

      Giving fluids to a normally hydrated woman, however, has not been shown to have an effect on preterm labor. If tocolysis is used, take care to avoid fluid overload to minimize the risk of pulmonary edema.

3. *Sedate the Patient*

Consider using morphine sulfate (5 mg intramuscularly or intravenously). This allows the patient to rest during this anxious period, and may reduce uterine activity.

4. *Provide Continuous External Monitoring of Fetal Heart Rate and Uterine Activity*

5. *Obtain Urinalysis and Urine Culture*

6. *Perform Sterile Speculum Examination*
   - Assess cervical dilatation, effacement, consistency, and position.
   - Determine whether there is ballooning of the lower uterine segment, from the appearance of bulging of the anterior vaginal wall.
   - Determine whether membranes are ruptured or intact.
   - Obtain
     - Cultures for group B streptococcus (GBS) (vaginal and rectal)
     - Sample to test for chlamydia and gonorrhea (cervical/vaginal)
     - Consider sampling cervicovaginal secretions for fetal fibronectin test (if membranes are intact, no bleeding is seen, and gestational age is 22 to 35 weeks.)

 Do not perform a digital examination if
   - *Membranes are ruptured (to avoid introducing infectious organisms into the uterus).*
   or
   - *Bleeding is present, until placenta previa has been ruled out (to avoid precipitating further bleeding).*

7. *Fetal Fibronectin*: Fetal fibronectin is present in maternal tissue and appears in cervicovaginal secretions as the cervix is remodeled in preparation for labor.

A sample of cervicovaginal secretions should be obtained ***before*** a digital examination is performed because a digital examination may cause increased fetal fibronectin in the cervical mucus and result in a falsely elevated value. The secretions need to be free of blood and amniotic fluid (membranes intact), as well as semen from recent intercourse (without a condom) because those substances may cause false-positive results. If a lubricant or antiseptic was used, it is recommended to wait 6 to 8 hours before sampling because those compounds may cause false-negative results. Cervical dilatation should be less than 3 cm.

Positive results are associated with preterm delivery but are not predictive of it. Negative results are more useful. Negative fetal fibronectin test results indicate delivery is unlikely to occur within the next 2 weeks.

This test is not recommended for routine screening of pregnant women. It is most useful in the evaluation of women who have signs or symptoms of preterm labor, with intact membranes.

8. *Recheck Pregnancy Dates, Fetal Size, and Gestational Age*

9. *Determine if Preterm Labor Is Present*

Preterm labor is commonly defined by
- Cervical changes that occur during the observation period

and/or
- Contractions that persist despite adequate hydration and sedation, and
  – Cervical dilatation of 2 cm or more

  or
  – Cervical effacement of 80% or more

If the woman does not have cervical changes or persistent contractions, and the membranes are not ruptured, there is no reason for her to stay in the hospital for continued observation. If membranes are ruptured, refer to Unit 6, Premature Rupture and/or Infection of the Amniotic Membranes, in this book.

Before the patient goes home, however, ultrasound examination may be used to obtain additional information about the likelihood of preterm labor occurring in the future.

10. *Ultrasound Examination*: If the membranes are intact, vaginal probe ultrasound examination may be used to assess cervical length and funneling of the lower uterine segment. Funneling refers to the shape created by the thinning and softening of the lower uterine segment and widening of the adjoining upper cervix. These changes allow the membranes to bulge into the upper cervix. If funneling is *not* present and/or the cervix is longer than 3 cm, there is a less than 5% chance that the woman will deliver before 35 weeks' gestation.

Funneling and/or a shortened cervix cannot, however, be used to predict if preterm labor will occur. Some women with funneling and/or a shortened cervix will go on to develop preterm labor, others will not. Only the *absence* of funneling is predictive of a low chance for preterm labor. The *presence* of funneling is not predictive.

Less than 1% of women who have an *absence* of funneling and an *absence* of fetal fibronectin in cervical mucus will develop preterm labor during the week following the examination.

B. Consider Consultation and Referral

If facilities for care of maternal, fetal, and/or expected neonatal condition are not present in your hospital, consider maternal/fetal transfer to a regional center, especially if the fetus is 34 weeks' gestation or younger or if there are any other complications. This allows the baby to be born in a hospital with a neonatal intensive care unit and avoids a family split between a mother in one hospital and a baby in another hospital.

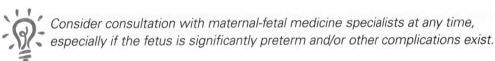 *Consider consultation with maternal-fetal medicine specialists at any time, especially if the fetus is significantly preterm and/or other complications exist.*

If transfer is indicated, it should be accomplished *early*, well before labor has progressed to the point where en route delivery might occur. Generally, therapy is started before transfer, and continued during transport, as appropriate to the individual circumstances.

C. Decide Whether to Attempt to Stop Labor

1. *Contraindications to Tocolysis*

   a. Tocolysis *should not* be used with
      - Acute nonreassuring fetal status
      - Dead fetus or lethal fetal anomaly

- Documented fetal lung maturity
- Maternal myasthenia gravis
- Severe fetal growth restriction, or other condition in which prolonging a pregnancy may jeopardize fetal or maternal health, such as
  - Intra-amniotic infection (chorioamnionitis)
  - Severe preeclampsia or eclampsia
  - Maternal physiologic instability (hemorrhage, severe medical illness, etc)

b. Tocolysis is *usually* not used with
- Maternal illness of mild or moderate severity, such as hypertension, heart disease, hyperthyroidism, diabetes mellitus, etc.
- Women with contractions but without cervical changes: Bed rest, adequate hydration, and close observation are recommended.

2. *Indications for Tocolysis*

The primary indication for tocolysis is treatment of preterm labor. As long as there is no evidence of infection, tocolysis may be used in the presence of ruptured membranes. This may allow safe transfer of the woman and her fetus to a higher level of care, as well as allowing more time for administration of corticosteroids. However, be aware that intra-amniotic infection, even subclinical infection, is often associated with preterm labor. Investigate the possibility of infection carefully.

The use of tocolytic medications is appropriate when
- Uterine contractions with cervical dilatation or effacement are present.
- Fetus is preterm and has not achieved pulmonary maturity.
- Pregnant woman is healthy.

Generally, all pregnancies with preterm labor at 34 weeks or less are treated with tocolytic medication (unless there are specific contraindications). Tocolysis, however, is usually *not* appropriate for preterm labor that occurs between 34 and 36 weeks.

In cases where cervical dilatation is advanced (≥4 cm), tocolytic therapy may still be used in an attempt to gain time for the administration of corticosteroids and, if appropriate, for safe transfer to a regional center.

 When gestational age is 34 weeks or less, prolonging a pregnancy for even a brief period can be extremely beneficial to fetal maturation and, hence, to neonatal survival and well-being.

D. Make a Plan of Care

In the absence of other complications, the main risks of preterm labor are the neonatal risks associated with preterm delivery. If complications are present, you will need to decide if the maternal and newborn risks are lower if the fetus remains in the uterus or if the fetus is delivered.

None of the drugs and other interventions used to treat preterm labor have been shown to be completely effective. In addition, tocolytic medications used to stop labor pose significant risk to both maternal and fetal health, particularly with prolonged administration. Significant fetal and neonatal benefits, however, may be obtained from tocolysis when it stops labor long enough to allow administration of corticosteroids.

Pediatric and obstetric physicians should discuss treatment options and associated risks for the woman and the baby with the family. The patient and her family should be involved in the deliberations regarding the use of tocolytics and have a thorough understanding of the purpose, possible risks, potential benefits, and limitations of the therapy. If the decision is made to attempt to halt labor and continue the pregnancy, tocolysis should be started *immediately*.

Self-test

Now answer these questions to test yourself on the information in the last section.

B1. If a woman is known to have cervical insufficiency, cerclage should be done at _____ weeks.

B2. Give 3 cervical changes that indicate possible preterm labor.

_____
_____
_____

B3. **True** **False** An attempt to stop labor should be made for *all* women who go into preterm labor.

B4. **True** **False** Preterm uterine contractions, without cervical changes, may stop with rehydration and bed rest.

B5. **True** **False** Every woman who goes into preterm labor should be checked for evidence of chorioamnionitis.

B6. **True** **False** Tocolysis is of no value when cervical dilatation is far advanced and delivery is likely to occur in less than 24 hours.

B7. **True** **False** The main risk of preterm delivery is the risk to the newborn of preterm birth, and the subsequent risks associated with prematurity.

B8. **True** **False** Prenatal care for women with a history of a previous preterm labor should include examination of the cervix every 1 to 2 weeks during the second trimester.

B9. What is a common definition of preterm labor?

_____
_____

B10. Which of the following should be included in the evaluation of preterm labor?

Yes	No	
____	____	Urinalysis
____	____	Discuss treatment options and risks and benefits with the woman and her family
____	____	Consider maternal/fetal referral for delivery at a regional center
____	____	Internal monitoring of fetal heart rate and uterine activity
____	____	Physical examination
____	____	Sterile speculum examination
____	____	Vaginal/rectal cultures

Check your answers with the list that follows the Recommended Routines. Correct any incorrect answers and review the appropriate section in the unit.

6. How Do You Treat Preterm Labor?

Ideally, preterm labor treatment will provide tocolysis that halts uterine contractions and cervical dilatation and allows the pregnancy to go to term. However, that is rarely possible. The goal of preterm labor treatment, therefore, is to delay delivery at least long enough to allow time for optimal administration of corticosteroids. Corticosteroids given to a pregnant woman threatened with preterm labor have been shown to accelerate fetal maturity and reduce the frequency of certain serious complications of prematurity.

A. Stop Contractions

 Tocolysis is most likely to be successful when there is rapid identification and prompt, aggressive intervention to stop preterm labor.

Regardless of the drug used, tocolysis therapy should
- Use the minimum amount of medication that will stop contractions.
- Monitor the woman and fetus for possible medication side effects.
- Monitor fetal heart rate and uterine activity continuously.
- Reduce (or stop) administration if significant side effects develop.
- If contractions continue after 12 to 18 hours of tocolytic therapy, reassess the situation. Decide if another drug should be tried, or if labor should be allowed to continue.

Magnesium sulfate is a commonly used tocolytic agent. Calcium channel blocking agents may also be used. Beta-mimetics are used less often than in the past, largely because of their side effects. Prostaglandin synthesis inhibitors and other tocolytic medications are also available. Sometimes one medication will not control uterine contractions, but switching from that drug to another tocolytic agent may prove to be effective.

The use of 2 drugs at the same time may be effective when neither medication alone was successful in stopping contractions. This generally carries a higher risk of maternal side effects. Certain combinations of drugs are safer than others. Consultation with maternal-fetal medicine specialists is recommended.

 All of the tocolytic agents have potentially devastating side effects.

Study Table 7.1 to learn about some commonly used tocolytic drugs and how you should monitor their administration.

B. Hasten Fetal Maturity*
1. *Indications and Benefits of Corticosteroids*
Corticosteroids accelerate fetal maturity. Antenatal corticosteroids are usually indicated whenever preterm delivery is likely to occur, either due to the spontaneous onset of labor or to complications that require early delivery.

---

*Recommendations in Section 6B are taken from *Effect of Corticosteroids for Fetal Maturation on Perinatal Outcomes.* NIH Consensus Statement. February 28-March 2, 1994;12(2) and *Antenatal Corticosteroids Revisited: Repeat Courses.* NIH Consensus Statement. August 17-18, 2000;17(2).

Table 7.1. Tocolytic Medications Commonly Used to Treat Preterm Labor

Medication	Contraindications	Dosage	Administration	Side Effects	Monitoring

Magnesium sulfate*	1. Myasthenia gravis
	
	2. Hypocalcemia
	
	3. Impaired renal function
	
	4. Concurrent use with nifedipine
		Loading dose: 4-6 g
		
		Continuous Infusion: 2-4 g/hour
		
		Adjust dose, as needed, to inhibit uterine activity and keep serum magnesium (Mg^{++}) level 6-8 mg/dL.
			Loading dose: Intravenously over 20 minutes
			
			Maintenance: Use piggyback intravenous infusion with pump to control rate.
			
			Duration: In general, intravenous therapy is used for approximately 24 hours
			
			CAUTION: *Use with nifedipine can cause neuromuscular blockade.*
				Maternal
				Transient flushing, headache, nystagmus, nausea, lethargy, dizziness, blurred or double vision are common, especially during loading dose.
				1. *Pulmonary edema risk is reduced with*
				  • Careful monitoring of intake/output
				  • Serum level kept 6-8 mg/dL
				2. *Hypocalcemia* (low serum calcium)
				Signs of Toxicity
				Loss of deep tendon reflexes at serum level 10-12 mg/dL
				At higher serum Mg^{++}
				• Respiratory depression
				• Severe hypotension
				• Tetany or paralysis
				• Cardiac arrest
				Neonatal
				Transient decrease in muscle tone, drowsiness in newborn may occur
					Check
					• *Urine output:* Mg^{++} excreted only by kidney
					• *Toxicity* risk increased when output <30 mL/hour
					• *Record Intake and output*
					• *Vital signs every hour*
					• *Deep tendon reflexes (DTR) every hour*
					• *Measure Serum Mg^{++} if DTRs diminish*
					• *Signs of pulmonary edema,* check breath sounds
					• *Fetal heart rate and pattern*
					Keep calcium gluconate available.
					Administer if signs of toxicity develop.

257

Table 7.1. Tocolytic Medications Commonly Used to Treat Preterm Labor (continued)

Medication	Contraindications	Dosage	Administration	Side Effects	Monitoring
Calcium channel blocker *Nifedipine*	1. Liver disease 2. Concurrent use with magnesium sulfate	*Loading dose:* 10 mg may be repeated 1-2 times, at 20-minute intervals, if contractions persist *Maintenance:* 10-20 mg, every 4-6 hours	*Route:* Oral *CAUTION: Use with magnesium sulfate can cause neuromuscular blockade.*	*Maternal* Vasodilatation: flushing, headache, transient heart rate increase, transient hypotension	*Check* • *Blood pressure* • *Fetal heart rate and pattern*
Beta-mimetic agent *Terbutaline*	1. Cardiac disease or rhythm disturbance 2. Poorly controlled • Hypertension • Diabetes mellitus • Thyrotoxicosis *Note:* Because of the risk of fluid retention, use D5W and avoid salt-containing intravenous fluids. For women with diabetes mellitus, however, 0.25% saline (1/4 normal) should be used to reduce the risk of hyperglycemia.	Obtain baseline information before first dose: maternal weight, complete blood count, electrolytes, blood glucose, urinalysis *Dose:* 0.25 mg Dose may be repeated 2 or 3 times at 30-minute intervals. If contractions stop, give 0.25 mg as maintenance dose every 3-4 hours.	*Route:* Subcutaneous, by intermittent dosing only, and for a maximum of 72 hours. Should be given in-hospital only, and under close observation, because of potential complications including arrhythmia and death.	*Maternal* 1. Pulmonary edema risk is *reduced with* • Intake limited • Intravenous fluids without salt • Maternal heart rate kept <130 bpm *Risk increased with* • Multifetal gestation • Cardiac disease • Maternal infection 2. *Cardiac ischemia,* arrhythmias, and/or severe hypotension 3. *Hyperglycemia* (high blood glucose) 4. *Hypokalemia* (low serum potassium) 5. *Maternal death* *Fetal* 1. *Tachycardia* 2. *Increased fetal heart rate variability*	*Check* • *Intake/output:* limit fluid to 2,500 mL/day • *Signs of pulmonary edema,* check breath sounds, use pulse oximeter to check Spo₂ • *Vital signs* every hour • *Serum potassium* levels every 4 hours • *Blood glucose* – Every 4 hours in nondiabetic women, especially if infusion for 12 hours or longer – Frequently in women with diabetes mellitus or abnormal glucose tolerance • *Fetal heart rate and pattern*

*Magnesium sulfate is on the Institute for Safe Medication Practices high-alert medication list of drugs creating a heightened risk of causing significant patient harm when used in error. Special precautions and protocols for administration can decrease the risk for error. (See http://www.ismp.org.)

The benefits of corticosteroid administration vastly outweigh the potential risks, even when preterm, premature rupture of membranes has occurred. These benefits include a reduction in

- The risk and/or severity of respiratory distress syndrome (RDS)
- The incidence of intraventricular hemorrhage (IVH)
- Mortality

 Treatment with corticosteroids should be considered for all pregnant women with fetuses between 24 and 34 weeks' gestation whenever preterm delivery threatens.

2. *Timing of Corticosteroid Administration*

Optimal benefits begin 24 hours after corticosteroid therapy is started and last for 7 days. While the greatest benefits are achieved if delivery occurs more than 24 hours after treatment is started, treatment with corticosteroids for less than 24 hours is also associated with significant reduction in neonatal mortality, RDS, and IVH. Unless imminent delivery is anticipated, antenatal corticosteroids should be given. Even an abbreviated course is likely to be beneficial to neonatal outcome.

 When use of antenatal steroids is appropriate, limited time until delivery should not inhibit their administration. Corticosteroids should be given unless immediate delivery is expected.

3. *Special Circumstances*

Antenatal corticosteroid use is recommended for women with preterm premature rupture of membranes at less than 32 weeks' gestation (some experts use <34 weeks' gestation).

Unless there is evidence of adverse effects for individual women, corticosteroid therapy should be given to women with pregnancies complicated by either high-risk maternal or fetal conditions in the same way it is provided to women with less complicated pregnancies.

4. *Repeated Doses of Corticosteroids*

Routine use of repeated doses of corticosteroids is not recommended. Although there is some evidence that repeated doses may be beneficial for improving lung function in babies born preterm, concerns have been raised about possible adverse effects on maternal and neonatal health, including possible inhibition of neurologic and physical growth in preterm fetuses. Until more evidence becomes available, repeated doses should be used cautiously in individual cases, and only after weighing the relative risks to the woman and the fetus, the degree of immaturity of the fetus, and the perceived likelihood of early delivery.

5. *Medication and Dosage*

Betamethasone: 2 doses, each 12 mg, given intramuscularly, 24 hours apart

7. How Do You Manage a Preterm Delivery?

If labor cannot be stopped or is allowed to continue due to maternal and/or fetal condition, consider maternal/fetal transfer to a regional center for delivery. If transfer is not appropriate, or if time does not allow safe transport, prepare for delivery and care of a preterm baby.

259

A. Discontinue Tocolytics

If used, tocolytic medication should be discontinued. This will allow maximum metabolism of the drug before delivery, minimizing possible adverse neonatal side effects.

B. Consider Intrapartum Antibiotics

Antibiotic therapy is recommended for any of the following situations:

- Labor occurs at 37 weeks' gestation or earlier, when GBS status is unknown.
- A previous baby had GBS disease.
- There was a positive vaginal/rectal culture for GBS obtained.
- An episode of GBS bacteriuria occurred during the current pregnancy.
- Amniotic membranes have been ruptured for 18 hours or longer.
- Maternal fever during labor is 100.4°F (38.0°C) or higher.

Antibiotics used

- *Preferred antibiotic* is penicillin. Penicillin G dose is 5 million units initially, intravenously, then 2.5 million units intravenously every 4 hours until delivery.
- *Alternative antibiotic* is ampicillin, 2 g first dose, intravenously, then 1 g intravenously every 4 hours until delivery.
- For penicillin-allergic women, see the GBS section in Unit 3, Perinatal Infections, in this book.

Whichever antibiotic is used, IV administration is preferred. Higher intra-amniotic concentrations are achieved with IV administration than with intramuscular administration.

C. Reduce Maternal Narcotics

If used, narcotic medication should be reduced. This is also to allow metabolism of the medication and thereby reduce the risk of newborn depression.

D. Choose Route of Delivery

1. Vertex presentation: The preterm fetus in vertex presentation may be delivered vaginally in the absence of any obstetric contraindication to vaginal delivery (such as active genital herpes, prior classical cesarean delivery, placenta previa, etc). The delivering provider should make every effort to achieve an atraumatic vaginal delivery. However, obstetric interventions, such as planned cesarean, "prophylactic" forceps delivery, or routine episiotomy, have not been shown to improve neonatal outcomes for preterm vertex fetuses, and should be reserved for specific indications, such as abnormal fetal heart rate patterns. Vacuum-assisted delivery is contraindicated in fetuses less than 35 weeks' gestation.

2. Non-vertex presentation: Preterm fetuses at a viable gestational age (>23 to 24 weeks) that are in breech presentation typically have better outcomes when delivered by cesarean than by vaginal delivery. This is in part related to the rare but serious complication of head entrapment in an incompletely dilated cervix. At the very threshold of viability, all preterm fetuses have a high neonatal mortality rate as well as a high complication rate among survivors; it is difficult to ascertain whether cesarean reduces these risks in the very smallest and youngest (23 to 24 weeks) babies. No prospective studies are available and none will likely be done. In certain circumstances, the delivering provider may determine that a vaginal delivery is the best route for a particular non-vertex fetus. This may be due to extreme prematurity with anticipated poor survival, co-existing major fetal anomalies, serious maternal illness (increasing the risk of maternal complications of surgery), or simply very rapid labor. Any time a vaginal breech delivery is anticipated, an essential element is the presence of an obstetrician skilled in breech delivery.

260

E. Be Prepared for Neonatal Resuscitation

Be prepared to resuscitate.

Gentle handling is especially important for small preterm babies because tiny babies have particularly fragile skin, lungs, and cerebral blood vessels.

Consider the following (review material in Book I: Maternal and Fetal Evaluation and Immediate Newborn Care, and Book III: Neonatal Care)

- Provide resuscitation.
- Observe for signs of respiratory distress. Use continuous positive airway pressure or intubate early if respiratory distress develops.
- Postnatal surfactant administration acts with antenatal corticosteroids to reduce RDS and mortality in extremely preterm newborns.
- Small preterm babies can be chilled *very* quickly. Warm the delivery environment and use plastic covering or chemical warming mattresses to facilitate thermal support.
- Check blood pressure and hematocrit.
- Screen for hypoglycemia. Start IV fluids and/or feedings early.
- Consider cultures and antibiotics if the baby is sick or if maternal risk factors for infection are present.

Self-test

Now answer these questions to test yourself on the information in the last section.

C1. **True** **False** Treatment with corticosteroids should be considered for *all* pregnant women with fetuses between 24 and 34 weeks' gestation when there is a threat of preterm delivery.

C2. **True** **False** Preterm fetuses in breech presentation have a higher survival rate with cesarean delivery than with vaginal delivery.

C3. **True** **False** Early, aggressive intervention may allow preterm labor to be stopped and the pregnancy to continue for days or weeks.

C4. In which of the following situations might the use of corticosteroids be appropriate?

Yes	No	
____	____	Healthy woman in labor at 30 weeks' gestation with intact membranes and 4-cm cervical dilatation, 60% effacement, receiving tocolytic medication
____	____	Woman in labor, following premature rupture of membranes at 30 weeks' gestation, without evidence of infection or other pregnancy complications, receiving tocolytic medication
____	____	Woman in labor at 37 weeks' gestation, with ruptured membranes and foul-smelling amniotic fluid, being treated with intravenous antibiotics
____	____	Healthy woman in labor at 28 weeks' gestation, with ruptured membranes, 8-cm cervical dilatation and 100% effacement
____	____	Healthy woman in labor, with intact membranes at 33 weeks' gestation, being treated with intravenous magnesium sulfate

C5. When preterm delivery is unavoidable, which of the following measures are appropriate?

Yes	No	
____	____	Consider maternal/fetal transfer to a regional center for delivery.
____	____	Rush the woman immediately to a regional center for delivery.
____	____	Discontinue tocolytics as soon as the decision to allow labor to proceed is made.
____	____	Cesarean delivery for *all* fetuses with estimated weight less than 1,500 g.
____	____	Provide anesthesia for pelvic relaxation during delivery.
____	____	Notify pediatric staff.

C6. Indicate whether the side effects and signs of toxicity listed below are associated with magnesium sulfate, beta-mimetic medication, or both.

Side Effect	Magnesium Sulfate	Beta-mimetic Medications
Pulmonary edema	____	____
Rapid heart rate	____	____
Chest pain with cardiac ischemia	____	____
Hyperglycemia (high blood glucose)	____	____
Loss of deep tendon reflexes	____	____
Hypokalemia (low serum potassium)	____	____
Respiratory depression	____	____

Check your answers with the list that follows the Recommended Routines. Correct any incorrect answers and review the appropriate section in the unit.

Preterm Labor

Recommended Routines

All the routines listed below are based on the principles of perinatal care presented in the unit you have just finished. They are recommended as part of routine perinatal care.

Read each routine carefully and decide whether it is standard operating procedure in your hospital. Check the appropriate blank next to each routine.

Procedure Standard in My Hospital	Needs Discussion by Our Staff	
_____	_____	1. Develop a system that allows outpatient evaluation, in an obstetrical care area, of women with questionable preterm labor, until it is determined that discharge home or hospitalization for continued treatment of preterm labor (or delivery) is appropriate.
_____	_____	2. Establish a protocol for prompt evaluation of preterm labor and, if appropriate, prompt intervention to stop labor.
_____	_____	3. Develop a system for appropriate consultation and referral of women at risk for preterm delivery.
_____	_____	4. Establish a system to ensure that all pregnant women with fetuses between 24 and 34 weeks' gestation are evaluated for treatment with corticosteroids, if preterm delivery becomes a threat.
_____	_____	5. Establish a system to notify nursery personnel whenever a preterm delivery is expected.

Self-test Answers

These are the answers to the self-test questions. Please check them with the answers you gave and review the information in the unit wherever necessary.

A1. Before the *start* of the 38th week of gestation (before the *end* of the 37th week)

A2. Prematurity accounts for approximately 75% of neonatal deaths that are not due to congenital malformations.

A3. Approximately 10% of babies born in the United States are born preterm.

A4. False.   Preterm labor often occurs in women who have no recognized risk factors.

A5. True

A6. True

A7. Abdominal cramping, change in vaginal discharge or onset of watery or mucoid discharge, low backache (intermittent or constant), and/or pelvic pressure, sense of heaviness in the vagina

A8. Yes   No

Yes	No	
X	____	Chorioamnionitis
X	____	Severe anemia
X	____	Gonorrhea
X	____	Maternal age 18 years or younger
X	____	Cocaine use
X	____	Cervical insufficiency
X	____	Absence of prenatal care
X	____	Preterm premature rupture of membranes

A9. Any 3 of the following:
- Previous preterm delivery
- Multifetal gestation
- Preterm premature rupture of membranes
- Infection, especially with chlamydia, gonorrhea, syphilis, and/or bacterial vaginosis

B1. 12 to 14 weeks

B2. Any 3 of the following cervical changes:
- Effacement
- Dilatation
- Softening
- Anterior position
- "Ballooning" of the lower uterine segment

B3. False.   Tocolysis is contraindicated in some situations. (See Section 5C1.)

B4. True

B5. True

B6. False.   Even when cervical dilatation is 4 cm or more, tocolysis might delay birth long enough for the fetus to benefit from corticosteroids given to the mother. While maximum benefits are gained when steroids are started more than 24 hours before delivery, administration for less than 24 hours is also of value to a preterm fetus, especially one of 34 weeks' gestation or younger. Tocolysis is appropriate unless imminent delivery is expected.

B7. True

B8. True

B9. Preterm labor is defined as persistent contractions (despite hydration and sedation) with cervical dilatation of 2 cm or more or effacement of 80% or more before the start of the 38th week of gestation and/or cervical changes that occur during the observation period.

B10. Yes   No

  X   ____ Urinalysis.

  X   ____ Discuss treatment options, risks, and benefits with the family.

  X   ____ Consider maternal/fetal referral for delivery at a regional center.

  ____   X Internal monitoring of fetal heart rate and uterine activity. (Even if the membranes are ruptured, use only external monitoring, unless decision made to allow labor to proceed. If labor is allowed, avoid internal monitoring when there is evidence of infection.).

  X   ____ Physical examination.

  X   ____ Sterile speculum examination.

  X   ____ Vaginal/rectal cultures.

C1. True

C2. True

C3. True

C4. Yes   No

  X   ____ Healthy woman in labor at 34 weeks' gestation with intact membranes and 4-cm cervical dilatation, 60% effacement, receiving tocolytic medication

  X   ____ Woman in labor, following premature rupture of membranes at 30 weeks' gestation, without evidence of infection or other pregnancy complications, receiving tocolytic medication

  ____   X Woman in labor at 37 weeks' gestation, with ruptured membranes and foul-smelling amniotic fluid, being treated with intravenous antibiotics

  ____   X Healthy woman in labor at 28 weeks' gestation, with ruptured membranes, 8-cm cervical dilatation, and 100% effacement (In this case, delivery is imminent.)

  X   ____ Healthy woman in labor, with intact membranes at 33 weeks' gestation, being treated with intravenous magnesium sulfate

C5. Yes   No

  X   ____ Consider maternal/fetal transfer to a regional center for delivery.

  ____   X Rush the woman immediately to a regional center for delivery. (Transfer should not be made if there is a risk of delivery en route or if maternal or fetal condition is unstable. Treatment, as appropriate, should be provided before and during transport. Prompt, efficient transport may be indicated but speed should never replace attention to patient stability and therapy. If transfer is appropriate, transport *early*.)

  X   ____ Discontinue tocolytics as soon as the decision to allow labor to proceed is made. (If it is appropriate to transfer the woman to a regional center for delivery, tocolysis would be continued during the transport process.)

  ____   X Cesarean delivery for *all* fetuses with estimated weight less than 1,500 g. (Cesarean delivery benefits small fetuses in breech presentation [except for the tiniest babies], but holds no advantage over vaginal delivery for small fetuses in vertex presentation.)

  X   ____ Provide anesthesia for pelvic relaxation during delivery.

  X   ____ Notify pediatric staff.

C6.

Possible Side Effect	Magnesium Sulfate	Beta-mimetic Medications
Pulmonary edema	X	X
Rapid heart rate		X
Chest pain with cardiac ischemia		X
Hyperglycemia (high blood glucose)		X
Loss of deep tendon reflexes	X	
Hypokalemia (low serum potassium)		X
Respiratory depression	X	

Unit 7 Posttest

If you are applying for continuing education credits, a posttest for this unit is available online. Completion of unit posttests and the book evaluation form are required to achieve continuing education credit. For more details, visit www.cmevillage.com.

Unit 8: Inducing and Augmenting Labor

Objectives

In this unit you will learn

A. When induction of labor is used, and when it should not be used

B. How to judge if an induction of labor is likely to be successful or not

C. When and how to use cervical ripening to facilitate induction of labor

D. When augmentation of labor is used, and when it should not be used

E. How oxytocin should be administered

F. How to determine when a normal contraction pattern has been achieved

G. What complications can occur with oxytocin administration

H. How to recognize and respond to complications of oxytocin administration

I. How long oxytocin should be given, and when it should be stopped

Unit 8 Pretest

Before reading the unit, please answer the following questions. Select the *one best* answer to each question (unless otherwise instructed). Record your answers on the test and check them against the answers at the end of the book.

1. **True   False**   According to the Bishop Scoring System (use the table below), labor induction is *un*likely to be successful in a woman whose cervix is of medium consistency, 20% effaced, midline position, and 2 cm dilated, with the fetus in vertex presentation at -3 station.

Bishop Scoring System

	0	1	2	3
Dilatation of cervix	Closed	1-2 cm	3-4 cm	5 cm
Effacement of cervix	0%-30%	40%-50%	60%-70%	80%
Station of presenting part	−3	−2	−1,0	+1, +2
Consistency of cervix	Firm	Medium	Soft	
Position of cervix	Posterior	Midline	Anterior	

2. **True   False**   Oxytocin dosage should be expressed in milliunits (mU) per minute delivered intravenously.

3. **True   False**   Although induction of labor is done to produce the artificial onset of labor, the contraction pattern achieved should resemble one that occurs with the spontaneous onset of labor.

4. **True   False**   For most patients, isotonic solutions are preferable to hypertonic solutions, when oxytocin is administered intravenously.

5. **True   False**   Six or more contractions within 10 minutes represents normal labor.

6. Induction of labor is usually appropriate in all of the following situations, *except* when
   A. A woman has severe preeclampsia.
   B. Herpes lesions are on the vulva.
   C. There is premature rupture of membranes at 36 weeks and the pregnant woman is afebrile.
   D. A fetus is post-term.

7. Possible complications of oxytocin infusion include all of the following, *except:*
   A. Uterine rupture
   B. Fetal heart rate abnormalities
   C. Tachysystole
   D. Chorioamnionitis

8. Which of the following should be ruled *out* before oxytocin is given for induction of labor?
   A. Post-term gestation
   B. Abnormal fetal presentation
   C. Premature rupture of membranes
   D. Maternal preeclampsia

9. Which of the following should you do *first* when uterine tachysystole occurs?
   A. Give a tocolytic drug to the woman to relax the uterus.
   B. Turn the woman on her left side and give oxygen by mask.
   C. Stop the oxytocin infusion.
   D. Perform a cesarean delivery.

10. When oxytocin is given for *induction* of labor, the rate of infusion should be gradually but steadily increased until
   A. Delivery occurs.
   B. Baseline uterine tone increases to 20 mm Hg or higher.
   C. Regular contractions, lasting 90 seconds or longer, become established.
   D. A contraction pattern that resembles normal labor is established.

11. Which of the following is a risk associated with prostaglandin cervical ripening medications?
   A. Neonatal sepsis
   B. Cervical bleeding
   C. Uterine tachysystole
   D. Maternal tachycardia

12. True   False   Maternal hyponatremia may be accompanied by mental confusion and seizures.

13. True   False   It is reasonable to give oxytocin augmentation of labor for 18 to 20 hours if it is needed to achieve a normal contraction pattern.

14. True   False   Labor induction with oxytocin infusion should proceed simultaneously with local application of a prostaglandin preparation to ripen the cervix.

1. What Is Induction and What Is Augmentation of Labor?

Induction of labor is the artificial initiation of labor before the spontaneous onset of labor. Induction may be accomplished by intravenous (IV) administration of oxytocin, administration of vaginal or oral prostaglandin, artificial rupture of membranes, membrane stripping, and nipple stimulation.

Labor is generally induced when

- The health of a woman and/or her fetus is in jeopardy and the situation can be expected to improve if the fetus is delivered.

AND

- Vaginal delivery is preferable to cesarean delivery.

Augmentation of labor is the further stimulation of labor that has already begun spontaneously. An indication for labor augmentation does not exist until it is clear that the natural labor process is not progressing normally, and that the risks of oxytocin are less than those for cesarean section.

2. When Is Induction of Labor Used?

Labor may be induced for a wide variety of reasons. None of them are absolute. Many factors must be taken into consideration when deciding either to induce labor, to undertake a cesarean delivery, or *not* to intervene in a high-risk pregnancy.

Induction of labor carries a higher rate of cesarean delivery than does spontaneous onset of labor, especially in nulliparous women with an unripe cervix. Nevertheless, inducing labor in the following situations is usually less risky than continuing a pregnancy:

- Abruptio placentae (Grade I with no fetal compromise or Grade III with fetal death, stable woman).
- Premature rupture of membranes, when delivery is indicated. (See Unit 6, Premature Rupture and/or Infection of the Amniotic Membranes, in this book.)
- Chorioamnionitis, regardless of gestational age.
- Complicated gestational hypertension and/or preeclampsia. (See Unit 1, Hypertension in Pregnancy, in this book.)
- Maternal medical illness with evidence of declining maternal and/or fetal health (unless fetal or maternal condition is such that cesarean delivery is deemed safer than labor and vaginal delivery).
- Fetal jeopardy as demonstrated by tests of fetal growth and/or well-being.
- Fetus approaching post-term gestation. (When dates are *certain,* consider induction in the 41st week of gestation.)
- Fetal death.
- Women at 39 or more weeks' gestation with a history of rapid labor(s) and geographic difficulties in reaching a hospital.
- Other. (Numerous uncommon indications for labor induction also exist. Consult with maternal-fetal medicine specialists regarding individual circumstances.)
- Labor may be induced electively if the pregnancy is well-dated with a gestational age greater than 39 weeks, and maternal consent. A favorable cervix is preferred, and the woman should understand the increased risk of cesarean delivery.

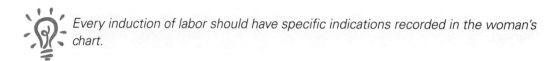 *Every induction of labor should have specific indications recorded in the woman's chart.*

3. When Should Induction of Labor *Not* Be Used?

The following conditions are *contraindications* to the induction of labor. Some exceptions may be reasonable, however, such as prolapsed umbilical cord with a dead fetus.

- Category III fetal heart rate pattern.
- Placenta previa.
- Vasa previa (uncommon, difficult to diagnose condition in which the umbilical vessels cover the cervical os). Occasionally, it may be possible to palpate the vessels or see them during a sterile speculum examination or with ultrasound. If found, cesarean delivery is indicated.
- Umbilical cord that is prolapsed or in front of the fetal presenting part. (The latter situation is described as funic presentation.)
- Active genital herpes lesions.
- Prior classical (vertical) cesarean incision.
- Fetopelvic disproportion, if known to be present prior to labor.
- Contracted maternal pelvis or bony abnormalities that encroach on the birth canal.
- Invasive cervical carcinoma.
- Abnormal fetal presentations (face, brow, compound, transverse lie, breech).

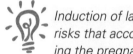 *Induction of labor is potentially hazardous. It should be undertaken only when the risks that accompany induction are lower than the risks associated with continuing the pregnancy or those associated with cesarean delivery.*

4. What Should Be Done Before Induction of Labor Is Undertaken?

Obtain informed consent. Explain to the woman and her family the reasons for an induction, how it will be done, and the accompanying risks. Discuss the possible need for repeat induction attempts and/or cesarean delivery. Nulliparous women with an unripe cervix who are being induced without a medical indication should be counseled about a 2-fold increased risk of cesarean delivery.

Assess fetal maturity, unless maternal and/or fetal condition mandates delivery, regardless of fetal maturity. A gestational age of 39 completed weeks should be established before an induction without a medical indication is undertaken. Fetal maturity criteria that should be fulfilled are given in Book I: Maternal and Fetal Evaluation and Immediate Newborn Care, Unit 2, Fetal Age, Growth, and Maturity.

Assess cervix, pelvis, fetal size, and presentation. Before an induction begins, the woman and fetus should be assessed to rule out the presence of contraindications to induction.

Prepare equipment and personnel to provide continuous electronic monitoring and possible surgical intervention. This is recommended due to the increased risk for uterine tachysystole when oxytocin is given. Oxytocin should be administered and monitored by nursing personnel knowledgeable and skilled in oxytocin administration. A physician capable of performing a cesarean delivery and corresponding personnel and support services should be readily available.

5. How Can You Tell if an Induction of Labor Is Likely to Succeed?

A. Examine the Woman

Natural preparation for the onset of labor is a gradual process, controlled by a multitude of poorly understood interactions of biochemical, biophysical, and hormonal systems. Softening and thinning (effacement) of the cervix occurs—a process termed ripening. The lower uterine segment thins as it is drawn toward the increasingly active myometrium of the fundus. This pulls the cervix from its normal position pointing posteriorly to an anterior position. In the anterior position the cervix can more readily be entered by an examining finger and seen during a speculum examination.

The closer to labor the patient is when examined, the more the
- Cervix will be pulled anteriorly.
- Cervix will be effaced and softened.
- Internal cervical os will be dilated.
- Uterine contractions will be felt by the patient and by the examiner.
- Uterine muscle (myometrium) will be more sensitive to oxytocin given intravenously.

B. Calculate a Bishop Score (Table 8.1)

The Bishop score indicates the likelihood an induction attempt will be successful. In general, a score of more than 8 suggests induction of labor will be successful, whereas a score of ≤6 is considered unfavorable.

Response to oxytocin is influenced by the degree of cervical dilatation, gestational age of the fetus, number of previous deliveries, and individual uterine sensitivity. *Uterine response to oxytocin is unpredictable and varies widely among women.*

The Bishop score should be used only as a guide to indicate which women are more likely to respond to oxytocin induction, and when administration of prostaglandins for cervical ripening is more likely to be helpful.

Example: Findings of a cervix 1 cm dilated (1), 50% effaced (1), medium consistency (1), posterior position (0), and fetal station of −3 (0) would receive a total score of 3.

6. What Do You Do if the Bishop Score Is Low?

A. Consider Cervical Ripening

In women who have an indication for delivery and no contraindications to induction, a low Bishop score (6 or less) indicates that cervical ripening should be considered.

Table 8.1. Bishop Scoring System					
	0	1	2	3	Score
Dilatation of cervix	Closed	1-2 cm	3-4 cm	5 cm	_____
Effacement of cervix	0%-30%	40%-50%	60%-70%	80%	_____
Station of presenting part*	−3	−2	−1, 0	+1, +2	_____
Consistency of cervix	Firm	Medium	Soft		_____
Position of cervix	Posterior	Midline	Anterior		
				Total score =	_____

*Using a −3 to +3 scale (not −5 to +5 scale).

Used with permission from Bishop EH. Pelvic scoring for elective inductions. *Obstet Gynecol.* 1964;24(2):266-268.

Preparation of the cervix with medication or mechanical dilatation increases the likelihood of successful induction of labor. These techniques and/or medications should be used only when induction of labor is indicated.

All cervical ripening techniques produce uterine contractions. Uterine contractions produced by a cervical ripening agent may, in some cases, go on to produce labor. In addition, prostaglandin preparations may make the uterus more sensitive to oxytocin.

There are several common methods used to promote cervical ripening.

1. *Stripping of the Membranes:* Manual separation of the membranes from the decidua (endometrium during pregnancy)

2. *Mechanical Techniques:* Dilatation of the cervix accomplished by inserting an osmotic dilator into the cervical canal, which swells as a result of absorbing fluid, or by inserting a 30 mL Foley catheter or a cervical ripening balloon through the cervical canal, inflating the balloon and leaving it inflated within the lower uterine segment

3. *Medication:* Topical application of one of several prostaglandin preparations

B. Contraindications and Risks of Cervical Ripening Techniques

 All techniques for cervical ripening carry risks. Their risks and indications should be explained to the woman and recorded in her chart.

1. *Stripping of the Membranes*
   Contraindications
   - Cervical infection
   - Active genital herpes
   - Recent unexplained vaginal bleeding
   - Placenta previa
   Risks
   - Infection
   - Premature rupture of membranes due to accidental amniotomy
   - Bleeding from an unidentified placenta previa

2. *Mechanical Techniques*
   Contraindications
   - Cervical infection
   - Ruptured membranes
   - Active genital herpes
   - Recent unexplained vaginal bleeding
   Risks
   - Infection
   - Premature rupture of membranes
   - Bleeding from an unidentified placenta previa

3. *Prostaglandins*
   Contraindications
   - Previous cesarean section or uterine surgery (increased risk of uterine rupture)
   - Presence of excessive uterine activity
   - Known hypersensitivity to prostaglandins
   - Recent unexplained vaginal bleeding

Relative contraindications
- Ruptured membranes
- Unexplained vaginal bleeding during this pregnancy
- Patients with a history of difficult labor and/or traumatic delivery
- Grand multiparity
- Multifetal gestation or suspected fetal macrosomia

Risks
- The onset of excessive force or frequency of uterine contractions is the primary risk of prostaglandin ripening agents.

Excessive uterine stimulation may involve
- *Tachysystole:* More than 5 contractions in 10 minutes
- *Tetany:* Contractions lasting longer than 2 minutes
- *Hypertonus:* Increase of 20 mm Hg or more above uterine resting tone

Tachysystole (or any type of excessive uterine activity) may reduce blood flow to the intervillous space within the placenta. At times, this may lead to fetal heart rate changes. Although rare, excessive uterine stimulation also may result in uterine rupture.

 Excessive contractions can occur with use of any prostaglandin preparation to ripen the cervix or oxytocin to induce or augment labor.

C. Cervical Ripening Techniques

1. *Stripping of the Membranes*

   Membranes are "stripped" by insertion of a gloved finger through the internal os and then sweeping the finger, in a circular motion, along the lower uterine segment. This separates the membranes from their attachment to the decidua, which, in turn, causes release of prostaglandins.

   Release of prostaglandins has a direct influence on cervical ripening, and causes the uterus to contract. Uterine contractions also promote the cervical changes that are associated with cervical ripening.

2. *Mechanical Technique*
   - Osmotic dilators used for mechanical dilatation of the cervix include natural seaweed *(Laminaria japonicum)* tents and several types of synthetic osmotic dilators. One to 4 dilators are inserted into the cervix during a sterile speculum examination. Generally, osmotic tents are inserted on an outpatient basis.
   - Insertion of a Foley catheter into the cervical canal, followed by inflation of the 30-mL balloon of the catheter, also has been used safely as a mechanical dilator. There are cervical dilation balloons currently available that are specifically designed for this use. This is usually done as an inpatient procedure.

     Both mechanical and biochemical methods of cervical ripening have been shown to be effective in ripening the cervix.

3. *Prostaglandins*

   Prostaglandin is abbreviated PG, with the specific form indicated by the letters and numbers that follow. Two are used for cervical ripening: PGE_2 and PGE_1.

   a. *Cervidil:* Each vaginal insert contains 10 mg of dinoprostone (PGE_2) in a sustained-release preparation (slower rate of release than Prepidil).
      - Store the inserts in a refrigerator. Warming before use is not necessary.
      - Avoid use of a lubricant during the insertion. If the insert becomes coated, release of dinoprostone may be hindered.

- Place the insert manually into the vagina, with the end containing the drug capsule placed across the posterior fornix and the woven tail left outside the vagina, for easy removal later.
- Leave the insert in place until the onset of labor or for 12 hours, whichever comes first. If ripening does not occur with the first insert, use of a second insert is *not* recommended.

b. *Prepidil:* This gel comes in prefilled syringes, which contain 0.5 mg of dinoprostone (PGE$_2$).

- Store the syringes in a refrigerator. Allow the gel to reach room temperature before use, but do *not* use an external heat source, such as a water bath or microwave, to warm the gel.
- Prepidil doses may be repeated 2 or 3 times, at 6- to 12-hour intervals, but should not exceed 1.5 mg of dinoprostone in 24 hours.
- Use a speculum for visualization while the gel is inserted into the cervical canal, using a shielded catheter supplied by the manufacturer. A disk (shield) surrounds the catheter, which blocks the opening of the cervix to minimize backflow of gel into the vagina. Size of shield used depends on the degree of cervical effacement. (See manufacturer's directions.)
- Select the length of catheter according to the length of the cervix. The tip of the catheter should protrude only a short distance beyond the shield into the cervical canal because the gel should be inserted *below* the internal os and away from the membranes (use with ruptured membranes is not recommended). If the cervix is long, use the catheter with the tip 2 cm beyond the shield; if the cervix is short, use the catheter with the 1-cm tip.

c. *Cytotec:* Each tablet contains 100 micrograms (µg) of misoprostol (an analog of PGE$_1$). This drug inhibits gastric acid secretion and is licensed for that purpose. It is not approved by the US Food and Drug Administration for use during pregnancy, but off-label use for cervical ripening and labor induction has been recognized by the American College of Obstetricians and Gynecologists as "safe and effective when used appropriately."[*]

- Each 100-µg tablet of Cytotec needs to be divided into 25 µg quarters. *Scoring and division of each tablet needs to be done with meticulous care and accuracy by skilled personnel.*
- Dosage is a 25-µg segment placed in the vagina every 4 to 6 hours or a 50-µg segment every 6 hours, for a maximum of 4 doses (total dosage is 100 to 200 µg over 16 to 24 hours). Dosing misoprostol every 6 hours may have a lower rate of uterine tachysystole. The 50-µg dose may be associated with a higher rate of fetal heart rate decelerations and uterine tachysystole.
- Misoprostol has been shown to be as effective as dinoprostone in producing cervical ripening. In addition, misoprostol more often goes on to produce labor, without the need for oxytocin infusion. Misoprostol carries a higher risk for adverse maternal and fetal responses with doses higher than 25 µg or given more frequently than every 3 to 6 hours.
- Misoprostol should *not* be used in women with a prior cesarean section or major uterine surgery. The safety of misoprostol use in women with multifetal gestation or fetal macrosomia is unknown.

---

[*]American College of Obstetricians and Gynecologists. Practice Bulletin. Number 107. August 2009.

D. Monitoring Prostaglandin Medications

Hospitalization is recommended for women undergoing cervical ripening attempt(s) with any of the prostaglandin medications. After placement of the ripening agent, a woman should rest on her side (sometimes the Trendelenburg position is used with dinoprostone gel) for 30 minutes after application. During this time, monitor her vital signs frequently.

The risk of excessive uterine contractions is greatest when the initial Bishop score was 5 or higher. If they develop, the onset of contractions that are too frequent or too strong most often occurs in the first 4 hours after application of a prostaglandin medication, but may not be seen for as long as 9 or 10 hours after application.

When using **Cervidil**, uterine activity and fetal heart rate should be monitored continuously for at least
- 30 minutes before application
- Throughout the period of cervical ripening
- 30 minutes following removal of the vaginal insert

When using **Prepidil** or **Cytotec**, uterine activity and fetal heart rate should be monitored continuously for at least
- 2 hours following the last dose of a cervical ripening agent and should be continued if regular uterine contractions persist

1. *If Excessive Contractions Develop,*
   a. *Remove vaginal insert, if Cervidil is being used*: Doing this may help to calm excessive contractions.
      Note: Only Cervidil can be removed. Cytotec dissolves and cannot be removed. Prepidil gel also cannot be removed, even by irrigation of the vagina. Vaginal irrigation has no value in treating excessive uterine activity.
   b. *Use in utero resuscitative measures*: Respond to excessive uterine activity and/or a change in the fetal heart rate pattern by providing such measures as turning the woman on her side and giving oxygen by mask. In most cases, a worrisome fetal heart rate pattern will resolve quickly as uterine tachysystole subsides. If it does not, manage as you would for any other episode of suspected fetal compromise.
   c. *Consider giving a tocolytic medication*: If the abnormal pattern does not quickly subside, consider giving
      - Terbutaline, 0.25 mg, subcutaneously

2. *If Labor Does Not Begin*

   Dinoprostone and misoprostol may initiate labor, as well as produce cervical ripening. Oxytocin may not be needed. If labor does not begin, allow a rest period before beginning induction of labor.

   The rest period should be *at least*
   - 30 to 60 minutes after removing a Cervidil vaginal insert
   - 6 to 12 hours after the last dose of Prepidil
   - 4 to 6 hours after the last dose of Cytotec

   In addition to increasing the likelihood of successful induction of labor, cervical ripening with prostaglandins has been associated with a reduction in the incidence of prolonged labor and in the amount of oxytocin needed.

   If labor has not begun by the end of the rest period, oxytocin infusion may then be started. Start with a low dose. The effects of prostaglandin on the myometrium generally increase uterine sensitivity to oxytocin.

Do not administer oxytocin too soon after use of any prostaglandin preparation. If labor has not started, wait the FULL rest period before beginning induction of labor with oxytocin.

7. What Do You Do if the Bishop Score Is Mid-Range?

If the Bishop score is 6 to 8, the need for delivery is high, and there are no contraindications to labor induction, consider cervical ripening before attempting to induce labor. Cervical ripening will increase the likelihood of successful induction and/or decrease the need for oxytocin.

If the cervix becomes ripe, proceed to oxytocin induction and/or amniotomy (described below) to induce labor.

If the cervix does not become ripe, oxytocin induction may still be successful. It should be considered before moving to cesarean delivery.

8. What Do You Do if the Bishop Score Is High?

If the Bishop score is 8 or higher, particularly if the woman is a multipara, labor induction by artificial rupture of membranes (amniotomy) may be successful, without requiring oxytocin infusion.

  A. Amniotomy Technique

   A sterile plastic hook, specifically designed for this purpose, is inserted through the cervix and used to rupture the membranes. Continuous fetal heart rate monitoring should be used before, during, and immediately following the procedure.

   Be sure the fetal head is well-applied to the cervix and the umbilical cord cannot be palpated. The head should not be moved during the procedure.

    Once the membranes have ruptured, delivery must occur. Unless you are willing to perform a cesarean delivery if an attempt at induction of labor fails, do NOT rupture the membranes.

   Note: When there is an urgent need for induction, amniotomy may be done together with oxytocin infusion, even if the Bishop score is low and cervical dilatation is minimal, in an effort to speed the onset of labor and reduce the time to delivery. This situation, however, increases the risk for abnormal fetal heart rate changes and intramniotic infection.

  B. Amniotomy Contraindications and Risks
   Contraindications
   • Nonvertex presentation
   • Head not well-applied to the cervix
   • Umbilical cord is presenting part (funis presentation)
   • Vasa previa
   • Group B streptococci colonization (relative contraindication)
   • Active genital herpes
   • Maternal human immunodeficiency virus infection (relative contraindication)
   • Unwillingness to discontinue induction or perform cesarean delivery if induction attempt fails

Risks

- Prolapsed or compressed umbilical cord
- Infection
- Umbilical cord compression
- Bleeding from an unidentified placenta previa or vasa previa

---

Self-test

Now answer these questions to test yourself on the information in the last section.

A1. All of the following are contraindications or relative contraindications to labor *induction, except:*
   A. Placenta previa
   B. Previous cesarean delivery with a classical incision
   C. Active herpes infection
   D. Post-term pregnancy

A2. Why is a Bishop score calculated?

A3. A Bishop score of 7 indicates

A4. What may be done to improve the likelihood of successful labor induction in a woman with a low Bishop score?

A5. Using Table 8.1, calculate a Bishop score for a woman whose cervix is
   A. Closed, soft, posterior position, and 50% effaced, with the fetus at -2 station

   B. 3-cm dilated, soft, anterior position, and 70% effaced, with the fetus at 0 station

A6. Give at least 2 situations when labor induction may be appropriate.

A7. Give at least 2 contraindications to stripping of the membranes.

A8. The main risk associated with cervical ripening is

A9. **True** **False** There is no limit on the number of attempts that may be made to ripen a cervix in preparation for oxytocin induction of labor.

A10. **True** **False** Oxytocin induction of labor may be started as soon as treatment with a prostaglandin cervical ripening agent has been inserted.

Check your answers with the list that follows the Recommended Routines. Correct any incorrect answers and review the appropriate section in the unit.

9. When Should Augmentation of Labor Be Considered?

Labor augmentation with oxytocin may be indicated in the following situations:

- Hypotonic uterine dysfunction
- Secondary arrest of labor

See Unit 9, Abnormal Labor and Difficult Deliveries, in this book, for further information about these conditions.

Note: In women requiring augmentation of labor, artificial rupture of membranes has *not* been shown to expedite the progression of labor.

10. When May Augmentation of Labor *Not* Be Appropriate?

A. When Normal Contraction Pattern Is Present

Uterine contractions with the following characteristics are considered normal:
- *Frequency:* 2 to 3 minutes apart (3 to 5 contractions within 10 minutes)
- *Duration:* 45 to 70 seconds each
- *Strength* (*intensity*)
  - "Strong" by palpation (difficult to indent uterine wall with your fingers at the height of a contraction)

OR

  - Peak pressure of 50 mm Hg or more (measured with an internal pressure monitor)

If labor progress has failed despite normal contractions, other reasons for lack of progress should be investigated.

 Normal contractions cannot be improved with oxytocin.

B. When Fetopelvic Disproportion Is Present

This occurs when the size or position of the fetus and the size or shape of a woman's pelvis does not allow passage of the fetus. This may be due to
- Contracted maternal pelvis
- Abnormal fetal presentation or abnormal position of the fetal head
- Fetal malformation or abnormal condition (hydrocephalus, hydrops fetalis, etc)
- Fetal macrosomia (large fetus, estimated weight more than 4,000 g [8 lb, 13 oz])

 Oxytocin should not be given when fetal malposition, malpresentation, or fetopelvic disproportion are known to be present.

C. When Contraindications or Cautions Exist for Oxytocin

Use of oxytocin to stimulate labor that began spontaneously is *contraindicated* with
- Prior classical (vertical) cesarean incision
- Transverse lie

Oxytocin should be *used with caution* in the following situations:
- Abnormal uterine distention (multifetal gestation, hydramnios)
- Presenting part above the pelvic inlet (more likely to be present with contracted pelvis and/or abnormal fetal presentation)
- Abnormal fetal presentations (face, brow, compound, breech)
- Grand multiparity (5 or more previous deliveries)
- Previous cesarean section or other uterine surgery

280

D. When Hypertonic Uterine Inertia Is Present

Oxytocin is not useful in the management of this uncommon disorder. See Unit 9, Abnormal Labor and Difficult Deliveries, in this book, for additional information.

E. When There Is Fetal Intolerance to Uterine Contractions

Although quick delivery is indicated when a Category II or Category III fetal heart rate pattern does not respond to the usual interventions (turning patient, increasing IV fluids, giving oxygen), stimulating even sluggish contractions with oxytocin is likely to make fetal condition worse. Strong, frequent contractions may not allow sufficient relaxation time between contractions for adequate placental perfusion. If placental blood flow is restricted, fetal oxygenation will be diminished, thus increasing the risk of fetal compromise.

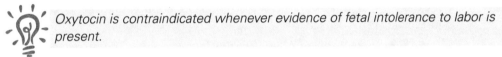
Oxytocin is contraindicated whenever evidence of fetal intolerance to labor is present.

11. How Should You Administer Oxytocin?

A. Prepare for Use of Oxytocin

While oxytocin is used frequently, and can be safely administered even in high-risk situations, risks do accompany the use of this drug. Those risks may be associated with the underlying maternal or fetal condition that indicates the need for oxytocin and/or with complications directly associated with the medication. Regardless of how low-risk a situation seems, adequate preparations should be taken *every* time oxytocin is given.

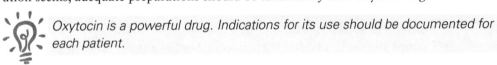
Oxytocin is a powerful drug. Indications for its use should be documented for each patient.

B. Use a Standard Protocol for Dosage and Rate Advancement

There are many acceptable protocols for the use of oxytocin. Use of *one* standard protocol, however, will help avoid confusion and errors that may accompany oxytocin administration. Whichever protocol your hospital uses, it is recommended that it be the same for all patients.

Use only IV administration of oxytocin for labor induction or augmentation. Buccal, nasal, or intramuscular administration of oxytocin should not be used to induce or to augment labor. Rate of uptake of the drug with these administration routes cannot be controlled or modified, and hyperstimulation is more common.

Things you should keep in mind when using oxytocin include

1. *Individualize Dosage*

Wide variation in response among patients to a given dose can be expected. Individualize dosage when oxytocin is first started, and throughout the infusion based on maternal and fetal response.

2. *Recognize Risk of Uterine Tachysystole*

Excessive uterine stimulation can have adverse consequences for a woman and her fetus. The risk of excessive stimulation is influenced by

- Dose of oxytocin (milliunit [mU] per minute rate of infusion)
- Frequency the infusion rate is increased
- Sensitivity of the myometrium

The faster the rate of infusion, and the more frequently the rate is increased, the higher the risk of overstimulating the uterus.

3. *Use Isotonic Solutions:* D5NS, D5LR, D51/2NS

   Oxytocin has antidiuretic effects, which promote fluid retention. For most women receiving oxytocin, use saline solutions for oxytocin dilution and for routine maintenance IV fluids.

4. *Use a Standard Dilution*

   Medication errors can be minimized by having only one concentration of oxytocin solution available on the labor and delivery unit. A pharmacy-prepared or manufacturer-prepared solution of 30 units of oxytocin in 500 mL of lactated Ringer's solution or normal saline results in a concentration where a pump setting of 1 mL/hour delivers an infusion rate of 1 mU/minute, and this 1:1 ratio is preserved with infusion rate increases. For example, with this oxytocin concentration, a 2-mL/hour infusion rate results in 2 mU/minute being delivered.

5. *Select Appropriate Route of Administration*
   - When used during the intrapartum period, oxytocin should be given intravenously and diluted before administration.
   - Intravenous administration of undiluted oxytocin can cause maternal hypotension and cardiac arrhythmia.
   - Intramuscular injection of undiluted oxytocin should be used *only* during the postpartum period, either before or after the placenta has been delivered based on a standard approach.

6. *Control Rate of IV Infusion*
   - Oxytocin should be provided in pre-mixed preparations, and then the IV tubing should be flushed with the mixture.
   - Connect the oxytocin solution with a side port, at a point near the patient, of the main IV infusion line.
   - Use an IV pump to control the rate of infusion.

7. *Control Rate of Dosage Increase*

   The initial effect of a given dose (mU per minute) of oxytocin may occur within a few minutes. The maximum effect of a specific dose, however, may not be fully developed for 30 to 45 minutes.

   Likewise, the initial effect of stopping an oxytocin infusion may be observed within a few minutes. Some effects, however, may last for 30 to 45 minutes after an oxytocin infusion is stopped or the rate is reduced.

   An initial infusion rate of 1 mU/minute (1 mL/hour) for both induction and augmentation of labor is recommended. This dose should be increased by 1 to 2 mU/minute every 30 to 60 minutes until a regular contraction pattern (contractions every 2 to 3 minutes) is achieved and sustained.

8. *Recognize Limits of Effectiveness*

   If a patient has not established a satisfactory labor pattern after sufficient oxytocin administration, the plan of care should be reevaluated with the patient.

Self-test

Now answer these questions to test yourself on the information in the last section.

B1. Which type of intravenous fluids should be given when oxytocin is administered?

_____

B2. **True** **False** In an emergency, an initial dose of oxytocin may be given by intravenous push, followed by a continuous infusion of dilute oxytocin.

B3. **True** **False** The more frequently the rate of oxytocin is increased, the more likely uterine tachysystole will occur.

B4. Thirty units oxytocin in 500 mL of normal saline was prepared by your hospital pharmacy. What initial intravenous pump setting should be set to deliver 1 milliiunit (mU)/minute?

_____

How should the rate be changed to deliver 1.5 mU/minute?

_____

B5. Normal labor has contractions with the following characteristics:
Frequency: _____
Duration: _____
Strength: _____

B6. Name at least 3 situations in which labor augmentation is _not_ appropriate.

_____
_____
_____

B7. List at least 3 things you should keep in mind when giving oxytocin.

_____
_____
_____

B8. Given a normal maternal pelvis and term gestation, all of the following are either contraindications or relative contraindications to labor _augmentation, except:_
   A. Hypotonic uterine dysfunction
   B. Face presentation
   C. Hydramnios
   D. Twins

B9. **True** **False** Fetal compromise is diagnosed when a laboring multiparous woman is at 8-cm cervical dilatation and the fetus is at 0 station. To speed delivery, you should start an oxytocin infusion at 2 mU/minute.

B10. **True** **False** Membranes should be ruptured so internal uterine pressure monitoring can be used whenever oxytocin is infused.

Check your answers with the list that follows the Recommended Routines. Correct any incorrect answers and review the appropriate section in the unit.

283

12. What Complications May Occur With Oxytocin Infusion?

A. Excessive Uterine Stimulation

1. *Cause*

Uterine tachysystole may develop because of prostaglandin medications used for cervical ripening or infusion of oxytocin for labor induction or augmentation.

During oxytocin infusion, excessive uterine stimulation may occur because

- A larger dose is given than is needed because either the dose is too high or the dose is increased too frequently. Most adverse responses to oxytocin infusion are dose related.

OR

- The myometrium becomes more sensitive to a previously satisfactory dosage of oxytocin.

Sometimes after a normal labor pattern has been achieved and a stable infusion of oxytocin has been used for an hour or more, tachysystole may develop unexpectedly. The myometrium becomes more receptive to oxytocin because more receptors, and corresponding muscle fibers, respond simultaneously to oxytocin. As a result, the same dosage of oxytocin may cause an increase in the number and/or strength of contractions. Many women will maintain active labor without the aid of oxytocin once active labor has been established.

2. *Risks*

a. *Maternal risks*

- Lacerations of the cervix, vagina, and/or perineum (results from rapid propulsion of the fetus through the birth canal)
- Uterine rupture (results from excessive strength of contractions; rare, particularly in the absence of a uterine scar)

b. *Fetal and neonatal risks:* Result from the forces that accompany rapid transit through the birth canal and/or reduced placental perfusion

- Restricted placental blood flow
- Fetal hypoxia
- Birth trauma
- Bruising
- Intracranial bleeding (rare, more likely in preterm babies)
- Need for resuscitation at birth

3. *Treatment*

If uterine tachysystole develops, labor may progress so rapidly that delivery will occur before the situation can be corrected. If recognized early, however, promptly stopping or reducing the oxytocin infusion may help. Immediate management depends on the fetal heart rate pattern.

a. Normal fetal heart rate pattern: *Reduce* the rate of the oxytocin infusion, usually by half.

b. Abnormal fetal heart rate pattern.

- STOP the oxytocin infusion.
- Consider administration of a tocolytic agent if excessive uterine activity and fetal heart rate pattern do not quickly resolve after other interventions.
  – Terbutaline (0.25 mg, subcutaneously)
- Provide other measures of in utero resuscitation: Turn woman onto her side or from one side to the other, give oxygen by mask, provide IV fluid bolus.

If contraction frequency decreases, uterine tonus returns to normal, and the worrisome fetal heart rate pattern disappears, oxytocin may be restarted at a slower rate. In general, the infusion is restarted at half the rate that was being used when the excessive uterine stimulation developed, and the interval between rate increases is lengthened.

B. Water Intoxication

As noted previously, oxytocin has an antidiuretic effect and should be mixed only in isotonic solutions. Although uncommon, if oxytocin is given in IV fluids containing glucose but no sodium, with prolonged administration of large doses, the antidiuretic effect of oxytocin may lead to retention of fluid without retention of sodium. The severe form of hyponatremia (low serum sodium) is water intoxication.

Clinical signs of water intoxication begin with decreased urinary output and headache, and may progress rapidly to mental confusion and seizures. These signs resemble the onset of eclampsia. The 2 signs can be differentiated by blood pressure (elevated in eclampsia) and serum sodium (low with water intoxication, normal in eclampsia).

Water intoxication should be avoided by
- Using only normal saline or a balanced salt solution for IV fluids
- Monitoring intake and output

If water intoxication occurs, severely restrict the volume of fluid given to the patient. Overly rapid correction of hyponatremia may lead to permanent neurologic damage. Consult with regional center specialists.

13. How Long Should You Continue an Oxytocin Infusion?

When oxytocin is used either to induce or to augment labor, the goal is to mimic the pattern of normal labor as closely as possible. Labor is normally *progressive,* with contractions becoming stronger and more frequent and lasting longer, as cervical dilatation and fetal descent progress.

Oxytocin primarily stimulates the frequency of uterine contractions. Usually, but *not* always, contraction strength and duration increase with increased contraction frequency. Uterine contractions that have the characteristics of normal labor represent an appropriate and adequate response to oxytocin.

A. Induction of Labor

1. *Establishment of Labor*

If oxytocin has been given for 12 to 18 hours without causing additional cervical effacement or dilatation, continuing the infusion is unlikely to produce labor. Reevaluate the clinical situation. If delivery needs to be accomplished without further delay, consider cesarean delivery.

If the indication for delivery is less urgent, discontinue the oxytocin and allow the woman to rest overnight. An attempt at induction may be repeated once or twice on successive days. If labor has not been established after 2 or 3 induction attempts, consider
- Sending the patient home
- Rupturing the membranes (if you are prepared for cesarean delivery if labor does not ensue)
- Performing a cesarean section

2. *Management After Labor Is Established*
- When contractions occur more frequently than every 2 minutes (from the start of one to the start of the next), their effectiveness in producing cervical effacement and dilatation is likely to diminish. As soon as contractions are occurring every 2 to 3 minutes, maintain the oxytocin infusion at that rate, increasing it further if the contraction frequency decreases.
- Generally, as labor progresses, less oxytocin is needed. The goal is to achieve the minimum effective dose of oxytocin. After 5- to 6-cm cervical dilatation has been reached and uterine activity is normal, consider reducing the rate of oxytocin infusion by approximately 10% to 25%.
- If labor progress continues satisfactorily after 30 to 60 minutes at a lower rate, reduce the rate of oxytocin infusion again. The aim is to continue this "stair-step" system of decreasing the oxytocin until the infusion is stopped entirely, with labor continuing on its own.
- Observe the uterine response carefully to be sure it does not decline. In some cases, reduction in the rate of oxytocin infusion will be accompanied by reduced labor quality. In this situation, the rate of oxytocin should be increased to the previous effective dosage.

B. Augmentation of Labor

When labor slows because of the development of hypotonic contractions, augmentation with an oxytocin infusion may be used. Adequate uterine response is usually seen promptly, but the response may be delayed for 2 to 4 hours. Most women promptly resume normal labor progress if there are no other problems.

If a normal labor pattern is not achieved after 2 to 4 hours of oxytocin infusion, reassess the woman's condition and be sure there is no other cause for failure to progress, such as fetopelvic disproportion or fetal malposition.

Augmentation should be considered unsuccessful if

- A normal contraction pattern cannot be achieved after 6 or more hours of oxytocin infusion. Consider use of an intrauterine pressure catheter to quantitatively assess contraction strength.

OR

- Progress is not made after 2 to 4 hours of oxytocin infusion with a normal labor pattern.

If no other cause exists for failure to respond adequately to oxytocin augmentation, consider

- A period of rest and hydration

OR

- Cesarean delivery

Self-test

Now answer these questions to test yourself on the information in the last section.

C1. When contractions occur more often than every 2 minutes, their effectiveness in producing cervical dilatation and effacement usually _____

_____ .

C2. Oxytocin primarily increases the _____ of contractions.

C3. **True** **False** When used for labor induction, the rate of oxytocin infusion should be increased every 15 minutes until 8-cm cervical dilatation is achieved.

C4. **True** **False** When labor is being augmented, if there is no progress after 2 to 4 hours of oxytocin administration in the presence of a normal contraction pattern, you should consider a cesarean delivery.

C5. Risks of excessive uterine stimulation include

Yes	No	
___	___	Uterine rupture
___	___	Birth trauma
___	___	Vaginal lacerations
___	___	Postpartum endometritis
___	___	Neonatal hypoglycemia
___	___	Intracranial bleeding in the newborn
___	___	Perineal tears
___	___	Fetal asphyxia

C6. What is the *first* thing you should do if uterine tachysystole develops?

_____

C7. What should you do if uterine tachysystole occurs when oxytocin is being infused?

_____

C8. **True** **False** When oxytocin is used to induce labor, it should be stopped after 12 to 18 hours if labor has not begun.

C9. **True** **False** In a patient undergoing oxytocin induction of labor, the dose that first brings about normal labor is the dose that should be maintained until delivery.

C10. **True** **False** Contraction strength and duration always increase when oxytocin is used to increase contraction frequency.

C11. **True** **False** Water intoxication is likely to occur if only balanced salt intravenous solutions are used with an oxytocin infusion.

C12. **True** **False** Whenever an oxytocin infusion is used, intake and output should be monitored.

Check your answers with the list that follows the Recommended Routines. Correct any incorrect answers and review the appropriate section in the unit.

Inducing and Augmenting Labor

Recommended Routines

All the routines listed below are based on the principles of perinatal care presented in the unit you have just finished. They are recommended as part of routine perinatal care.

Read each routine carefully and decide whether it is standard operating procedure in your hospital. Check the appropriate blank next to each routine.

Procedure Standard in My Hospital	Needs Discussion by Our Staff	
_____	_____	1. Establish a protocol for patient care and monitoring when prostaglandins are used for cervical ripening.
_____	_____	2. Establish a system to identify and record the reasons for the use of oxytocin, and the evaluation done to rule out contraindications, whenever labor is induced or augmented.
_____	_____	3. Establish protocols for the use of oxytocin that include • Uniform dilution of oxytocin for intravenous administration • Standard interval for the rate of intravenous oxytocin infusion change (both increase and decrease) • Administration of oxytocin only by the intravenous route for labor induction or augmentation
_____	_____	4. Establish a flow sheet for the administration of oxytocin that shows the dosage rate of oxytocin (mU per minute), and every change in the rate, with the corresponding • Time • Maternal vital signs • Fetal heart rate and pattern • Contraction frequency, duration, and strength • Uterine tonus

_____   _____   5. Establish guidelines for staffing and personnel availability whenever oxytocin is given, including
- Nurse:patient ratio
- Attending physician or certified nurse midwife
- Surgical and anesthesia staff
- Continuous electronic fetal heart rate and uterine contraction monitoring

_____   _____   6. Establish guidelines for the response to uterine tachysystole.

_____   _____   7. Develop a system whereby an emergency cesarean delivery can be started within 30 minutes of the decision to operate, at any time of the day or night.

Self-test Answers

These are the answers to the self-test questions. Please check them with the answers you gave and review the information in the unit wherever necessary.

A1. D

A2. A Bishop score is calculated to indicate the likelihood that an attempt at induction of labor will be successful and to indicate when cervical ripening is likely to be most helpful.

A3. It is likely an induction of labor will be successful.

A4. Cervical ripening with a prostaglandin preparation, stripping of membranes, mechanical dilators

A5. a. Cervix is closed = 0, soft = 2, posterior position = 0, 50% effaced = 1; -2 station = 1: *total score* = 4
    b. Cervix is 3 cm dilated = 2, soft = 2, anterior position = 2, 70% effaced = 2; 0 station = 2: *total score* = 10

A6. Any 2 of the following:
- Premature rupture of membranes, when delivery is indicated
- Chorioamnionitis
- Complicated gestational hypertension, and/or preeclampsia
- Maternal medical illness with evidence of declining maternal and/or fetal health
- Fetal jeopardy as demonstrated by tests of fetal growth and/or well-being
- Abruptio placentae (Grade I with no fetal compromise or Grade III with fetal death and a stable woman)
- Fetus approaching post-term gestation. (When dates are *certain*, consider induction in the 41st week of gestation.)
- Fetal death
- Women at 39 or more weeks' gestation, with a history of rapid labor(s) and geographic difficulties in reaching a hospital
- Other, various, uncommon individual indications

A7. Any 2 of the following:
- Cervical infection
- Active genital herpes
- Recent unexplained vaginal bleeding

A8. Uterine tachysystole

A9. False. Repeated use of Cervidil vaginal insert is not recommended. Prepidil gel may be repeated 2 or 3 times (with 6 to 8 hours of rest between applications), but total dose should not exceed 1.5 mg in 24 hours.

A10. False. A period of rest should follow use of any of the prostaglandin cervical ripening agents.

B1. Isotonic solutions—Normal saline or other fluid containing sodium

B2. False. Intravenous push of undiluted oxytocin can cause maternal hypotension and cardiac arrhythmia.

B3. True

B4. Initial intravenous rate = 1.0 mL/hour; rate to deliver 1.5 milliunits (mU)/minute = intravenous rate of 1.5 mL/hour

B5. Normal labor has contractions every 2 to 3 minutes (3 to 5 in 10 minutes), each lasting 45 to 70 seconds, that are strong by palpation (or 50 mm Hg measured with an internal monitor)

B6. Any 3 of the following:
- When labor is normal
- When fetopelvic disproportion is present
- Generally, for any of the situations when labor induction is not recommended
- When hypertonic uterine inertia is present
- When there is fetal intolerance to labor

B7. Any 3 of the following:
- Individualize dosage.
- Recognize risk of uterine tachysystole.
- Use a standard dilution.
- Use isotonic solutions.
- Select appropriate route of administration.
- Control rate of intravenous infusion.
- Calculate intravenous rate for mU per minute dosage.
- Control rate of dosage increase.
- Recognize limits of effectiveness.

B8. A. Hypotonic uterine dysfunction is an *indication*.

B9. False. Oxytocin will increase the frequency, and usually the strength and duration, of contractions. Any or all of these effects may limit placental blood flow and, thereby, worsen fetal response. Oxytocin should *not* be used when there is evidence of fetal compromise.

B10. False. Prolonged rupture of membranes increases the risk of infection for both the woman and the newborn. Artificial rupture of membranes should not be done unless you are willing and prepared to perform a cesarean delivery if the induction attempt fails. Intrauterine pressure monitoring should only be used when indicated. It is not required for all patients receiving oxytocin.

C1. Decreases or diminishes

C2. Frequency

C3. False. The dose should be increased by 1 to 2 mU/minute every 30 to 60 minutes until a regular contraction pattern (contractions every 2 to 3 minutes) is achieved and sustained.

C4. True

C5.

Yes	No	
X	____	Uterine rupture
X	____	Birth trauma
X	____	Vaginal lacerations
____	X	Postpartum endometritis
____	X	Neonatal hypoglycemia
X	____	Intracranial bleeding (especially in preterm fetuses)
X	____	Perineal tears
X	____	Fetal asphyxia

C6. Stop the oxytocin.

C7. Immediately reduce the rate of oxytocin infusion, usually by half. Maternal hydration, administration of oxygen, and lateral positioning also may be useful.

C8. True

C9. False. Generally, less and less oxytocin is needed once labor becomes established. After 5- to 6-cm cervical dilatation is achieved, you should begin to reduce the amount of oxytocin infused. In most cases, but not all, the oxytocin can be reduced in increments until it is stopped completely, with labor progressing on its own. Occasionally, labor quality declines and oxytocin needs to be continued until delivery occurs. You should observe uterine response closely and use the minimum amount of oxytocin that maintains a normal labor pattern.

C10. False. Oxytocin works primarily by increasing contraction frequency. Contraction strength and duration usually, but *not always*, increase with increased contraction frequency.

C11. False. Only normal saline or balanced salt solutions should be used with oxytocin infusion to *avoid* the possibility of water intoxication.

C12. True

292

Unit 8 Posttest

If you are applying for continuing education credits, a posttest for this unit is available online. Completion of unit posttests and the book evaluation form are required to achieve continuing education credit. For more details, visit www.cmevillage.com.

Unit 9: Abnormal Labor Progress and Difficult Deliveries

Objectives

In this unit you will learn

A. How to determine the difference between true, false, and prodromal labor

B. What maternal, fetal, and neonatal risks accompany abnormal labor

C. How to recognize normal and abnormal labor progress

D. When and how to investigate abnormal labor progress

E. How to treat the causes of abnormal labor

F. When forceps or vacuum extractor are used and how to ensure their safe application

G. How to respond to emergent, or potentially emergent, fetal conditions, including
   - Meconium-stained amniotic fluid
   - Fetal heart rate abnormalities
   - Complications of maternal analgesia or anesthesia
   - Prolapsed umbilical cord
   - Shoulder dystocia

H. How to identify and manage an abnormal third stage of labor

Unit 9 Pretest

Before reading the unit, please answer the following questions. Select the *one best* answer to each question (unless otherwise instructed). Record your answers on the test and check them against the answers at the end of the book.

1. Shoulder dystocia is associated with all of the following, *except:*
   A. Fetal macrosomia
   B. Brachial plexus injury
   C. Maternal thigh flexion
   D. Vaginal birth after cesarean delivery

2. You see the sudden onset of severe variable decelerations on a fetal heart rate tracing. Of the following, what is the *first* thing you should do?
   A. Check for umbilical cord prolapse.
   B. Check the woman's blood pressure.
   C. Prepare to give a tocolytic medication.
   D. Prepare for emergency cesarean delivery.

3. **True   False**   With meconium-stained amniotic fluid, suctioning of a baby's mouth and nose after delivery of the head, but before delivery of the shoulders, is no longer recommended as a routine procedure.

4. **True   False**   Narcotics given to a laboring woman may cause minimal or absent fetal heart rate variability.

5. **True   False**   Face presentation puts a baby at risk for spinal cord injury.

6. **True   False**   The fetal head should be engaged before a forceps delivery is attempted.

7. **True   False**   Once normal fetal size, presentation, and position, and adequate pelvic size have been determined, oxytocin augmentation is the treatment of choice for hypertonic uterine dysfunction.

8. **True   False**   When cord prolapse occurs, one appropriate way to elevate the presenting part off the cord is to fill the woman's bladder with 500 mL of sterile saline and have her assume knee-chest position.

9. **True   False**   Contraction quality is poor, but baseline tonus is usually elevated with hypotonic uterine dysfunction.

10. Which of the following should *always* be present before forceps or vacuum extraction delivery is attempted?

Yes	No	
____	____	Estimated fetal weight of 4,000 g (8 lb, 13 oz) or more
____	____	Maternal anesthesia
____	____	Complete cervical dilatation
____	____	Evaluation of fetal size, presentation, and position
____	____	Oxytocin augmentation of labor

297

11. In which of the following situations is oxytocin augmentation of labor most likely to be useful (assuming normal fetal size, presentation, and position, and normal pelvic size is present)?

Yes	No	
____	____	Arrested second stage with normal contraction pattern
____	____	Hypotonic uterine dysfunction during the active phase
____	____	Hypertonic uterine dysfunction during the latent phase
____	____	Maternal fatigue with weak pushing efforts but normal labor pattern

12. Maternal risks of precipitate labor include all of the following *except*

A. Postpartum hemorrhage

B. Postpartum endometritis

C. Lacerations of the birth canal

D. Uterine atony

13. Which of the following are appropriate interventions when there is rapid cervical dilatation and precipitate labor is suspected?

Yes	No	
____	____	Begin broad-spectrum antibiotics.
____	____	Investigate for abruptio placentae.
____	____	Check cervical dilatation every 15 to 30 minutes.
____	____	Prepare for delivery.
____	____	Anticipate need for neonatal resuscitation.
____	____	Place the woman in reverse Trendelenburg position.
____	____	Administer large doses of narcotic analgesia to the laboring woman.

14. Which of the following are associated with vaginal breech delivery?

Yes	No	
____	____	Abruptio placentae
____	____	Birth trauma
____	____	Growth-restricted fetus
____	____	Prolapsed umbilical cord

15. True   False   If there is excessive bleeding during the third stage of labor, oxytocin should be given to cause the uterus to contract and expel the placenta.

16. True   False   The second stage of labor normally lasts 6 hours or longer.

17. True   False   Oxytocin infusion may be appropriate treatment for second-stage arrest of labor.

18. True   False   If delivery of the placenta does not occur within 30 minutes of delivery of the baby, but there is no evidence of vaginal bleeding, it is best to wait for spontaneous delivery of the placenta.

19. True   False   Ultrasound estimation of fetal weight is less accurate when the fetal head is deep in the pelvis.

20. True   False   The hallmark of true labor is contractions with progressive cervical dilatation.

21. **True** **False** Goiter and tumors of the neck are associated with an increased likelihood of a fetus being in face or brow presentation.

22. **True** **False** The most common cause of prolonged labor is breech presentation.

23. **True** **False** A woman is exhausted and can no longer push effectively. The fetus is vertex, right occiput posterior, at +3 station. Manual rotation of the head and low forceps delivery is one appropriate approach to this situation.

24. **True** **False** Artificially rupturing the membranes to stimulate labor in a woman with prolonged latent phase will require a cesarean delivery if labor does not progress.

25. **True** **False** When fetal gestational age is 34 weeks or less, and an operative vaginal delivery is indicated, a vacuum extractor is preferred to forceps.

26. Which of the following is *most* likely to be a cause of prolonged latent phase?
  A. Fetal malformation
  B. Uterine fibroids
  C. Excessive maternal sedation
  D. Grand multiparity

27. Which of the following is the *best* indication of true labor?
  A. Regular contractions
  B. Rupture of membranes
  C. Painful contractions
  D. Cervical dilatation

28. Once labor becomes established, clues to abnormal progress include all of the following, *except:*
  A. Cervix becomes edematous
  B. Presenting part remains unengaged
  C. Contractions every minute
  D. Cervical dilatation averaging 1.5 cm/hour

29. Evaluation of prolonged active phase reveals fetal hydrocephalus. The fetus is vertex, with a reassuring fetal heart rate pattern. Which of the following are appropriate actions to take?

Yes	No	
____	____	Begin oxytocin augmentation.
____	____	Drain the hydrocephalus with a needle and monitor labor for fetal descent.
____	____	Advise the parents that hydrocephalus is a fatal malformation.
____	____	Perform cesarean delivery.

1. How Do You Know When True Labor Is Present?

During the last few weeks of pregnancy, there is a gradual increase in uterine activity that leads to true labor. Pregnant women associate the onset of labor with an increase in regularity and strength, with the addition of pain, to the irregular contractions they have been feeling. Obstetric caregivers document the presence of true labor with progressive cervical dilatation, almost always accompanied by painful and palpable uterine contractions. A woman whose cervix is 5 cm or more dilated on arrival at a hospital can be assumed to be in true labor.

Women with less than 5 cm cervical dilatation may or may not be in true labor. True labor may be difficult to distinguish from false or prodromal labor when painful contractions are present but little or no cervical dilatation has occurred. A period of observation is needed. The general characteristics of false, prodromal, and true labor are listed in Table 9.1.

If contractions continue, but the cervix has not changed after observation and monitoring for 1 to 2 hours, administration of a mild sedative may help differentiate between true and false labor.

False labor was present if contractions stopped after mild sedation. *Prodromal labor* may be present if contractions continue after sedation and 3 to 4 hours of observation, but without cervical change. The contractions of prodromal labor are often associated with little or no discomfort. Prodromal labor may stop (in which case, it was actually false labor), or may progress into true labor over a period of several hours or days.

Patients with false or prodromal labor usually do not need to be observed continuously in a health care setting. Unless there are specific risk factors or other contraindications, these women may be discharged, with instructions for changes that should prompt them to return to the hospital.

Table 9.1. Characteristics of False, Prodromal, and True Labor		
False Labor	**Prodromal Labor**	**True Labor**
Uterine Contractions		
• Usually irregular • Duration varies • Strength varies • Usually stopped by sedation • May be painful	• Usually irregular • Duration varies • Strength varies • Usually *not* stopped by sedation • Usually little pain	• Increasingly regular • Increasing duration • Increasing strength • Usually *not* stopped by sedation • Usually painful
Cervical Dilatation		
• No change	• No change	• Progresses

2. What Is the Normal Progress of Labor?

    A. Time of Onset

       The exact time at which labor begins is often difficult to determine. Establishing the time of labor onset is important only when it is needed to determine that labor is prolonged. In most cases, the time of hospital admission is used as the time of the onset of labor.

    B. Contraction Pattern

       Normal contraction frequency, duration, and strength is described in Unit 8, Inducing and Augmenting Labor, in this book.

C. Stages of Labor

Normal labor is progressive with a predictable pattern. Uterine contractions become more frequent, last longer, are accompanied by more discomfort, and are associated with certain identifiable changes in the maternal cervix and fetal station.

1. *First Stage of Labor*

   The first stage of labor is divided into 2 well-defined phases that, together, span the time from the onset of labor until the cervix is completely dilated.

   a. *Latent phase*: This begins with the onset of regular contractions and ends when the next phase, the active phase, begins. Most of the work of uterine contractions during the latent phase goes to softening and effacing the cervix. The length of the latent phase varies widely among women.

   Hospital admission often occurs during the latter part of the latent phase.

   b. *Active phase*: This begins when the cervix starts to dilate at a progressive rate and ends either with complete dilatation of the cervix or the beginning of the deceleration phase. Most of the work of uterine contractions during the active phase goes to cervical dilatation. In primigravidas, cervical dilatation normally progresses at a rate of 1.2 to 3 cm/hour, while cervical dilatation in multiparas normally progresses at a rate of 1.5 to 6 cm/hour.

   In some women, particularly primigravidas, the rate of cervical dilatation may slow near the end of the active phase. This is sometimes called the *deceleration phase*.

   Fetal descent is usually minimal during the first stage of labor, quite often just 1 to 2 cm. Most women will not feel the urge to push until the cervix is fully dilated and the second stage of labor has been reached. Some women will have an urge to push earlier, late in the first stage. Strong pushing efforts prior to full cervical dilatation are to be avoided, as they can lead to cervical edema and subsequent laceration, as well as maternal exhaustion.

    The critical feature of progress in the first stage of labor is cervical dilatation.

2. *Second Stage of Labor*

   This stage begins with complete dilatation of the cervix and ends with delivery of the baby.

   a. *Descent*: Cervical dilatation is said to be *complete, full,* or *10 cm* when an examining finger can no longer feel any cervix around the presenting part. With the resistance of the cervix gone, fetal descent is more rapid because maternal pelvic structures are less resistant to pressure applied to the presenting part. With the continued pressure of uterine contractions, plus the added force of maternal pushing efforts, the presenting part descends deeper and deeper into the pelvis.

   b. *Rotation*: The fetal head normally enters the true pelvis in a flexed position, with the chin close to the chest. The posterior fontanel and the sagittal suture running from it are the landmarks most easily felt on vaginal examination.

The occipitofrontal ("front-to-back") diameter of the fetal head is greater than the biparietal ("side-to-side") diameter. Because the maternal pelvis usually is wider from side to side at the inlet, the head enters the pelvis with the sagittal suture oriented transversely ("running from side to side") and the posterior fontanel oriented toward either the left or right side of the pregnant woman's pelvis.

The pelvis becomes narrower below the inlet, with the narrowest part being between the ischial spines. At that point, the pelvis is widest from the symphysis to the sacrum (front to back). This creates a twisting funnel through which the fetus must pass. As fetal station approaches the level of the ischial spines, the downward pressure on the fetus forces the longer part of the head to rotate to the largest diameter of the maternal pelvis. Thus, the head rotates 90°, to either *occiput anterior* or to *occiput posterior*. The sagittal suture is now oriented anterior-posterior rather than transverse. This process of the fetal head turning, as labor progresses, to accommodate the size and shape of the maternal pelvis is referred to as internal rotation.

As long as contractions remain strong and the woman pushes well, rotation and descent will progress if the size of the pelvis and the fetus, and the position of the presenting part allow it.

Some women do not feel the urge to push until after the cervix has been dilated fully for some time. Waiting for a woman to get the urge to push will allow her pushing to be more effective.

 The critical feature of progress in the second stage of labor is descent of the presenting part.

3. *Third Stage of Labor*
   This stage begins after the birth of the baby and ends when the placenta is delivered.
   Delivery of the placenta usually occurs 5 to 10 minutes after delivery of the baby. If it does not occur spontaneously within 30 minutes, manual removal of the placenta will be needed.

4. *Fourth Stage of Labor*
   The fourth stage is not a classic stage of labor, but is used to identify the period that begins after delivery of the placenta and ends an hour later.
   During this time, the uterus normally contracts to prevent excessive postpartum bleeding. It is the time postpartum hemorrhage occurs most often and, therefore, is the time after delivery when careful observation and monitoring of maternal condition is especially important.

3. What Constitutes Abnormal Labor?

Abnormal labor can be either extremely slow or excessively rapid. It is most often associated with slow progress. Delay of labor progress poses risks for a woman and her fetus. Labor can become

- *Protracted* (slow rate of progress)
- *Prolonged* (long time for progress to occur)
- *Arrested* (progress stops)

Although much less common than delayed labor progress, *precipitate labor* (very rapid labor) is also abnormal. Precipitate labor, which also carries risks for a woman and her fetus, occurs when the entire labor process from the first contraction to delivery takes less than 3 hours.

A. First Stage/Cervical Dilatation
   Dilatation may be protracted if the cervix fails to dilate at a normal rate, prolonged if dilatation fails to progress within a specified period of time, or arrested if dilatation stops entirely.

B. Second Stage/Fetal Descent
   Descent is considered arrested if there is no progress in descent for a 2-hour period with adequate maternal effort. For most women, the second stage of labor lasts less than 2 hours. Longer durations of the second stage may be acceptable, as long as progress (fetal descent) is being made and the woman and fetus remain stable, with a reassuring fetal heart rate pattern.

Table 9.2 lists the characteristics of labor, including the normal rate of progress and length of each stage and phase, and defines when progress becomes abnormally slow.

4. What Are the Risks of Abnormal Labor?

All labor carries risks of morbidity and mortality for the woman and the fetus. When labor progresses normally, the risks are minimal. When labor progress is delayed, or is extremely fast, the risks increase.

Manipulation of the process of labor, however, also carries risks. The risks that accompany medical manipulation must be weighed against the risks that accompany continued observation of suspected abnormal labor. The goal of medical intervention on the process of labor should be to reduce the risks to the woman and the fetus.

When labor progress is abnormal, particularly when it is abnormally slow, there may be more than one cause. When more than one cause is present, the effect of each abnormality is magnified and the likelihood of successful vaginal delivery is significantly reduced.

				Time	
Period	**Defining Event(s)**	**Cervical Dilatation**		**Primipara**	**Multipara**
Stage I	*DILATATION OF THE CERVIX* Onset of labor until complete cervical dilatation (10 cm)				
Latent phase	Onset of contractions until beginning of active phase. (Note: If contractions stop, the patient was in false labor.)	0 → 3-5 cm	Normal Prolonged	Up to 20 hours >20 hours*	Up to 14 hours >14 hours*
Active phase	Dilatation progresses at 1.2-3 cm/hour until complete dilatation.	3-5 → 8-10 cm	Normal Prolonged Protracted Arrested	Up to 6 hours >6 hours from 5 → 10 cm Dilatation at >1.2 cm/hour† No progress in 6 hours	Up to 6 hours >6 hours from 5 → 10 cm Dilatation at >1.5 cm/hour† No progress in 6 hours
Stage II	*DESCENT OF PRESENTING PART*				
	From full cervical dilatation until delivery of the baby (Note: Assuming the woman and fetus are well, and as long as labor progress is being made, up to 5 hours in the second stage does not increase maternal or neonatal morbidity or mortality, and may reduce operative deliveries.)		Normal *Usual Acceptable* Arrested	2 hours Up to 5 hours No descent in 2 hours	1 hour Up to 5 hours No descent in 2 hours
Stage III	*IMMEDIATE POSTPARTUM PERIOD*				
	From delivery of the baby until delivery of the placenta		Normal Abnormal	Up to 30 minutes >30 minutes	Up to 30 minutes >30 minutes
Stage IV	*FIRST HOUR AFTER PLACENTAL DELIVERY*				
	Not a true stage of labor, but is the time postpartum hemorrhage is most likely to occur				

*When labor is induced, the latent phase may be longer than this.
†Rate of dilatation calculated at 2-hour intervals, or longer.
Protracted refers to a slow rate of progress. *Prolonged* refers to an abnormally long length of time for progress to occur. In many cases, protracted labor becomes prolonged labor.

Self-test

Now answer these questions to test yourself on the information in the last section.

A1. **True** **False** The contractions of false labor usually stop after mild sedation.

A2. **True** **False** If a woman enters a hospital with contractions and cervical dilatation of 5 cm or more, she can be assumed to be in true labor.

A3. An active phase of labor with cervical dilatation progressing at a rate of 0.8 cm/hour would be called a _____ active phase.

A4. An active phase that lasted longer than 6 hours would be called a _____ active phase.

A5. When the cervix is completely dilated, but fetal station does not change during a 2-hour period, it is called _____.

A6. Describe the stages of labor.

The first stage of labor starts with the onset of true labor and continues until _____

_____.

The second stage of labor starts with _____ and continues until _____.

The third stage of labor starts following _____ and ends with

_____.

The "fourth stage" of labor starts following _____ and ends _____. It is the time when the risk of postpartum hemorrhage is the _____.

A7. Normal cervical dilatation during the *active phase* for a primipara is _____ cm/hour and for a multipara it is _____ cm/hour.

A8. Normal duration of the *active phase* of labor in primigravidas is _____ hours or less and in multigravidas is _____ hours or less.

A9. Usual duration of the *second* stage of labor in primigravidas is _____ hours or less and in multigravidas is _____ hours or less.

A10. The critical feature of progress in the first stage of labor is _____ , and in the second stage of labor it is _____.

Check your answers with the list that follows the Recommended Routines. Correct any incorrect answers and review the appropriate section in the unit.

5. When Should You Suspect Abnormal Labor?

A. Clinical Clues

If prolonged labor occurred in one pregnancy, it is likely to recur in subsequent pregnancies. There is also an increased risk for precipitate labor to recur. While the risk for recurrence of abnormal labor is increased, it does not always happen, and subsequent labor(s) may be entirely normal.

Once labor starts, signs of difficult labor may be found long before a diagnosis can be established. Recognizing the clues enables you to anticipate that labor may not progress well, to identify a problem early, and to prepare for treatment that may be needed.

The following 7 factors are clues to a potentially difficult labor:
- *Poor application of head to the cervix:* Suggests fetopelvic disproportion (FPD)
- *Deflexed head:* Suggests FPD may be present
- *Unengaged head:* Suggests FPD or placenta previa may be present
- *Poor contractions:* Suggests hypotonic uterine dysfunction may be present
- *Continuous contractions, seemingly without letup:* Suggests hypertonic dysfunction

305

- *Edema of the cervix:* Suggests FPD with the head compressing the cervix against the pelvic bones, thus limiting lymphatic return in the lower portion of the cervix
- *Pushing uncontrollably before complete dilatation:* Suggests occiput posterior, with the occiput pushing the rectum against the sacrum, thus giving the woman the sensation of an urge to push

B. Labor Progress Curve

The labor of any woman may be plotted on a graph ("partogram") that shows a normal labor pattern (primigravidas and multiparas plotted separately, on their respective normal curve). If the resulting curve deviates significantly from the general, normal pattern, further investigation into the progress of labor is recommended.

Normal labor patterns are shown in Figure 9.1. For most women, labor begins before the time of hospital admission; therefore, much of the latent phase may not be included in the graph.

Figure 9.2 shows another normal labor curve for a primigravida, plus plots for 3 abnormal labors. This graph shows hospital admission earlier in the course of labor than is shown in Figure 9.1. Therefore, more of the latent phase is seen.

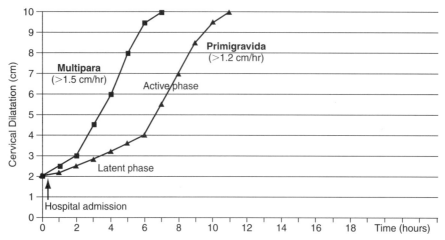

Figure 9.1. Labor Curves: Normal Progress, First Stage of Labor.

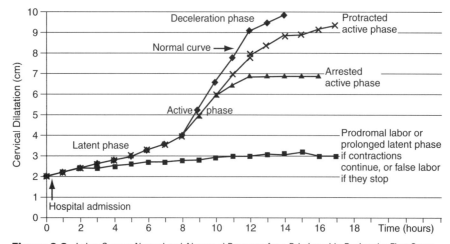

Figure 9.2. Labor Curves: Normal and Abnormal Progress for a Primigravida During the First Stage of Labor.

6. What Are the Causes of Abnormal Labor?

Approximately 90% of failures of dilatation or descent can be attributed to a problem, or combination of problems, with

- Maternal pelvic size or shape (passage)
- Fetal size, position, or presentation (passenger)
- Contraction strength and effectiveness (power)

 Keep the 3 Ps in mind.
- *Passage*
- *Passenger*
- *Power*

Some factors can cause delay in labor progress at more than one point in labor. In addition, it is common for a combination of factors to be responsible for abnormal progress. For example, slightly large fetal size and a mild degree of pelvic contraction may, together, result in arrest of descent.

It is not always possible, however, to determine which factor, or combination of factors, is the cause of abnormal labor. Approximately 10% of abnormal labors never have a clear cause identified.

The *fourth "P," for psyche*, is important in how a woman perceives her accomplishments in labor and to the actual physical progress of labor.

A woman's attitude is influenced by her

- Level of fear
- Understanding of the labor process
- Confidence in her ability to cope with labor and parenthood
- Support she receives from her family
- Response she receives from health care givers and the labor environment

For women who feel completely overwhelmed by labor, the psychological stress, added to the physical stress, may interfere with normal labor progress.

 Despite normal pelvic size, normal fetal position and size, and normal uterine contractions, labor in some women will fail to progress.

Possible causes of delayed labor progress are listed in Table 9.3, along with the period of labor in which they are likely to occur. Psychological influences, although important, are difficult to isolate or quantify and are not listed.

7. How Should You Investigate Abnormal Progress During Labor?

 Investigate all causes. More than one cause of abnormal labor may be present.

307

A. *Power* → Assess Uterine Contractions

Power relates to uterine contractions and, in the second stage, to maternal pushing efforts.

- Is *true* labor present? If not, Section 1 for the management of false or prodromal labor.
- If labor is in the *latent phase,*
  - Is the woman *excessively sedated*? If so, allow the sedation to wear off while monitoring the status of her labor.
  - Was the *labor induced*? If so, this phase may take longer than when labor has a spontaneous onset, and some portion occurs before hospital admission.
- Is *contraction quality* normal?
  - *If yes*, investigate other causes of abnormal labor.
  - *If no*, determine whether hypotonic or hypertonic uterine dysfunction is present (Table 9.4) and treat accordingly.
  - *If uncertain* and membranes are *already* ruptured, and there are no contraindications to internal monitoring, consider inserting an intrauterine pressure catheter to allow more precise evaluation of uterine function.

Table 9.3. Causes of Delay in Labor Progress				
Period	Uterine Dysfunction (Power)	Fetopelvic Disproportion (Passage)	Fetal Position (Passenger)	Other Causes
Stage I: Cervical Dilatation				
Prolonged *latent phase*	Hypotonic (uncommon) or hypertonic (uncommon)	Uncommon	Uncommon	False labor; excessive sedation; induced labor
Prolonged or arrested *active phase*	Hypotonic (common) or hypertonic (uncommon)	Common	Uncommon	Uterine over-distension: check for hydramnios, twins
Prolonged *deceleration phase*	Hypotonic (common) or hypertonic (rare)	Common	Common*	Occiput posterior
Stage II: Fetal Descent				
Prolonged or arrested *descent*	Hypotonic (uncommon) or Hypertonic (rare)	Common	Common*	Inadequate pushing; excessive sedation or anesthesia; fetal malposition or malformation (rare)

*Fetopelvic disproportion (FPD) (smaller pelvis and/or larger fetus) is the cause in about half of the patients who develop delay in labor progress at this point. Fetal malformations or tumors also may obstruct passage through the birth canal (hydrocephalus is the malformation most often associated with FPD).

Note: Uterine dysfunction delays cervical dilatation. Fetopelvic disproportion and abnormal fetal positions primarily interfere with descent of the presenting part. Uterine dysfunction and FPD may be present at the same time.

Table 9.4. Characteristics of Uterine Dysfunction		
	Hypotonic (Common)	**Hypertonic (Rare)**
Contractions	Poor quality, low intensity, irregular	Poor quality; low intensity; irregular; may be nearly continuous—difficult to time onset and end; often do not match with patient's perception of pain
Baseline tonus	Normal	Usually elevated
Pain	Minimal	Continuous, usually felt in the back; often out of proportion to contraction strength
Fetal distress	Rare	Common
Oxytocin	Usually helpful in achieving normal labor	Not useful

 Do not rupture the membranes artificially unless you are committed to delivery at this time. You must be prepared to perform a cesarean delivery if labor does not progress after intervention.

- If *hypotonic contractions* are present, is the uterus overdistended? Check for twins or hydramnios.
- Is the fetus in vertex presentation with the *occiput posterior*? Occiput posterior may be associated with a prolonged deceleration phase late in the first stage and/or delay in descent during the second stage of labor.
- If labor is in the *second stage,*
  - Is *epidural or spinal anesthesia* (may slow second stage) being used?
  - Is there *excessive maternal sedation*?
  - Is maternal *pushing inadequate*?

B. *Passenger* → Determine Size and Position of the Fetus

When there is significant delay in the progress of labor, reevaluate the size, presentation, and position of the fetus. Look for findings that might have been overlooked in earlier examination(s), and for things that might have changed.

Fetal lie refers to the position of the fetus in relationship to the woman, using the spinal columns as reference points. Longitudinal lie is when the spines of the woman and the fetus are parallel to each other, and is present with a fetus in either vertex or breech presentation. Transverse lie is when the fetal spine is at right angles to the maternal spine and the fetus appears to lie across the woman's abdomen.

Presentation refers to the part of the fetus that leads into the pelvis. The general term for a fetus headfirst in the pelvis is called cephalic or vertex presentation, but may be made more specific if the brow or face is the presenting part. Buttocks first is called a breech presentation, but also may be labeled more specifically as frank, complete, footling, or double footling, depending on the exact presentation.

Position refers to the relationship of the presenting part to the maternal pelvis. For example, a normal vertex presentation may be left occiput anterior, right occiput anterior, or left occiput posterior, etc.

1. *Clinical Evaluation*
   a. *Palpate the maternal abdomen.*
      • Recheck Leopold's maneuvers to determine fetal lie and presentation.
      • Reassess the size of the fetus.
   b. *Perform digital vaginal examination* to help identify the presenting part and its position, and determine fetal station. Be especially careful if an abnormal presentation is suspected.

 While vertex presentation, with the occiput being the leading part, is the most common presentation by far, genitalia, hand, face, foot, or the umbilical cord also can be the presenting part.

2. *Ultrasound Examination*
   Ultrasound is useful in determining
   • Fetal lie, presentation, and position
   • Estimation of fetal weight, with these limitations
     – When the head is deep in the pelvis, the fetal biparietal diameter cannot be measured accurately, thus significantly reducing the accuracy of fetal weight estimates.
     – Oligohydramnios reduces the accuracy of fetal weight estimation.
     – The accuracy of fetal weight estimation decreases as the fetal weight increases.
   • Presence of fetal malformation that may obstruct labor progress (eg, hydrocephalus) or lethal anomaly that might preclude a cesarean delivery (eg, anencephaly)
   • Location of placenta

C. *Passage* → Determine Maternal Pelvic Size
   1. *Clinical Evaluation*
      Pelvic abnormalities can contribute to delay of labor progress. Clinical estimation of the size of the pelvis will help determine if any gross abnormalities in the shape of the midpelvis or pelvic outlet are present. The diagonal conjugate provides an estimate of the anterior-posterior dimension of the pelvis (Figure 9.3). Although the transverse diameter (width from side to side) may be narrow with a normal anterior-posterior size, this is uncommon. In most cases, if the diagonal conjugate is normal, the transverse diameter of the pelvis is normal too.

 If there is any suspicion of a placenta previa, do not perform a digital pelvic examination until an ultrasound has ruled it out.

The distance between the tip of the middle finger on the sacral promontory (P) and the point where the hand meets the symphysis pubis (S) is the diagonal conjugate, as shown in illustration A.

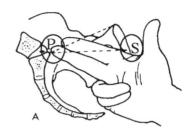

Often, the middle finger cannot reach the sacral promontory (P), as shown in illustration B. When this happens, the diagonal conjugate can be assumed to be 12.5 cm or more.

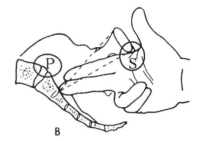

Figure 9.3. Clinical Pelvimetry: Measurement of Diagonal Conjugate.

a. *Obtain the diagonal conjugate measurement.*
  - Insert your index and middle finger into the vagina.
  - Hold these 2 fingers together and trace the anterior surface of the sacrum until your middle finger reaches the sacral promontory (most prominent portion of the upper sacrum).
  - Keep your middle finger firmly in place on the sacral promontory and pivot your hand upward until the web of your thumb reaches the symphysis pubis.
  - Mark the point on the lateral surface of your hand where it touches the symphysis.
  - Withdraw your hand and measure the distance between the mark and the tip of your middle finger.

b. *Interpret the diagonal conjugate measurement.*
  - *Diagonal conjugate less than 11.5 cm*: When the diagonal conjugate is less than 11.5 cm, the obstetric conjugate (distance between the sacral promontory and the *inside* edge of the symphysis pubis, which represents the space available to the fetus) will average less than 10 cm. This represents a pelvis too small to allow easy passage of an average-sized, term fetus.
  - *Diagonal conjugate greater than 11.5 cm*: A pelvic inlet of this size is adequate for the birth of most fetuses. A diagonal conjugate close to 11.5 cm, however, may not be adequate for a very large fetus.

D. Summarize Your Findings

Make a summary of your findings after *systematically* evaluating

- Quality of the uterine contractions
- Size, presentation, and position of the fetus
- General size of the pelvis
- Other factors that may be considered
  - Placental location (particularly if there is a reason to suspect placenta previa)
  - Presence/absence of major fetal malformation (particularly if there is a reason to suspect fetal hydrocephalus)
  - Uterine over-distension (multifetal gestation, hydramnios)
  - Level of maternal sedation and/or anesthesia
  - Adequacy of maternal pushing (if in second stage); maternal exhaustion
  - Ability of woman to cope with labor
  - Fetal status

Identify the probable cause(s) of the delayed progress of labor and document these in the patient's chart.

Self-test

Now answer these questions to test yourself on the information in the last section.

B1. Which of the following are associated with *prolonged first stage* of labor?

Yes	No	
_____	_____	Fetopelvic disproportion
_____	_____	Large fetus
_____	_____	Post-term pregnancy
_____	_____	Hydramnios
_____	_____	Uterus that is contracting poorly
_____	_____	Malpositioned fetus
_____	_____	Woman addicted to cocaine

B2. Which of the following are associated with *prolonged second stage* of labor?

Yes	No	
_____	_____	Fetopelvic disproportion
_____	_____	Inadequate pushing
_____	_____	Fetal malposition
_____	_____	Hypotonic uterine dysfunction

B3. The graph to the right shows a _____ _____ of labor.

B4. **True** **False** With thorough investigation, a clear cause, or causes, of abnormal labor can always be determined.

B5. **True** **False** Hypertonic uterine dysfunction is uncommon, but hypotonic uterine dysfunction is common.

B6. **True** **False** Fetopelvic disproportion may be due to a small pelvis, a large fetus, or a combination of both factors.

B7. Name at least 4 of 7 early clues to abnormal labor.

_____

_____

_____

_____

B8. Match the following characteristics with the corresponding type of uterine dysfunction.
a. Hypotonic
b. Hypertonic
___ Minimal pain
___ Usually responds well to oxytocin treatment
___ Elevated baseline tonus
___ Fetal distress more common
___ Normal baseline tonus
___ Nearly continuous contractions

B9. All causes of abnormal labor relate to p_____ , p_____ , and/or p_____ , and sometimes p_____ .

Check your answers with the list that follows the Recommended Routines. Correct any incorrect answers and review the appropriate section in the unit.

8. How Should You Respond to Abnormal Labor?

Treatment of a particular cause of abnormal labor may vary, depending on the point in labor when the problem arises. In addition, more than one factor may be responsible for delayed labor progress. When more than one cause for abnormal labor is identified, cesarean delivery may be indicated by the combination of factors, even when no individual factor, by itself, would warrant cesarean section.

Evidence of non-reassuring fetal status at any point during labor requires immediate reevaluation of labor and delivery management and may necessitate intervention in the interest of the fetus, regardless of labor quality or progress.

A. Uterine Dysfunction
   1. *Hypertonic Uterine Dysfunction*
   This rare type of uterine dysfunction occurs when the uterus does not relax between contractions or contracts in an uneven, uncoordinated pattern. If it develops, it almost always does so during the latent phase of labor. Hypertonic uterine dysfunction is separate from uterine hypertonus, which may follow excessive oxytocin administration.

   If oxytocin is being used to induce or augment labor, and hypertonic uterine dysfunction develops, the oxytocin should be stopped and the labor progress should be observed for up to 1 hour. At that time, respond to whatever pattern is present after the period of observation. Many times, after discontinuing oxytocin in such a situation, a normal labor pattern will develop.

313

Another cause of hypertonic dysfunction can be placental abruption. Be sure an abruption has been ruled out before proceeding with the care outlined in the following text.

a. *Provide therapeutic rest.*

- Give enough medication to allow the patient to sleep for at least 4 hours. Any of several parenteral analgesics, sedatives, or tranquilizers are appropriate, including the following combination:

  – Morphine sulfate, 8 to 15 mg (depending on patient's weight), intramuscularly with

  – Promethazine, 25 mg, intramuscularly, to decrease nausea

  OR

- Provide lumbar epidural anesthesia (intrathecal narcotics may be used instead of epidural anesthesia) and intravenous (IV) fluid hydration. Give enough fluids to produce 30 to 50 mL/hour of urine.

Most women (about 85%) with prolonged latent phase due to hypertonic uterine dysfunction, who are treated with therapeutic rest, will awaken in the active phase and continue with normal labor progress.

b. *Consider cesarean delivery.*

If normal labor does not follow the rest period, low-dose oxytocin augmentation may be attempted. There is an increased risk, however, that hypertonic uterine dysfunction will recur. In that case, cesarean section may be associated with less risk of fetal compromise and newborn depression than continued augmentation of labor.

2. *Hypotonic Uterine Dysfunction*

After true labor has been established, as documented by uterine contractions with progressive cervical dilatation, hypotonic uterine dysfunction may develop. This occurs when contractions become ineffective because they become less frequent, of lower intensity, and/or of shorter duration.

a. *Begin oxytocin augmentation.* (See Unit 8, Inducing and Augmenting Labor, in this book).

When the pelvis is normal and the fetus is of normal size, presentation, and position, oxytocin augmentation is successful in correcting abnormal labor progress in about 80% of women with hypotonic uterine dysfunction.

b. *Be prepared to perform cesarean delivery* if oxytocin augmentation fails.

3. *Secondary Arrest of Labor*

Progress during labor can simply stop. If contractions are normal but progress has been stopped for 2 hours or longer, investigate other causes of abnormal labor and consider cesarean delivery.

If contractions have diminished, consider augmentation of labor.

a. *Begin oxytocin augmentation.*

b. *Be prepared to perform cesarean delivery* if oxytocin augmentation fails.

 Whenever abnormal labor develops, consider the possibility that fetal malpresentation, malposition, and/or fetopelvic disproportion is present.

B. Fetal Presentation or Position

An abnormal presentation detected during pregnancy may have corrected itself by the time labor begins. Many times, however, malpresentation is not recognized until it is revealed through investigation of poor labor progress.

If malpresentation is found, evaluate maternal pelvic size (if not already done) and placental location. A contracted pelvis and a low-lying placenta may be associated with abnormal presentation.

Management depends on the specific abnormal presentation or position.

1. *Brow or Face Presentation*

With this much deflexion, most often the fetal head cannot pass through the pelvis (Figure 9.4). Sometimes, with a large pelvis and good labor, the head may be forced to flex with the pressure from above. The result will be a vertex presentation, which can be expected to deliver vaginally.

   a. *Management*

   - *Avoid* internal fetal heart rate monitoring. Accurate placement of a fetal scalp electrode is more difficult, and inaccurate placement may result in damage to the fetal face or eye.
   - Brow and face presentations prior to labor may flex into normal vertex presentation during early labor. Some will not, and some brow presentations will change to face presentations.
   - Nuchal teratomas and goiters are associated with an increased risk of face and brow presentation.
   - If the mentum (chin) is posterior (with face presentation) and does not rotate spontaneously to anterior with descent, vaginal delivery is contraindicated because of the risk of spinal cord trauma to the abnormally extended fetal neck and the risks associated with forceps rotation.
   - If a brow presentation does not flex to become vertex, or a face presentation does not rotate to become mentum (chin) anterior within 2 hours of the onset of the second stage, a cesarean delivery is usually necessary.
   - If a cesarean section is necessary, special attention should be given to gentle delivery of the deflexed head; this will help avoid fetal spinal cord injury.

   b. *Neonatal risks*

   - If a nuchal teratoma or goiter is present, emergency care at delivery, particularly endotracheal intubation, may be needed.
   - Severe facial and laryngeal edema may occur with face presentation. Endotracheal intubation may be needed to maintain an open airway.
   - Check for spinal cord trauma.
   - Severe facial bruising may occur. Check bilirubin levels.

2. *Compound Presentation*

This occurs when an extremity presents alongside the presenting part. For example, a fetus in vertex position may have a hand in front of or beside the head.

   a. *Management*

   - Do not attempt to replace the extremity into the uterus because trauma to the woman or fetus, or prolapse of the umbilical cord, may occur.

315

With face presentation, vaginal delivery cannot be accomplished safely, unless the fetus's chin rotates to anterior with descent (Figure 9.5).

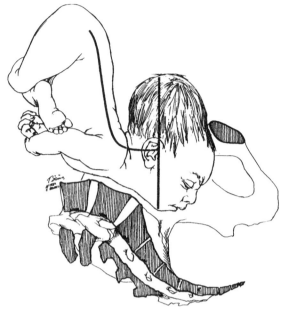

Figure 9.4. Face Presentation with Mentum (Chin) Posterior. Reproduced with permission from Cunningham FG, MacDonald PC, Gant NF, et al. *Williams Obstetrics*. 20th ed. Stamford, CT: Appleton & Lange; 1997:445.

Spontaneous rotation from right mentum posterior to mentum anterior during descent. This allows vaginal delivery, with the chin coming directly under the symphysis pubis.

Rotation is shown in 45° increments.

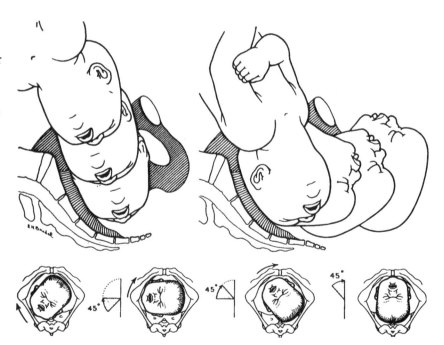

Figure 9.5. Spontaneous Rotation of Face Presentation During Descent. Reproduced with permission from Cunningham FG, MacDonald PC, Gant NF, et al. *Williams Obstetrics*. 20th ed. Stamford, CT: Appleton & Lange; 1997:444.

- If a compound presentation is present early in labor with a fetus in vertex presentation, most babies can be delivered vaginally. As labor progresses, the hand usually will retract into the uterus.
- If a compound presentation occurs with a fetus in non-vertex position or is associated with delay of labor progress, cesarean delivery is recommended.

b. *Neonatal risks*
- These depend on presentation (vertex or breech, etc), route of delivery, and other risk factors, if any.
- Bruising or trauma to the presenting extremity may occur. Examine carefully. If bruising is severe, check bilirubin levels. A fracture can occur, but is rare.

3. *Transverse Lie*

This occurs when the body of the fetus lies horizontally in the uterus, across the birth canal entrance. It is associated with contracted pelvis, placenta previa, uterine fibroids, abnormal uterine shape, high parity (several previous deliveries), and certain congenital malformations in the fetus, particularly hydrocephalus.

a. *Management*
- In most cases, transverse lie detected earlier in pregnancy will have changed spontaneously to vertex, or sometimes to breech, presentation by the time labor starts.
- If transverse lie persists, the fetus appears normal, and placenta previa is not present, consider external cephalic version (turning the fetus) at approximately 34 to 36 weeks' gestation.
- If transverse lie is first detected early in labor, a *gentle* attempt at external version may be successful. After the active phase has begun, external version is not recommended.
- If transverse lie cannot *easily* be changed to vertex, a cesarean section is needed for safe delivery. In most cases, a vertical incision (classical cesarean) is used because the larger incision generally allows an easier delivery of the fetus than the extraction process that would be necessary with a low transverse incision.
- Postdelivery, check for maternal fibroids or uterine duplication.

b. *Neonatal risks*
- Check for malformations that may have influenced fetal position.
- If the uterus is malformed, check for fetal positional deformities that may have resulted from a cramped position in utero.

4. *Breech Presentation*

This occurs when one foot or both feet (footling or double footling), or the buttocks (frank or complete breech, depending on whether the legs are extended or flexed at the knees) are the presenting parts. The risk of asphyxia, umbilical cord prolapse, and birth trauma are increased with vaginal breech delivery.

 Recent reports have documented an increase in perinatal morbidity and mortality in planned vaginal breech delivery. Many obstetricians have not been trained in the skills of vaginal breech delivery. Consideration should be given to cesarean delivery for all viable fetuses in breech presentation.

There is also a risk of fetal head entrapment after the body is delivered. Because the width of the fetal body is generally smaller than the width of the head, particularly in preterm fetuses, the cervix can trap the after-coming head. Preterm fetuses, especially those weighing less than 2,500 g, are at highest risk for fetal head entrapment, which can be fatal.

a. *Vaginal versus cesarean delivery decision factors*
  - A fetus in breech position early in pregnancy will, almost always, turn spontaneously to vertex. If not, and conditions are favorable, consider external cephalic version at approximately 34 to 36 weeks.
  - Vaginal breech delivery is controversial. A trial of labor may be considered if, and only if, all the following conditions are met:
    – Fetal gestational age of 35 weeks or older
    – Frank or complete breech (buttocks present first, not feet)
    – Adequate maternal pelvic size
    – Flexed fetal head (as documented with x-ray or ultrasound)
    – No maternal or fetal distress
    – Good labor progress (oxytocin augmentation is controversial)
    – Availability of continuous fetal monitoring
    – Availability of physician experienced and skilled in vaginal breech delivery
    – Capability (staff and equipment) for rapid cesarean section
    – Prior vaginal delivery
  - Consider a *cesarean delivery* if *any* of the following conditions exist:
    – Fetal gestational age of 34 weeks or younger
    – Footling breech (one or both feet present first, not buttocks)
    – Contracted pelvis by clinical pelvimetry
    – Hyperextended fetal head by ultrasound, sometimes described as a "stargazing fetus" (significantly increases likelihood of traumatic delivery and risk to the fetus's neck and spinal cord)
    – Abnormal fetal heart rate pattern
    – Secondary arrest of labor progress
    – Lack of availability of physician experienced and skilled in vaginal breech delivery
    – Absence of anesthesia personnel and facilities for immediate cesarean delivery throughout second stage of labor

b. *Management*
A general rule for management of breech presentation during labor is: *If anything goes wrong, perform a cesarean delivery.*
  - Avoid artificial rupture of membranes, because there is an increased risk of umbilical cord prolapse with breech presentation (especially complete or footling breech).
  - If membranes rupture spontaneously, examine the woman to be sure cord prolapse has not occurred.
  - If internal fetal heart rate monitoring is used, determine placement of the electrode carefully to avoid damage to the genitalia or anus.
  - Decide delivery route. Once the legs or buttocks have been delivered, a cesarean delivery cannot be safely carried out.

 The decision to deliver a fetus in breech presentation vaginally or by cesarean section must be made before the delivery process begins.

If vaginal delivery is undertaken.

- Allow spontaneous delivery to the umbilicus, then use *gentle* assistance to deliver the arms and head.
- Generally, one person is needed to support the baby's legs and thorax while the second person delivers the head.

c. *Neonatal risks:* Anticipate need for resuscitation and evaluation.

5. *Occiput Posterior*

While this is one of the normal positions for a vertex presentation, it is much less common than occiput anterior, and is often associated with hypotonic uterine dysfunction and deflexion of the fetal head (head in neutral, non-flexed position).

a. *Management*
- If labor is normal, observation for 2 to 3 hours may be all that is needed for a fetus in occiput posterior position to rotate to occiput anterior and deliver.
- If hypotonic uterine dysfunction is present, but there is no evidence of fetopelvic disproportion, a trial of oxytocin augmentation is warranted.
- If oxytocin is used, follow the guidelines in the Unit 8, Inducing and Augmenting Labor, in this book, starting with a low dose (0.5 milliunits [mU]/minute) and increasing cautiously. If progress is not made after 2 hours of normal labor (if in first stage of labor) or 1 hour (if in second stage of labor), deliver by cesarean section.
- Attempt manual rotation when the head reaches the perineum (consider low forceps or vacuum extraction delivery). The vacuum extractor should never be used to effect rotation of the fetal vertex; spontaneous rotation may occur with descent during traction. If this fails or is difficult, deliver by cesarean section.
- Serious lacerations of the birth canal, including fourth-degree perineal tears (laceration extends into the woman's rectum), may result from spontaneous delivery of the fetus in occiput posterior position or from operative vaginal delivery. (See Section 9.)

b. *Neonatal risks:* These depend on course of labor, type of delivery (spontaneous or operative vaginal deliveries) and other risk factors, if any.

C. Congenital Malformation

Investigation of delayed progress in labor sometimes reveals a fetal malformation or condition (hydrocephalus, hydrops, etc) that obstructs descent. These situations often require cesarean delivery.

Not all fetal malformations necessitate cesarean delivery. A lethal malformation that does not obstruct fetal descent, such as anencephaly, does not require cesarean delivery. In these situations, cesarean delivery has no benefit to the fetus, but has the risks of surgery and anesthesia for the woman.

The management of other malformations (such as meningomyelocele, encephalocele, gastroschisis, omphalocele, etc) should be discussed with specialists at a regional center.

In some cases, the route of delivery may affect neonatal outcome. In addition, even the smoothest neonatal transport may be more traumatic for a baby than maternal/fetal transfer would be. Delivery at a hospital that can provide full evaluation and surgical treatment of the baby also allows the mother to be with her baby. Consider referral of a woman for delivery at a regional center if a fetal malformation is identified before labor or during *early* labor.

319

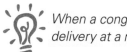 *When a congenital malformation is identified, maternal/fetal referral for delivery at a regional center is often preferable to neonatal transport.*

D. Fetopelvic Disproportion

Incompatibility in size between the fetus and the pelvis, whether it is due to a small maternal pelvis, large fetal size, and/or fetal anomaly, is also sometimes called cephalopelvic disproportion.

Clinical pelvimetry, estimation of fetal size, and determination of fetal position are used together to decide if FPD is present.
- Does the pelvis seem small enough to cause or contribute to the delay in labor?
- Does the fetus seem large enough to cause or contribute to the delay in labor?
- Is an abnormal presentation or fetal malformation present? If so, is it responsible for the delay in labor?

If FPD is found, it is managed by cesarean section.

E. Excessive Sedation, Narcotic Analgesia, or Anesthesia

Heavy doses (or the cumulative effect of several smaller doses) of medication may cause or contribute to delay of labor progress, particularly early in labor, during the latent phase. Simply allow the medication effects to wear off.

Slowing of labor progress may occur with epidural or spinal anesthesia. Oxytocin augmentation may be appropriate, or the medication may be allowed to wear off.

F. Inadequate Pushing

Complete cervical dilatation does not bring the urge to push in all women. Encouraging a woman to push as soon as cervical dilatation is complete may exhaust her and reduce the effectiveness of her efforts. As long as a woman and a fetus are well, and the fetal heart rate pattern is reassuring, it is reasonable to wait up to 1 to 2 hours for the woman to develop the urge to push. Provided that fetal descent continues, waiting for a woman to feel ready to push may lengthen the second stage but also may reduce the need for operative delivery.

In rare situations, a woman may need to avoid pushing (certain maternal cardiac or cerebrovascular diseases). Other than this rare situation, management options include the following:

1. *Consider That Medication May Be Responsible for Ineffective Pushing.* Consider allowing epidural or spinal analgesia or narcotic analgesia to wear off.

2. *Consider Providing a Period of Rest.* Sometimes a woman becomes exhausted or uncooperative after a long, difficult labor and lengthy second stage with the need for active pushing over an extended period. If the woman is well, the fetal heart rate pattern is reassuring, and the arrest of descent is due to the inability of the woman to push any more, consider a rest period with sedation or conduction anesthesia and hydration.

    Many times, a woman will be able to push more effectively after a period of rest. Duration needed for recuperative rest varies, but a period of approximately 2 hours is often adequate.

3. *Consider a Trial of Forceps or Vacuum Extraction Delivery.* Be prepared for cesarean delivery if the trial does not proceed *easily*. Operative deliveries are presented later in this unit.

4. *Consider Delivering the Baby by Cesarean Section.*

Table 9.5. Suggested Response to Delay of Labor Progress*

Consider the Ps: *passage, passenger, power.* Investigate each as a possible cause of abnormal labor (more than one may contribute to a delay). Consider the woman's *psyche* too. Depending on your findings, provide treatment for the cause(s), or proceed directly to cesarean delivery.

Period of Labor	Actions to Take[†]
First Stage (cervical dilatation)	
Prolonged	1. Allow excessive sedation to wear off. Alternatively, if a woman is not overly sedated, providing analgesia and/or sedation to produce therapeutic rest (sleep) may be beneficial.
	2. If, after therapeutic rest, contractions persist but fail to produce adequate progress, investigate for fetopelvic disproportion, malposition, and malpresentation. Deliver by cesarean section if • Fetopelvic disproportion is found. or • Fetal indications are present.
	3. If maternal pelvis is considered adequate and there are no fetal contraindications, consider oxytocin[‡] augmentation. The goal is to achieve at least 2 hours of a normal contraction pattern.
Prolonged or arrested active phase	1. If due to hypotonic uterine dysfunction, consider oxytocin[‡] augmentation to achieve at least 2 hours of normal contraction pattern.
	2. Deliver by cesarean section if • Fetopelvic disproportion is found or • Fetal indications are present or • Oxytocin trial fails to produce labor progress after 2 to 4 hours of normal contractions.
Second Stage (Fetal Descent)	
Prolonged or arrested	1. If contractions have been normal and maternal pushing has been strong for 2 hours but without progress, and the fetus is at +1 station or higher, deliver by cesarean section.
	2. If due to hypotonic uterine dysfunction, consider oxytocin[‡] augmentation to achieve 1 hour of normal contraction pattern.
	3. Consider allowing narcotic sedation or epidural/spinal anesthesia to wear off.
	4. If maternal exhaustion prevents effective pushing, consider hydration and sedation or conduction anesthesia. (Two hours of rest is usually adequate.)
	5. Consider trial of forceps or vacuum extraction if the vertex position is at +2 station or below.
	6. Deliver by cesarean section if • Fetopelvic disproportion is found or • Fetal indications are present or • Oxytocin trial fails to produce labor progress after 2 hours of normal contractions or • Trial of forceps or vacuum extractor does not proceed *easily*

Fetal well-being is assumed. Evidence of fetal distress at any point requires immediate reevaluation, and possible revision, of management plan.

[†]Whenever abnormal labor develops, consider the possibility that fetal malpresentation, malposition, and/or fetopelvic disproportion is present.

[‡]See Unit 8, Inducing and Augmenting Labor, in this book, for information about oxytocin use.

G. Summarize Your Plan

Earlier, you summarized your findings regarding the probable cause(s) of delay in labor progress for a patient. Now you should expand that summary to include an outline of your management plan. Discuss this plan with the woman and her family.

If your initial plan does not proceed as expected, you will need to review your findings, reconsider your plan, and outline a revised plan. Keep the woman and her family informed regarding the expected and actual course of events. Discuss any revisions in your management plan with them.

At each junction in therapy, you should *systematically* review your findings and revise your plan as the situation changes. It is important that you approach the management of abnormal labor in a systematic way, as well as document your findings, your actions, and the maternal and fetal response to each step as care is given.

Management of abnormal labor is summarized in Table 9.5. Review the steps for each period of labor.

Self-test

Now answer these questions to test yourself on the information in the last section.

C1. **True** **False** Breech presentation is associated with increased risk for umbilical cord prolapse.

C2. **True** **False** Quite often, more than one factor contributes to abnormal progress of labor.

C3. **True** **False** Although occiput posterior is a normal vertex presentation, it is associated with hypotonic uterine dysfunction and with an increased likelihood of birth canal lacerations.

C4. **True** **False** Hypertonic uterine dysfunction is treated with therapeutic rest.

C5. **True** **False** Maternal exhaustion and inadequate pushing may be an indication for cesarean delivery.

C6. **True** **False** Maternal exhaustion and inadequate pushing may be an indication for forceps or vacuum extraction delivery.

C7. **True** **False** Maternal exhaustion and inadequate pushing may be an indication for a period of sedation or conduction anesthesia, hydration, and rest.

C8. **True** **False** Evaluation of abnormal labor should be followed by a summary, written in the patient's chart, of suspected cause(s) and subsequent management plan.

C9. **True** **False** Face presentation, with the chin posterior, is an indication for cesarean delivery.

C10. Compound presentation occurs when _____.

C11. Hypertonic uterine dysfunction occurs when _____.

C12. Which of the following is *not* indicated when abnormal fetal position is detected early in labor?
   A. Prepare for immediate cesarean delivery.
   B. Evaluate size of maternal pelvis.
   C. Evaluate fetus for congenital malformations.
   D. Determine location of placenta.

C13. Cesarean delivery is performed more frequently for breech presentation than for vertex presentation because
   A. The cervix may not allow passage of the head after delivery of the body.
   B. The risk of asphyxia and birth trauma are higher with vaginal breech delivery.
   C. Fewer physicians are skilled in breech delivery than in cesarean delivery.
   D. All of the above.

C14. Before oxytocin augmentation of labor is started, _____ and _____ should be ruled out.

C15. In which of the following situations may oxytocin augmentation of labor be appropriate?

Yes	No	
___	___	Hypertonic uterine dysfunction during the active phase
___	___	Secondary arrest of labor
___	___	Hypotonic uterine dysfunction during the deceleration phase
___	___	Hypotonic uterine dysfunction during the active phase

C16. **True** **False** If external version cannot *easily* convert a transverse lie to vertex, a cesarean section is needed for safe delivery.

C17. **True** **False** A 30-year-old woman who easily delivered 3 healthy term babies, and is now pregnant at 39 weeks with the fetus in breech position, represents a high-risk pregnancy.

Check your answers with the list that follows the Recommended Routines. Correct any incorrect answers and review the appropriate section in the unit.

9. What Are Operative Vaginal Deliveries?

Operative vaginal delivery refers to one that is assisted by use of obstetric forceps or a vacuum extractor (VE).

 Training, skill, and experience are ESSENTIAL for either safe forceps or safe VE delivery.

1. *Forceps*

   There are many types of obstetric forceps. All have metal "blades" shaped (in different ways) to fit on either side of the fetal head. They are slid into place separately and then locked together before traction is applied. This technique requires proper application of the forceps, then rotation and traction maneuvers, which change progressively according to fetal station and descent. Traction and rotation should be *gentle*, and coordinated with uterine contractions and maternal pushing.

   Figure 9.6 shows the proper application of obstetric forceps to the fetal head for an outlet forceps delivery. The technique shown is with the fetus in vertex, occiput anterior presentation and crowning. Techniques are somewhat different for other fetal presentations and for low or midforceps application.

After the left blade (Simpson forceps are shown) is in place, the right blade is applied. The 2 blades are then interlocked at the handles and *gentle* traction is applied.

Correct positioning of both blades is essential.

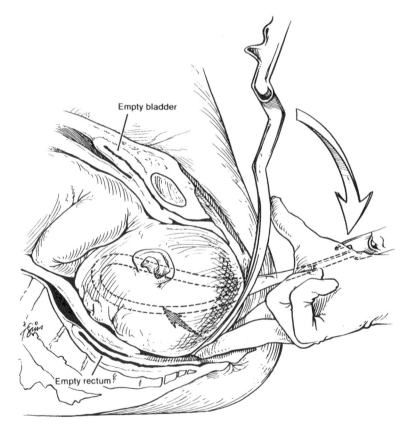

Empty bladder

Empty rectum

Figure 9.6. Application of Forceps Blades for an Outlet Delivery.
Reproduced with permission from Cunningham FG, MacDonald PC, Gant NF, et al. *Williams Obstetrics*. 20th ed. Stamford, CT: Appleton & Lange; 1997:478.

2. *VE*

   A soft or rigid suction cup (metal cups are no longer commonly used) is placed on the fetal occiput, in the midline, away from the fontanels. The center of the cup should be about 3 cm (1 to 1.5 inches) in front of the posterior fontanel and over the midline (sagittal) suture. Correct placement is generally straightforward when the fetal position is occiput anterior, but can be much more difficult with other vertex positions. Care should be taken to avoid trapping maternal tissue (vaginal or cervical) under the cup edges. Once the cup is applied, do not attempt to twist it in an effort to rotate the fetal head because lacerations of the fetal scalp may result.

   Traction should be coordinated with uterine contractions and simultaneous maternal pushing. Rotation will occur naturally as the descending head follows its normal course through the birth canal. Descent of the fetal head should occur with each uterine contraction and application of traction, so that the head is completely delivered within 15 minutes or less of when the cup was applied (usually in 3 pulls).

3. *Types of Forceps or VE Deliveries**

   The following definitions use the system that describes station as the level of the leading point of the skull in centimeters, using a scale of -5 to +5, with 0 being the level of the maternal ischial spines.

   a. *Outlet forceps or VE:* This procedure has the same risk of perinatal morbidity and mortality as spontaneous delivery. It is defined by the following:
      - Fetal scalp is visible without manually separating the labia.
      - Fetal skull has reached the pelvic floor.
      - Sagittal suture is in the anterior-posterior diameter of the pelvis or in the right or left occiput anterior or posterior position (ie, no more than 45° from vertical).
      - Rotation does not exceed 45° from the vertical midline.

   b. *Low forceps or VE:* The leading point of the fetal skull at station +2 station or lower, but not on the pelvic floor.
      Use of forceps is divided into 2 categories.
      - *Rotation 45° or less:* Left or right occiput anterior rotated to occiput anterior or left or right occiput posterior rotated to occiput posterior.
      - *Rotation more than 45°:* Rotation and delivery with forceps requires much skill and experience, is more likely to be unsuccessful, and is associated with increased neonatal morbidity. A VE is not used in this situation. See Section 10.

   c. *Midforceps or VE:* The fetal head is engaged in the pelvis, but the leading part of the fetal skull is above station +2. It is associated with a higher likelihood of maternal and/or fetal morbidity, and is more likely to be unsuccessful but, in skilled hands, may still be of lower morbidity than a cesarean delivery.

   d. *High Forceps or VE:* The fetal head is unengaged. It is associated with an unacceptable degree of risk to the woman and fetus and is not performed in modern obstetrics.

---

*Adapted with permission from American College of Obstetricians and Gynecologists. *Operative Vaginal Delivery.* Practice Bulletin #17. June 2000.

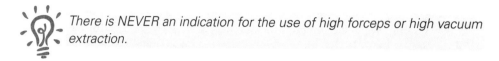

There is NEVER an indication for the use of high forceps or high vacuum extraction.

10. When Are Operative Vaginal Deliveries Used and What Can You Do to Make Them Safe?

Obstetric forceps and VE are valuable tools for obstetric care. The potentially serious risks associated with these tools can be minimized with adequate preparation, clear indications for use, and recognition that cesarean delivery is preferable to a traumatic assisted vaginal delivery. When the instruments cannot be applied smoothly, or when rotation or traction does not produce the desired results with minimum effort, the attempt should be stopped and a cesarean delivery should be performed.

Application of forceps or suction cup should be EASY; rotation of the head should be EASY; traction should EASILY result in fetal descent.

A. Meet Basic Requirements

Before either forceps or VE delivery is considered, the following need to be ensured:

1. *Maternal Informed Consent* for the procedure

2. *Physician Trained, Experienced, and Skilled* in the use of forceps and/or VE

3. *Adequate Anesthesia* given to the woman; anesthesia personnel should be continuously available if either midforceps or mid-VE is attempted

4. *Capability to Perform Cesarean Section Immediately* if an attempt at forceps or VE delivery does not proceed easily

5. *Fully Dilated Cervix*

6. *Engaged Fetal Head*

7. *Empty Maternal Bladder*

8. *Thorough Assessment of Fetal Presentation and Position, Fetal Size, Gestational Age, and Maternal Pelvic Size* to be certain vaginal delivery is possible and advisable, and for accurate application of forceps or suction cup

9. *Safe Fetal Age, Size, Position, and Presentation*

   a. *Forceps or VE delivery is **not** advisable* in the following situations:
      • There is a suspected or known fetal coagulation defect.
      • There is a known or suspected demineralizing fetal skeletal condition (eg, osteogenesis imperfecta).
      • Any non-vertex presentation, including face or brow presentation.
      • Position of the presenting part cannot be identified.

   b. *Vacuum extraction also should be avoided* when
      • Gestational age is 34 weeks or less (risk of intracranial hemorrhage is increased in preterm fetuses).
      • Rotation is required to effect delivery.

Forceps or VE should never be applied unless there is complete cervical dilatation and the fetal head is engaged.

B. Use Only When Indicated

1. *Evidence of Non-reassuring Fetal Status or Maternal Compromise*

   If the need for rapid delivery develops at a time when the fetal head is deep in the maternal pelvis, low forceps (or even midforceps/mid-VE) may be faster and safer than a "crash" cesarean section. Preparations for cesarean delivery should continue while forceps or VE delivery is attempted, in case the trial does not proceed easily and must, therefore, be abandoned.

2. *Arrested Descent During the Second Stage*

   Slow rate of fetal descent is acceptable as long as the woman and fetus show no signs of distress. When there is *no* fetal descent for 2 hours, with a normal labor pattern, there are 2 management options. Depending on fetal station, perform

   - *Cesarean delivery*

   OR

   - *Forceps or VE delivery*

3. *Inadequate Voluntary Pushing*

   In certain situations, a woman should not push (cardiac or cerebrovascular disease). In other cases, a woman may not be able to push effectively due to exhaustion or excessive sedation or anesthesia. (See Sections 8E and 8F.)

C. Select the Appropriate Technique

1. *Vacuum Extraction*

   Use of VE is appropriate whenever use of forceps also would be considered, as long as the gestational age is greater than 34 weeks. A VE may be safer than forceps when the

   - Fetal head is rotated 45° or more from the midline. This situation can be a difficult forceps delivery, but with VE, the head may rotate naturally when traction is applied to the suction cup.

   Increase suction gradually within the cup. Control suction to stay within the recommended limit. Follow manufacturers' recommendations for the specific cup used in your hospital.

2. *Low or Outlet Forceps or VE*

   Use of either of these techniques is appropriate whenever an operative vaginal delivery is indicated.

   - Fetal distress or maternal compromise is best treated by a prompt vaginal delivery
   - Delayed or arrested second stage of labor without FPD, malpresentation, or malformation
   - Ineffective maternal pushing

3. *Midforceps or Mid-VE*

   This technique has very limited uses. The higher the fetal head is in the pelvis, the more difficult and dangerous operative vaginal delivery becomes.

   Midforceps or mid-VE may, however, be appropriate when

   - There is arrest of descent above +2 station but below 0 station, in the apparent absence of FPD. (This situation most often develops when there is ineffective maternal pushing.)
   - Abnormal fetal heart rate patterns or maternal compromise dictate delivery sooner than it can be expected to occur spontaneously, and midforceps or mid-VE seem preferable to cesarean delivery.

When application of the VE or forceps is easy and subsequent rotation and/or traction occurs with minimal force, delivery is usually successful without trauma to the fetus or the woman. When the application, rotation, or traction require an inordinate amount of force, it is usually better to abandon the attempt and perform a cesarean delivery.

Every attempt at delivery with midforceps or mid-VE should be considered a trial.

If the attempt does not proceed easily, you should be willing and prepared to abandon it and promptly perform a cesarean delivery.

D. Prepare Adequately

Each of the following items should be ensured before operative vaginal delivery is attempted.

1. *Prepare the Woman*
   - Bladder empty
   - Buttocks overhang bed or table slightly
   - Perineum not excessively stretched (associated with episiotomy extensions)
   - Legs supported in stirrups but not restrained (due to possible shoulder dystocia)

2. *Provide Anesthesia*
   - Outlet and low forceps or VE deliveries usually can be performed under pudendal nerve block or local infiltration.
   - Midforceps or mid-VE deliveries require major conduction (spinal or epidural) anesthesia or, occasionally, inhalation anesthesia, with anesthesia personnel in attendance during the procedure.

3. *Organize Personnel and Equipment*
   An operative vaginal delivery should be treated like any other operative procedure, with indications, maneuvers to bring about application of the forceps or suction cup and the delivery, and the postdelivery condition of the woman and the newborn recorded in the chart.

Whenever a midforceps or mid-VE is undertaken, it is preferable to use an operating room and table where an unsuccessful attempt can be followed promptly by a cesarean section.

Abdominal surgery setup, with surgical and anesthesia staff present during the midforceps or mid-VE trial, is recommended.

4. *Anticipate Care for the Newborn* (See also Section 12.)
   - Risk for birth trauma, including fractures and intracranial bleeding, is increased.
   - Need for resuscitation may be increased.

Self-test

Now answer these questions to test yourself on the information in the last section.

D1. True False The *only* reason to use low forceps is to speed delivery when there is evidence of fetal compromise.

D2. True False Midforceps or mid-vacuum extraction delivery are higher risk than low forceps or low vacuum extraction delivery.

D3. True False Outlet forceps is an unnecessary procedure that is associated with a high risk of fetal morbidity.

D4. True False When a vacuum extractor is used, traction on the fetal head should be coordinated with uterine contractions and maternal pushing.

D5. True False When low forceps is used, rotation of the fetal head more than 45° requires considerable skill and is associated with an increased risk of trauma to the fetus.

D6. When a vacuum extractor is used, all of the following statements are correct, *except:*
  A. The traction cup should be centered over the anterior fontanel.
  B. Delivery should occur within 15 minutes after the cup is applied.
  C. Descent of the fetal head should occur with each contraction and simultaneous application of traction with the vacuum extractor.
  D. In certain situations, vacuum extraction may be safer than forceps.

D7. Every midforceps or mid-vacuum extractor delivery attempt should be considered a
_____. If the procedure does not proceed _____, you should be willing and prepared to perform a cesarean delivery promptly.

D8. Forceps or vacuum extractor should *never* be applied unless
  1. _____ and
  2. _____.

D9. Match the procedures in the left column with the best choice from the right.
  ___ Low forceps   a. Contraindicated before 35 weeks' gestation
  ___ Midforceps   b. Fetal head is below +2 station
  ___ Vacuum extraction   c. Use is seldom indicated

Check your answers with the list that follows the Recommended Routines. Correct any incorrect answers and review the appropriate section in the unit.

11. What Are the Maternal Risks of Prolonged Labor or Difficult Delivery?

Maternal and fetal risks may not end with birth of the baby. You should anticipate possible complications, and continue to monitor the woman and newborn after delivery.

A. Prolonged Labor

Prolonged labor carries an increased risk of infection. Keep digital examinations to a minimum and monitor for signs of maternal infection, including postpartum endometritis.

Review the indications for intrapartum antibiotics. (See Unit 3, Perinatal Infections, in this book, in particular the group B beta-hemolytic streptococci section.)

B. Prolonged Labor or Difficult Delivery

1. *Lacerations of the Birth Canal*

Lacerations of the cervix, vagina, and/or perineum, with tears that may extend into the rectum or parametrium (area around the cervix and lower uterus), may occur. After delivery, visually inspect the birth canal.

329

2. *Postpartum Hemorrhage*

This is more common when

- Long labor leads to a fatigued uterus, which may fail to contract well after delivery.
- Second stage of labor was delayed due to hypotonic uterine dysfunction.
- Chorioamnionitis was present
- Forceps or VE were used.

3. *Maternal Exhaustion*

This may interfere with a woman's ability to interact with and care for her newborn.

4. *Macrosomic Fetus*

Excessively large fetuses are associated with prolonged labor. Delivery of a macrosomic fetus carries additional risks. (See Book I: Maternal and Fetal Evaluation and Immediate Newborn Care, Unit 6, Gestational Age and Size and Associated Risk Factors; and Book II: Maternal and Fetal Care, Unit 4, Various High-Risk Conditions, and Unit 5, Abnormal Glucose Tolerance.)

C. Cesarean Delivery

If required, cesarean delivery carries the risks associated with any surgery and use of anesthesia.

12. What Are the Fetal and Neonatal Risks of Prolonged Labor?

A. Prolonged Labor Risks

By itself, lengthy labor usually does not cause fetal harm but may increase the risk of neonatal infection.

- Review the baby's risk for infection; consider obtaining blood cultures.
- Observe and monitor for sign of infection.
- Begin antibiotics, if appropriate, based on risk factors and/or clinical condition. (See Book III: Neonatal Care, Unit 8, Infections.)

B. Management of Intervention Risks

1. *Oxytocin Augmentation*

This is associated with more frequent onset of abnormal fetal heart rate patterns, which is often related to uterine tachysystole.

2. *Operative Deliveries*

Mid-VE or midforceps deliveries are sometimes associated with shoulder dystocia, but neither is a cause of shoulder dystocia. Failure of fetal descent may be the cause for both the use of the instruments and the shoulder dystocia.

a. *Vacuum extraction*

Any of the following may occur as a result of a VE applied to the fetal scalp:

- Caput succedaneum
- Cephalohematoma
- Subgaleal hemorrhage (rare)
- Scalp avulsion or bleeding (rare)
- Intracranial bleeding (rare, but higher if gestational age is <34 weeks)

b. *Forceps delivery*

Any of the following may occur with a forceps delivery:
- Cephalohematoma
- Facial bruises or abrasions
- Subgaleal hemorrhage (rare)
- Facial nerve palsy (rare)
- Skull fracture (rare)
- Intracranial bleeding (rare)

3. *Maternal Medication*

Narcotics given to the woman close to delivery may cause the baby to be depressed at birth.

13. How Do You Recognize and Treat Precipitate Labor?

A. Risk Factors and Recognition

Precipitate labor cannot be predicted, although it is more often associated with high parity (several previous births) and oxytocin infusion during labor. If precipitate labor happened in one pregnancy, it is more likely to happen in a subsequent pregnancy, but it does not always recur. The onset of precipitate labor also may be triggered by placental abruption.

Rapid or tumultuous labor produces very strong contractions with very little relaxation time between contractions, accompanied by rapid cervical dilatation and rapid fetal descent. Because of the extremely forceful and frequent uterine contractions, fast labors are often accompanied by abnormal fetal heart rate patterns, stillbirth, and newborn depression. The rapid, forceful passage through the birth canal also may result in maternal trauma.

1. *Maternal*
   - *During labor:* Patients often complain of severe, nearly constant pain. Cervical dilatation progresses at a rate of 3 to 4 cm/hour, or faster. Uterine rupture can occur from the strong and frequent contractions.
   - *Postpartum*
     - Hemorrhage due to uterine atony
     - Lacerations of the birth canal and/or perineum
     - Disseminated intravascular coagulation, if abruptio placentae was the cause of the rapid labor

2. *Fetal*
   - Strong contractions in quick succession exert strong pressure, and rapid changes in pressure, on the fetal head.
   - Compression of placental blood flow may reduce oxygen exchange and lead to fetal compromise.
   - Rapid fetal descent and explosive delivery may lead to birth trauma.

3. *Neonatal*
   - Anticipate the possible need for neonatal resuscitation and, if needed, monitor for post-resuscitation complications.
   - Consider computed tomography scan to evaluate for subarachnoid, subdural, or intraventricular hemorrhage.
   - Assess for birth trauma, including bruising and/or fractures of the skull, humerus, or clavicles.

B. Treatment: If labor seems to be progressing with excessive speed,

1. *Discontinue Oxytocin* infusion *immediately* if being used.

2. *Monitor the Fetus* continuously.

3. *Provide In Utero Resuscitative Measures* if fetal distress develops.

4. *Check Cervical Dilatation* every 15 to 30 minutes.

5. *Consider Use of Tocolytic Agents.*
    If there is evidence of fetal compromise, tocolytic medication may be used to relax the uterus and decrease the frequency of uterine contractions. Appropriate medications include
    *   Terbutaline, 0.25 mg, subcutaneously
    OR
    *   Magnesium sulfate 6 g *slow* IV push (over 20 minutes), followed by IV infusion of 1 to 2 g/hour
    Tocolytic medications are particularly important when fetal compromise is present, during preparation for emergency vaginal or cesarean delivery.

6. *Consider Possibility of Abruptio Placentae.*
    Placental abruption may irritate the uterus and cause tumultuous labor. Refer to evaluation and management of abruption in Unit 2, Obstetric Hemorrhage, in this book.

7. *Prepare for Delivery.*
    There often is little that can be done to slow precipitate labor. Anticipate the possible complications the woman and the newborn may have, and be prepared to treat them.

Self-test

Now answer these questions to test yourself on the information in the last section.

E1. With precipitate labor, fetal distress may develop due to _____

_____.

E2. Which of the following risks are increased with *precipitate* labor?

Yes	No	
____	____	Facial nerve palsy
____	____	Maternal pulmonary edema
____	____	Fetal intracranial hemorrhage
____	____	Fetal distress
____	____	Broken clavicle
____	____	Uterine rupture
____	____	Perineal tears

E3. Which of the following risks are increased with *prolonged* labor?

Yes	No	
____	____	Postpartum hemorrhage
____	____	Postpartum endometritis
____	____	Birth canal lacerations
____	____	Neonatal infection
____	____	Abruptio placentae
____	____	Disseminated intravascular coagulation
____	____	Maternal hypertension

E4. Which of the following risks are increased with *forceps or vacuum extractor* deliveries?

Yes	No	
___	___	Fetal intracranial hemorrhage
___	___	Cephalohematoma
___	___	Birth canal lacerations
___	___	Neonatal infection
___	___	Facial nerve palsy
___	___	Postpartum hemorrhage

E5. Which of the following actions should be taken when precipitate labor is identified?

Immediately	Within Several Minutes	Not Indicated	
___	___	___	Check maternal blood pressure.
___	___	___	Stop oxytocin, if infusing.
___	___	___	Check cervical dilatation.
___	___	___	Check fetal station.
___	___	___	Perform emergency cesarean delivery.
___	___	___	Check fetal heart rate pattern.

Check your answers with the list that follows the Recommended Routines. Correct any incorrect answers and review the appropriate section in the unit.

14. How Should You Handle Emergent, or Potentially Emergent, Conditions During Labor?

A. Obstetric Hemorrhage (See Unit 2, Obstetric Hemorrhage, in this book.)

B. Meconium-Stained Amniotic Fluid

1. *Risk for Meconium Aspiration*
   - May occur in normal pregnancies and labors.
   - Is more common with breech presentation and in post-term pregnancies.
   - May be associated with a hypoxic event, which may cause relaxation of the rectal sphincter and release of meconium.

   Regardless of the reason meconium came to be in the amniotic fluid, its presence places the baby at risk for meconium aspiration. Severe neonatal respiratory distress may result from meconium aspiration.

2. *Warning Sign for Possible Fetal Distress*
   If meconium-stained fluid is seen when the membranes rupture, begin fetal heart rate and uterine contraction monitoring, if not already initiated. Anticipate possible fetal distress and need for neonatal resuscitation.

3. *Management at Delivery*
   Previous guidelines recommended that the upper pharynx of a baby born from meconium-stained fluid be suctioned after delivery of the head, but before delivery of the shoulders. A recent multicenter randomized trial showed that this practice did not result in lowering the incidence of neonatal meconium aspiration syndrome. Therefore, national guidelines no longer recommend this practice as a routine

procedure.* However, clearing meconium from a baby's nose and mouth is still a good practice, as long as it does not delay handing the newborn to the pediatrics team for further management.

See Book I: Maternal and Fetal Evaluation and Immediate Newborn Care, Unit 5, Resuscitating the Newborn, for additional, *essential* information about delivery room management. For nonvigorous babies, endotracheal suctioning is indicated to suction the trachea directly and help prevent meconium aspiration syndrome.

C. Fetal Heart Rate Abnormalities (See Book I: Maternal and Fetal Evaluation and Immediate Newborn Care, Unit 3, Fetal Well-being.)

1. *Provide In Utero Resuscitation*

Whenever there is a non-reassuring fetal heart rate pattern, quickly provide in utero resuscitative measures.

- Turn off oxytocin, if used.
- Position the woman on her left side (if already on left side, turn to right side or put in knee-chest position).
- Give 100% oxygen by mask.
- Increase rate of IV fluid infusion.
- Check maternal blood pressure.
- Perform a vaginal examination to assess labor progress and determine whether umbilical cord prolapse is present.

Employ other measures, according to individual situation.

- Elevate fetal head off prolapsed cord.
- Consider tocolytic drugs to relax the uterus.
- Ask the woman to stop pushing.

2. *Prepare for Emergency Delivery and Neonatal Resuscitation*

If a non-reassuring or ominous pattern continues, proceed with emergency cesarean section, or assisted vaginal delivery, depending on fetal station and the speed with which a vaginal delivery can safely be accomplished. Be prepared for resuscitation of the newborn.

D. Maternal Analgesia and/or Anesthesia

1. *Medications, Dosage, and Timing of Administration*

Use the least amount of analgesic needed to make the woman comfortable. Recommended medications include

- Meperidine (Demerol): 25 to 50 mg, intravenously, every 1 to 2 hours, or 50 to 100 mg, intramuscularly, every 2 to 4 hours
- Butorphanol tartrate (Stadol) 1 to 2 mg, intramuscularly or intravenously, every 2 to 4 hours
- Fentanyl 50 to 100 mcg, intravenously, every 1 to 2 hours

For all these medications, dosage and frequency of administration should be determined according to each woman's individual response to them. Analgesia, with small, patient-controlled, IV boluses, is often used.

---

*Kattwinkel J, Perlman JM, Aziz K, et al. American Heart Association guidelines for cardiopulmonary resuscitation and emergency cardiovascular care of pediatric and neonatal patients: neonatal resuscitation guidelines. *Circulation.* 122:S909-S919;2010.

Narcotics given to a laboring woman can cause neonatal depression, particularly if multiple doses are given over time or large doses are given close to delivery. Although these drugs readily cross the placenta, the time of peak fetal tissue concentration does not occur until 2 or 3 hours after administration of the medication to the woman. Therefore, avoid giving large doses of narcotics if delivery is anticipated to occur within 2 to 3 hours.

2. *Consider Possibility of Maternal Substance Use:* Excessive need for narcotic analgesia may indicate drug addiction.

3. *Effects on Laboring Woman*
   Heavy narcotic analgesia early in labor may result in a prolonged latent phase. Late in labor, heavy narcotic analgesia or epidural or spinal anesthesia may result in a prolonged second stage. In addition, narcotic analgesia may depress maternal respirations.

4. *Effects on Fetus and Newborn*
   Small amounts of narcotics given to a laboring woman usually do not depress a healthy fetus, unless multiple doses are given over a long labor. They do, however, cause diminished fetal heart rate variability.

   Epidural, spinal, or general anesthesia generally do not, by themselves, adversely affect the fetus. However, if anesthesia causes maternal hypotension (low blood pressure), the fetus may be compromised by poor blood flow to the placenta with subsequent fetal distress.

   If the baby is depressed at birth,
   - Assist ventilation, as necessary; give oxygen, as appropriate.
   - *After* the baby is stable and well-oxygenated, consider use of naloxone HCl (Narcan) to reverse the effects of narcotics given to the mother. Narcan is *not* a resuscitation drug and should be used only after a depressed baby is resuscitated. (See Book I: Maternal and Fetal Evaluation and Immediate Newborn Care, Unit 5, Resuscitating the Newborn.)
   - Be cautious about the use of naloxone if maternal drug addiction is suspected. In this situation, naloxone administration may precipitate acute withdrawal reaction in the baby.

E. Prolapsed Umbilical Cord

   1. *Risk Factors*
      Prolapse of the umbilical cord cannot be predicted, but certain conditions increase the risk of occurrence. The possibility of cord prolapse should be considered and/or investigated if any of the following risk factors are present:
      - Cord presentation
      - Preterm labor
      - Spontaneous premature rupture of membranes
      - Artificial rupture of membranes before the presenting part is engaged
      - Non-vertex presentation
      - Hydramnios
      - Multifetal gestation

2. *Diagnosis*

- Variable fetal heart rate decelerations are associated with cord compression, which can occur when the cord is compressed between a fetal part and the uterine wall. The sudden onset of deep variable fetal heart rate declarations is often the first sign of cord prolapse.
- Prolapse may be visible or hidden. A prolapsed cord may be felt in the vagina or it may be palpable, through intact membranes, in front of the presenting part (cord presentation).

3. *Management*

 Umbilical cord prolapse is a fetal emergency. Fetal asphyxia can occur. Prompt intervention is essential to preserve or restore fetal health.

- If the diagnosis is clear, continue external fetal monitoring and perform emergency cesarean delivery as soon as possible.
- If fetal heart rate monitoring indicates fetal compromise, elevate the fetal presenting part off the prolapsed cord until a cesarean delivery can be performed.
- The following maneuvers may lift the presenting part off the cord without compressing the cord in the vagina:
  - Insert a gloved hand into the woman's vagina and hold the presenting part off the cord.
  - Insert a Foley catheter into the woman's bladder, fill it with 400 to 500 mL of sterile saline, and put the patient in knee-chest position.

4. *Neonatal Care:* Be prepared for prompt and aggressive resuscitation. If resuscitation is needed, monitor for possible post-resuscitation complications.

F. Shoulder Dystocia (impaction of the fetal shoulders after delivery of the head)

1. *Risk Factors*

Risk increases as fetal weight increases, but does not always occur, even with the largest babies, and is possible with all but the smallest fetuses. Large fetal size, therefore, increases the risk, but is not predictive of the occurrence of shoulder dystocia.

Women who gave birth to one macrosomic baby are more likely to have macrosomic babies in subsequent pregnancies. Women with abnormal glucose tolerance or diabetes mellitus are also more likely to have large babies. Many large babies, however, are born to women with no known risk factors.

Neither estimated fetal weight nor labor progress is a good predictor of shoulder dystocia. Pregnancy and labor may be uncomplicated until the shoulders become impacted after delivery of the head. The majority of shoulder dystocia deliveries occur in women without apparent risk factors.

 Shoulder dystocia is unpredictable. You should be prepared for the possibility of shoulder dystocia with every delivery.

2. *Diagnosis*

The baby's head delivers and promptly "snaps back" against the woman's perineum. The usual traction on the head does not produce delivery of the anterior shoulder. At this point, care must be taken to avoid excess traction on the head because undue force may injure the brachial plexus (bundle of nerves in the neck) and result in temporary or permanent paralysis of the arm on the injured side.

3. *Management**

When shoulder dystocia occurs, it suddenly poses immediate and grave danger to the fetus.

 Urgent and coordinated action is needed. If the shoulders remain trapped, severe damage or fetal death may result from asphyxia within minutes of delivery of the head.

Summon additional help to the delivery room immediately, including nursing, anesthesiology, and a pediatrics team prepared for resuscitation.

Systematically and quickly carry out the following steps, until delivery is accomplished.

Primary Maneuvers

a. *Thigh flexion (McRoberts maneuver)*
   • With her legs out of stirrups, help the woman flex her hips by pulling her thighs onto her abdomen and chest, so her knees are near her breasts. Ask the woman to grasp tightly behind her knees to hold this position (Figure 9.7).

b. *Suprapubic pressure*
   • One person then applies pressure on the baby's anterior shoulder by pressing downward and laterally on the woman's abdomen, just above the symphysis pubis (suprapubic pressure), while another person exerts gentle downward traction on the baby's head (not shown).

Often, McRoberts maneuver and suprapubic pressure result promptly in delivery of the anterior shoulder. If delivery does not occur, however, proceed quickly to

Secondary Maneuvers

Secondary maneuvers are those that require intravaginal manipulation of the baby's position to rotate the shoulders out of the vertical orientation. The order in which secondary maneuvers are applied is dictated by the orientation of the baby (right vs left occiput transverse), by the amount of space available within the vagina for manipulation and, to some extent, by the "handedness" of the operator (right vs left).

a. *Woods screw maneuver*
   • To rotate the shoulders into an oblique orientation, pressure is applied by the operator against the clavicle of the posterior shoulder to effect rotation. In some

*Many of the techniques described here are shown in a video developed at Dartmouth-Hitchcock Medical Center and available from that institution (www.dhmc.org/goto/regionalprogram, click on Best Practices & Protocols) or through the American College of Obstetricians and Gynecologists Bookstore. William Young, MD. *Shoulder Dystocia Drill.* 1995 Updated version pending.

337

Sharp flexion of the maternal hips increases the useful size of the pelvic outlet. Note the change in relationship of the pelvic bones with full hip flexion.

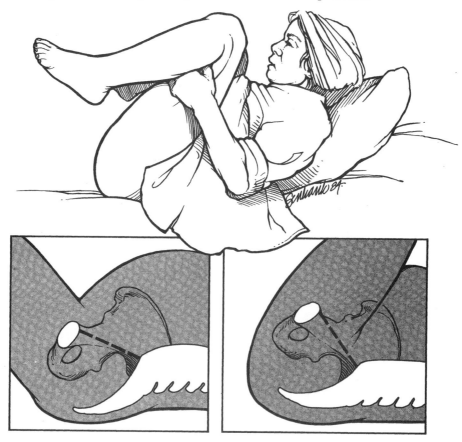

Figure 9.7. Thigh Flexion for Treatment of Shoulder Dystocia.
Reproduced with permission from Gabbe SG, Niebyl JR, Simpson JL, eds. *Obstetrics: Normal and Problem Pregnancies.* 3rd ed. New York, NY: Churchill Livingstone; 1996:492.

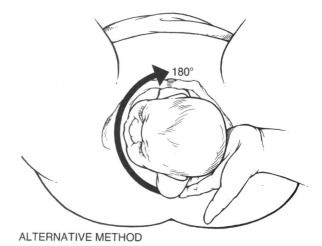

ALTERNATIVE METHOD

Forward rotation of the posterior shoulder is more likely to compress the shoulder girdle (reducing its size) than backward rotation.

Figure 9.8. Shoulder Rotation for Treatment of Shoulder Dystocia.
Reproduced with permission from Gabbe SG, Niebyl JR, Simpson JL, eds. *Obstetrics: Normal and Problem Pregnancies.* 3rd ed. New York, NY: Churchill Livingstone; 1996:493.

cases, it is necessary to rotate the posterior arm and shoulder 180° so that the posterior shoulder becomes the anterior shoulder. This is done by pushing the posterior shoulder forward (Figure 9.8).

b. Rubin maneuver

- Either alone, or in conjunction with Woods maneuver, pressure is applied to either the anterior or posterior scapula, again attempting to rotate the shoulders into an oblique orientation.

- Simultaneously, a second person applies suprapubic pressure on the anterior shoulder (wedged against the symphysis pubis) by pressing on the lower maternal abdomen (not shown).

If shoulder rotation was not successful, proceed immediately to

c. *Delivery of the posterior arm (Barnum maneuver)*

Often, it is only the anterior shoulder that is impacted. The posterior pelvis may be roomy. Delivery of the posterior arm is almost always successful in freeing the shoulders, but is more likely to be accompanied by fracture of the humerus or clavicle than the shoulder rotation maneuver (Figure 9.9).

A: Insert your hand into the vagina, posterior to the baby, grasp the posterior arm from the shoulder to the elbow, and slide it across the baby's chest.

B: Then grasp the hand.

C: Bring the hand and arm forward out of the vagina.

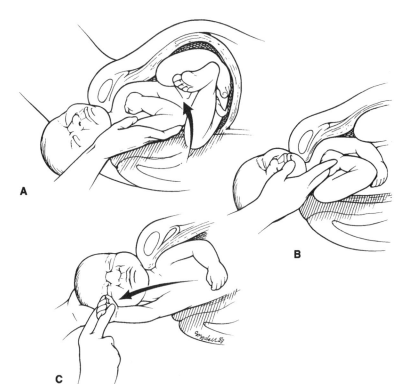

Figure 9.9. Delivery of the Posterior Arm.
Reproduced with permission from Cunningham FG, MacDonald PC, Gant NF, et al. *Williams Obstetrics.* 20th ed. Stamford, CT: Appleton & Lange; 1997:453.

If the baby is still not delivered, proceed to

    d. *Cephalic replacement (Zavanelli maneuver):* Replace the fetal head into the pelvis before delivering the baby by cesarean section.

- Occasionally, by grasping the head and turning it from side to side (rotation should not exceed 90° in either direction), the head will retract into the vagina.
- Do *not* push the head inward. If it is going to retract, it will do so by itself, from the upward pull of the extended shoulders.
- Perform an immediate cesarean section.
- Continue to monitor the fetal heart rate while waiting for cesarean delivery. If fetal bradycardia occurs, cord compression may be present and may be relieved by

    – Further elevation of the head by putting the woman in knee-chest position AND/OR

    – Administration of tocolytic drugs to diminish uterine contractions

      o Terbutaline, 0.25 mg, subcutaneously

      OR

      o Magnesium sulfate 4 to 6 g, intravenously over 20 minutes

4. *Postdelivery Considerations*

    Maternal: Check for vaginal, cervical, perineal, and/or rectal lacerations.

    Neonatal

- Be prepared for prompt and aggressive resuscitation. If needed, monitor for possible post-resuscitation complications.
- Obtain x-ray(s) if there is reason to suspect fracture of the humerus or clavicle.
- Evaluate for brachial plexus nerve injury (Erb palsy).

15. How Should You Manage an Abnormal Third Stage of Labor?

The third stage of labor lasts from delivery of the baby to delivery of the placenta, which is normally a period of less than 30 minutes. After delivery of the baby, the placenta usually separates from the uterine wall because of continued uterine contractions. Once separated, it descends into the cervix and is then expelled from the vagina by the pushing efforts of the woman.

When the placenta has not been delivered within 30 minutes after delivery of the baby, it should be removed manually. The clinical situations fall into 2 main categories: excessive bleeding and little or no bleeding.

 Do not give oxytocin until the placenta has been delivered.

A. Excessive Bleeding (See Unit 2, Obstetric Hemorrhage, in this book.)

While there is normally a gush of blood from the vagina immediately following separation of the placenta from the uterine wall, continued uterine contractions stop excessive blood flow. If heavy bleeding persists, life-threatening hemorrhage can result. If the placenta separates but is not expelled from the uterus, the bulk of the placenta prevents the uterus from contracting enough to close off the bleeding arteries and veins.

Take the following steps to deliver the placenta:

1. *Insert One Hand Into the Vagina and Explore the Cervix.* If the placenta can be felt, grasp it and pull it out. Puncturing the placenta with your fingers is appropriate if you need to do so to get a grip on it.

2. *If the Placenta Cannot Be Felt in the Cervix, Continue Upward Into the Uterus.* Grasp the placenta and pull it out of the uterus.

3. *Inspect the Placenta* carefully for missing pieces. If fragments are missing, explore the uterus again for the remaining pieces.

   If available, anesthesia should be given to the mother. If the bleeding is profuse, however, there may not be time to wait for anesthesia personnel. In this case, IV sedation with narcotics and/or tranquilizers may be helpful.

B. Little or No Bleeding

Examine the vagina and cervix for the placenta. If it is not there, *do NOT enter the uterus.* The placenta has not separated from the uterine wall and manually separating it may cause hemorrhage. General anesthesia will probably be required to relax the uterus enough to get your hand inside.

1. *Make the Following Preparations Before Attempting to Remove the Placenta:*
   a. *Summon anesthesia personnel.*
   b. *Send blood for crossmatching.* Ask that at least 2 units be set up.
   c. *Start an IV line or increase the infusion rate of an existing IV line.*

2. *As Soon as Blood is Available and the Woman Has Been Anesthetized*
   a. *Explore the uterus and find the placental edge.*
      If a distinct placental edge can be felt, systematically loosen the adhered areas of the placenta. Once separated, grasp the placenta and pull it out of the uterus.
      - Place one hand on the abdomen to hold the fundus in place.
      - Insert your other hand into the uterus. Using your fingertips held together, with the palm of your hand facing the inside of the uterus (back of your hand against the uterine wall), begin to work your fingers under the edge of the placenta.
      - Proceed until the placenta separates completely.
   b. *If a distinct placental edge cannot be found, STOP.*
      Placenta accreta may be present. Placenta accreta occurs when the tissue of the placenta invades the uterine wall, making separation of the placenta impossible. Massive hemorrhage may result, particularly if efforts to separate the placenta continue and uterine rupture occurs. Because the placenta has grown into the uterus and cannot be separated from it, an abdominal hysterectomy is almost always required to remove it.

Self-test

Now answer these questions to test yourself on the information in the last section.

F1. Which of the following factors are associated with increased risk for umbilical cord prolapse?

Yes	No	
____	____	Maternal obesity
____	____	Premature rupture of membranes
____	____	Non-vertex presentation
____	____	Multifetal gestation
____	____	Preterm labor
____	____	Hydramnios
____	____	Growth-restricted fetus

F2. When an umbilical cord prolapses, what should you do in the time between diagnosis and emergency cesarean delivery?

_____

_____

F3. **True** **False** Meconium in the amniotic fluid always indicates that an episode of fetal compromise has occurred.

F4. **True** **False** If a woman received large or frequent doses of narcotic medication during labor, and the baby is born depressed, naloxone HCl (Narcan) should be given *immediately* in the delivery room.

F5. **True** **False** Only babies weighing 4,000 g or more are at risk for shoulder dystocia.

F6. **True** **False** If maternal anesthesia causes hypotension, the fetus may be compromised because of poor blood flow to the placenta.

F7. **True** **False** If a woman is addicted to narcotics, drug withdrawal reaction in the baby may be brought on by administration of neonatal naloxone.

F8. **True** **False** There is an increased risk of umbilical cord prolapse with vaginal delivery of twins.

F9. **True** **False** Delivery of the placenta should occur spontaneously within 30 minutes of the birth of the baby.

F10. Meconium in the amniotic fluid

Yes	No	
____	____	May be a sign of fetal compromise
____	____	Occurs more frequently in post-term pregnancies
____	____	May lead to meconium aspiration
____	____	May be a normal finding

F11. Describe the McRoberts maneuver: _____

_____

F12. **True** **False** When umbilical cord prolapse occurs, the fetal heart rate pattern seen most often is sudden development of *late* decelerations.

F13. **True** **False** Severe neonatal respiratory distress may result from meconium aspiration.

F14. **True** **False** Unless shoulder dystocia is treated and the baby is delivered within minutes, death or severe asphyxia may occur.

F15. **True** **False** Placenta accreta is best managed by separation of the adherent areas of the placenta with your fingertips.

F16. Which of the following events can be predicted before they occur?
- **A.** Umbilical cord prolapse
- **B.** Precipitate labor
- **C.** Shoulder dystocia
- **D.** All of the above
- **E.** None of the above

F17. Which of the following options are part of in utero resuscitative measures that should be taken whenever a non-reassuring fetal heart rate pattern develops?

Yes	No	
____	____	Turn off oxytocin infusion, if being used.
____	____	Check for prolapsed umbilical cord.
____	____	Check maternal blood pressure.
____	____	Give the woman 100% oxygen by mask.
____	____	Turn the woman onto her side.
____	____	Obtain vaginal culture, then begin broad-spectrum antibiotics.
____	____	Give fentanyl, 50 micrograms (μg), intravenously.

Check your answers with the list that follows the Recommended Routines. Correct any incorrect answers and review the appropriate section in the unit.

343

Abnormal Labor Progress and Difficult Deliveries

Recommended Routines

All the routines listed below are based on the principles of perinatal care presented in the unit you have just finished. They are recommended as part of routine perinatal care.

Read each routine carefully and decide whether it is standard operating procedure in your hospital. Check the appropriate blank next to each routine.

Procedure Standard in My Hospital	Needs Discussion by Our Staff	
_____	_____	1. Establish a protocol for the assessment of women in questionable labor, including documentation of • Cervical dilatation • Fetal presentation • Contraction characteristics • Care provided • Response to therapy
_____	_____	2. Establish guidelines for the augmentation of labor (see also Unit 8, Inducing and Augmenting Labor in this book), including documentation of • Factors that indicate the need for oxytocin • Evaluation done to rule out contraindications to the use of oxytocin • Uniform dilution for oxytocin • Standard interval for the rate of infusion change
_____	_____	3. Establish guidelines for the use and application of forceps and vacuum extractor. For midforceps or mid-vacuum extractor, establish guidelines for personnel and readiness for immediate cesarean delivery if the trial fails.
_____	_____	4. Establish guidelines for response to precipitate labor.
_____	_____	5. Establish guidelines for response to emergent or potentially emergent, fetal situations, including • Meconium-stained amniotic fluid • Fetal heart rate abnormalities • Complications of maternal anesthesia or narcotic analgesia • Prolapsed umbilical cord • Shoulder dystocia
_____	_____	6. Develop a system whereby an emergency cesarean delivery can be started within a maximum of 30 minutes, at any time of the day or night.

345

Self-test Answers

These are the answers to the self-test questions. Please check them with the answers you gave and review the information in the unit wherever necessary.

A1. True

A2. True

A3. Protracted

A4. Prolonged

A5. Arrest of descent or arrested second stage

A6. The first stage of labor starts with the onset of true labor and continues until *the cervix is fully dilated.* The second stage of labor starts with *full cervical dilatation* and continues until *delivery of the baby.* The third stage of labor starts following *delivery of the baby* and ends with *delivery of the placenta.* The "fourth stage" of labor starts following *delivery of the placenta* and ends *an hour later.* It is the time when the risk of postpartum hemorrhage is the *greatest.*

A7. 1.2 to 3 cm/hour for primipara, 1.5 to 6 cm/hour for multipara

A8. *Active phase:* primigravidas: up to 6 hours (6 hours or less), multigravidas: up to 6 hours (6 hours or less)

A9. *Second* stage *usual length:* primigravidas = 2 hours or less, multigravidas = 1 hour or less (5 hours is *acceptable* as long as the woman and fetus are well and labor progress [fetal descent] is being made).

A10. First stage of labor = cervical dilatation; second stage of labor = fetal descent

B1.

Yes	No	
X	___	Fetopelvic disproportion
X	___	Large fetus
___	X	Post-term pregnancy
X	___	Hydramnios
X	___	Uterus that is contracting poorly
X	___	Malpositioned fetus
___	X	Woman addicted to cocaine

B2.

Yes	No	
X	___	Fetopelvic disproportion
X	___	Inadequate pushing
X	___	Fetal malposition
X	___	Hypotonic uterine dysfunction

B3. *Protracted* (cervical dilatation has progressed at <2 cm/hour = slow rate for a primigravida, <1.5 cm/hour = slow for a multipara) and *prolonged* (>6 hours since 5-cm dilatation, and 10 cm not yet reached) *active phase* (See Table 9.2.)

B4. False.   In about 10% of labors with abnormal progress, a clear cause is never found.

B5. True

B6. True

B7. Any 4 of the following:
- Application of head to the cervix is poor
- Deflexed head
- Unengaged head
- Poor contractions
- Continuous contractions, seemingly without letup
- Edema of the cervix
- Pushing uncontrollably before complete dilatation

B8. a Minimal pain
    a Usually responds well to oxytocin treatment
    b Elevated baseline tonus
    b Fetal distress more common
    a Normal baseline tonus
    b Nearly continuous contractions

B9. Passage, passenger, and/or power, and sometimes psyche

C1. True

C2. True

C3. True

C4. True

C5. True

C6. True

C7 True

C8. True

C9. True

C10. An extremity presents alongside the presenting part.

C11. The uterus does not relax between contractions or contracts in an uncoordinated way.

C12. A

C13. D

C14. Fetal malposition or malpresentation; fetopelvic disproportion

C15.

Yes	No	
___	X	Hypertonic uterine dysfunction during the active phase
X	___	Secondary arrest of labor
X	___	Hypotonic uterine dysfunction during the deceleration phase
X	___	Hypotonic uterine dysfunction during the active phase

C16. True

C17. True

D1. False. Use of low forceps is appropriate to speed delivery when there is evidence of fetal distress, for delayed or arrested second stage (no fetopelvic disproportion or malposition), or for ineffective maternal pushing.

D2. True

D3. False. Outlet forceps delivery has the same risk of perinatal morbidity as spontaneous vaginal delivery.

D4. True

D5. True

D6. A

D7. Trial; easily or smoothly

D8. 1. Cervix is completely dilated 2. Fetal head is engaged.

D9.
b	Low forceps	a. Contraindicated before 35 weeks' gestation.
c	Midforceps	b. Fetal head is below +2 station.
a	Vacuum extraction	c. Use is seldom indicated.

E1. Frequent and strong compression of the placenta, which can interfere with normal oxygen exchange

E2.
Yes	No	
	X	Facial nerve palsy
	X	Maternal pulmonary edema
X		Intracranial hemorrhage
X		Fetal distress
X		Broken clavicle
X		Uterine rupture
X		Perineal tears

E3.
Yes	No	
X		Postpartum hemorrhage
X		Postpartum endometritis
X		Birth canal lacerations
X		Neonatal infection
	X	Abruptio placentae
	X	Disseminated intravascular coagulation
	X	Maternal hypertension

E4.
Yes	No	
X		Fetal Intracranial hemorrhage
X		Cephalhematoma
X		Birth canal lacerations
	X	Neonatal infection
X		Facial nerve palsy
X		Postpartum hemorrhage

E5.
Immediately	Within Several Minutes	Not Indicated	
	X		Check maternal blood pressure.
X			Stop oxytocin, if infusing.
	X		Check cervical dilatation.
	X		Check fetal station.
		X	Perform emergency cesarean delivery.
X			Check fetal heart rate pattern.

F1.
Yes	No	
	X	Maternal obesity
X		Premature rupture of membranes
X		Non-vertex presentation
X		Multifetal gestation
X		Preterm labor
X		Hydramnios
	X	Growth-restricted fetus

F2. Elevate fetal presenting part off the prolapsed cord by

1. Inserting gloved hand into the vagina and elevating the presenting part

OR

2. Placing a Foley catheter into the bladder and infusing 400 to 500 mL of sterile saline, then positioning the patient in knee-chest position

F3. False. Meconium in the amniotic fluid MAY indicate fetal distress and should be considered a warning sign for possible distress. In utero passage of meconium also may occur in uncomplicated pregnancies and labors and is more common with post-term gestation and breech presentation.

F4. **False.** If a baby is depressed at birth, resuscitative measures should be done FIRST. After the baby is stabilized, it may be appropriate to give Narcan, if excessive maternal narcotic analgesia is the likely reason for the baby's depression.

F5. **False.** Shoulder dystocia is unpredictable and can occur with delivery of all but the smallest babies.

F6. True

F7. True

F8. True

F9. True

F10.

Yes	No	
X	____	May be a sign of fetal distress
X	____	Occurs more frequently in post-term pregnancies
X	____	May lead to meconium aspiration
X	____	May be a normal finding

F11. Sharp flexion of the woman's hips by maximal flexion of her thighs onto her abdomen; used to free the anterior shoulder when shoulder dystocia occurs

F12. **False.** Variable decelerations are associated with compression of the umbilical cord. When cord prolapse occurs, the fetal heart rate pattern seen most often is *sudden onset* of *deep variable* decelerations.

F13. True

F14. True

F15. **False.** Attempts to separate a placenta accreta are likely to result in severe hemorrhage and/or uterine rupture. A hysterectomy is almost always the only way to remove the placenta.

F16. E. None of the above. (While each condition listed is associated with certain risk factors, and is more likely to occur in pregnancies with those corresponding factors, none can be predicted and each may occur in any pregnancy.)

F17.

Yes	No	
X	____	Turn off oxytocin infusion, if being used.
X	____	Check for prolapsed umbilical cord.
X	____	Check maternal blood pressure.
X	____	Give 100% oxygen by mask.
X	____	Turn the woman onto her side.
____	X	Obtain vaginal culture, then begin broad-spectrum antibiotics.
____	X	Give fentanyl, 50 µg, intravenously.

Unit 9 Posttest

If you are applying for continuing education credits, a posttest for this unit is available online. Completion of unit posttests and the book evaluation form are required to achieve continuing education credit. For more details, visit www.cmevillage.com.

Unit 10: Imminent Delivery and Preparation for Maternal/Fetal Transport

Objectives

In this unit you will learn

Imminent Delivery

A. What actions to take, and not take, when delivery is about to occur unexpectedly

B. How to assist the woman in achieving a safe delivery with
- Vertex presentation
- Breech presentation

C. What to do after the baby is born

D. What to do, and not do, for delivery of the placenta

E. How to recognize and respond to an abnormal third stage of labor

Preparation for Maternal/Fetal Transport

A. Which pregnant women may benefit from transport

B. Primary goals for preparing a pregnant woman for transport

C. Which pregnant women should not be transported

D. How to prepare a pregnant woman for transport

Unit 10 Pretest

Before reading the unit, please answer the following questions. Select the *one best* answer to each question (unless otherwise instructed). Record your answers on the test and check them against the answers at the end of the book.

1. If the head of a baby delivers and the woman gives several strong pushes, but the shoulders do not deliver, you should

Yes	No	
___	___	Move the woman immediately to the operating room.
___	___	Ask the woman to grasp her legs behind the knees and pull them to her chest.
___	___	Tell the woman to rest and try pushing again in several minutes.
___	___	Put the head of the bed flat.
___	___	Press down on the woman's abdomen, just above the symphysis pubis, while gentle downward traction is placed on the baby's head by a second person.

2. All of the following indicate delivery of a baby is imminent, *except:*

A. A sudden gush of blood

B. Anus dilates and anterior wall of the rectum becomes visible

C. Perineum bulges

D. Woman states that the baby is coming

3. Which of the following is appropriate when imminent delivery is recognized?

Yes	No	
___	___	Tell the woman that she will need to push, or stop pushing, as you direct.
___	___	Ask the woman to assume knee-chest position until her physician arrives.
___	___	Call for help, but do not leave the woman.
___	___	Assist the woman to deliver where she is.
___	___	Move the woman immediately to a delivery room.

4. True   False   When a woman with a known placenta previa, at 30 weeks' gestation, and on bed rest in your hospital, begins to have bright red spotting, she should be transferred immediately to the regional perinatal center for delivery.

5. True   False   A gush of blood from the vagina normally follows placental separation.

6. True   False   If a baby is in breech presentation, you should wrap a dry towel around the baby's legs and hips and begin to pull gently but steadily.

7. The *first* thing to do after the baby's head delivers is to
   A. Begin delivery of the shoulders
   B. Suction the baby's nose
   C. Tell the mother to stop pushing
   D. Check for a nuchal cord

8. If the placenta does not separate within 30 minutes after birth of a baby, and there is no bleeding, which of the following should you do *first*?
   A. Pull gently but steadily on the umbilical cord.
   B. Do nothing while you wait for spontaneous separation.
   C. Call for anesthesia staff and start an intravenous line.
   D. Insert a gloved hand into the vagina, through the cervix, and into the uterus to remove the placenta.

9. True   False   Immediately after a baby is born, you should tug firmly on the placental end of the umbilical cord to begin delivery of the placenta.

10. True   False   It is best to transport a woman with severe preeclampsia for delivery at a regional perinatal center as soon as her blood pressure elevation of 190/110 is noted.

11. True   False   It would generally be considered safe to transport a woman in early labor at 32 weeks' gestation, 4 cm dilated, and 80% effaced to a regional center an hour away for delivery at the center.

Imminent Delivery

1. What Is an Imminent Delivery?

An imminent delivery is one that is about to occur unexpectedly.

There are no emergent conditions, such as maternal hemorrhage or fetal bradycardia. It is simply a matter of labor progressing more quickly than anticipated.

Help should be sought as soon as the situation of imminent delivery is recognized. If maternal complications develop, or the baby requires resuscitation or is significantly preterm, prompt and aggressive intervention may be needed immediately and would require additional personnel. Management of those situations is not covered in this unit, but is covered in other maternal and fetal care and/or neonatal care units in the Perinatal Continuing Education Program series.

The material in this unit covers care of the woman and baby during a very short period. If delivery and the third stage of labor are uncomplicated, and the newborn is a healthy, term newborn, little additional care will be needed.

2. How Do You Know That Delivery Is Imminent?

Delivery will generally occur within moments when the

- Presenting part is visible in the vagina (almost always the baby's scalp and hair)
- Perineum bulges
- Anus dilates, and the anterior wall of the rectum is visible
- Woman cries out that the baby is coming

3. What Do You Do When You Recognize That Delivery Is Imminent?

A. Allow the Woman to Deliver Where She Is
You can be helpful to the woman and assist her with the delivery only if you respond to the situation where it occurs. You cannot help with the birth or care of the baby if you are pushing the bed to a delivery room.
If she is in a labor-delivery-recovery room, and the bed is in the "labor" position, leave it there. There is no need to convert it to the "delivery" configuration. If the woman is in the delivery room, leave the foot of the delivery table extended, like a bed. There is no need to put the woman's legs in stirrups.

 Call for help but stay with the patient.

Talk with the woman about what you and she need to do together to ensure a safe delivery. Calmly explain the situation to the woman with clear, direct instructions regarding her assistance.

B. Allow the Woman to Deliver the Baby Without Interference
If your call for help yielded a second person, that person should bring a kit for imminent delivery (KID) to the room where you are, and open the kit.
A KID is a packaged bundle of sterile supplies that is kept readily available in the labor area at all times and contains
- Two to 4 pairs of sterile gloves
- Bulb syringe, large-bore suction catheters, and meconium aspirator

- Two Kelly clamps or cord clamps (for clamping the cord)
- Scissors (to cut the cord)
- Box of sterile 4 × 4 gauze squares (to blot blood)
- Two towels (to dry the baby)
- Two baby blankets
- Stocking cap
- Resuscitation equipment and supplies for the baby

Depending on experience, one person becomes first assistant and the other becomes second assistant to the delivering woman. Inform the woman of what to expect and what she needs to do. Tell her she may need to push or to stop pushing, as directed. Reassure her that she will be able to do everything you ask her to do.

Delivery will occur. Do *not* try to delay it by crossing the woman's legs or pushing in against the baby's head. Work with the woman to accomplish a safe delivery.

4. What Do You Do When the Head Crowns?

As little as possible. An episiotomy is rarely necessary. Unless you have considerable skill and experience, allow the natural process to proceed without interference. In nearly all cases, the head will deliver spontaneously with minimal risk to either the woman or the baby.

If it is clear that the next push will be very forceful, tell the woman to push less vigorously and with more control. Ask her to breathe or "pant" and to stop pushing. She can push again with the next contraction. This will help keep the delivery from becoming explosive.

5. What Do You Do After the Head Delivers?

A. Check for a Nuchal Cord
- If the umbilical cord is wrapped around the baby's neck, see if you can pull out the loop. If you can, pull that over the baby's head and go on with the delivery.
- If the cord is tight and will not loosen easily, ask the mother not to push until the cord is free.
- Be very hesitant to clamp and cut the umbilical cord before delivery of the shoulders. If shoulder dystocia occurs, several minutes may elapse before the baby is delivered, and clamping the cord will have completely interrupted feto-placental blood flow and gas exchange.

B. Monitor Delivery of the Shoulders
- Encourage the woman to push, in control. Anytime it seems the baby is coming too fast, ask her to stop pushing.
- In the situation of spontaneous, unexpected delivery, the shoulders almost always will deliver unaided and without difficulty.
- If the shoulders do not deliver after 3 to 5 strong pushes, there may be shoulder dystocia. (See Unit 9, Abnormal Labor and Difficult Deliveries, in this book.)
Quickly do the following:
- Put the head of the bed flat (if not already flat).
- Have the woman grasp behind her knees and pull them to her chest (McRoberts maneuver).

These actions, by themselves, usually will bring about delivery of the shoulders.

If not, the perineum must be elevated far enough off the bed to allow gentle downward traction on the head by one person, while another person exerts pressure on the anterior shoulder by pressing on the woman's abdomen, just above the symphysis pubis. Elevation of the perineum will not be needed if the woman is in a bed that can be instantly split to "delivery" configuration. That configuration allows room for gentle downward traction on the baby's head.

6. What Do You Do if the Baby Is Breech?

As little as possible. Babies in breech presentation, either full-term or preterm, that come this fast usually deliver easily and do well. Let the woman push the body of the baby out as far as she can.

 Do not, at any time, pull on the baby.

A. Delivery Up to the Umbilicus

Do *not* pull on the baby's body. Pulling on the baby may cause the arms and neck to extend (deflex the head), thereby impeding delivery. Pulling on the baby also may cause severe trauma to the spine and spinal cord. Until the body is delivered past the umbilicus, the baby is getting enough blood flow through the cord to provide adequate oxygenation.

B. Delivery Beyond the Umbilicus

1. Let the Woman Deliver the Baby

   If the woman can push the rest of the baby out within 5 minutes, let her. Do not intervene unless delivery is delayed beyond 5 minutes. Five minutes can seem like an eternity, but avoid interfering until it is clear that the woman cannot accomplish the delivery by herself.

2. If the Woman Cannot Deliver the Baby Within 5 Minutes

   • Wrap a dry towel around the baby. Hold the baby's legs and body together with both hands (Figure 10.1, towel not shown).
   Do *not* pull on the baby's legs, hips, or lower trunk.

   • Support the baby's body off the bed as rotation naturally occurs. Do not, however, attempt to rotate the baby. Just provide support as the natural process occurs.

   • **Lift,** but do *not* pull, the baby's hips and trunk upward as the arms and shoulders are being delivered.

   • Continue to support the baby's body in a vertical position, with the back held (not pressed) against the woman's symphysis. (See Figure 10.1.) Continue to lift, but do *not* pull, the baby while the woman pushes. The head will deliver promptly.

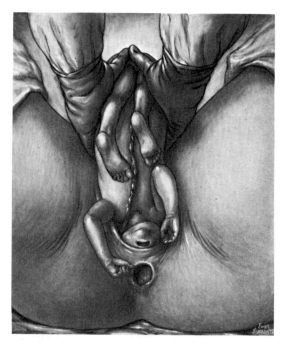

Figure 10.1. The Bracht Maneuver. The Bracht maneuver may seem as if it would hurt the baby, but is actually the safest technique to use for a breech delivery in bed.
Reprinted with permission from Plentl AA, Stone RE. The Bracht maneuver. *Obstet Gynecol Surv.* 1953;8:313.

7. What Do You Do After the Baby Is Delivered?

A. One Person Takes Care of the Baby

1. Assess the Baby's Condition

Remember the ABCs of resuscitation (Book I: Maternal and Fetal Evaluation and Immediate Newborn Care, Unit 5, Resuscitating the Newborn). Follow standard neonatal resuscitation procedures to assess and ensure

- Airway
- Breathing
- Circulation

Suction first the baby's mouth and then the nose with the bulb syringe from the KID. If meconium is present, follow standard procedure for neonatal resuscitation.
Then

- *Dry baby:* During your initial assessment, you already should have started to dry the baby. Now be sure the baby is completely dry, including the hair.

Then

- *Clamp umbilical cord:* After you have assessed and dried the baby, clamp and cut the cord. Clamp the cord in 2 places, close together, and cut it between the Kelly clamps or cord clamps.

2. Provide Warmth for the Baby

The way this is done will depend on the baby's gestational age and condition. Keep in mind, however, even a healthy, term baby can become chilled extremely quickly after delivery.

In most cases, after the baby has been dried, maternal body heat can be used to help keep a term baby warm by having the mother hold her newborn on her chest, skin-to-skin. Cover the baby's head with the stocking cap and the exposed side of the baby with the baby blankets. Be sure you can assess the baby's color and breathing.

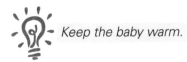 *Keep the baby warm.*

B. One Person Takes Care of the Mother

1. Wait for the Placenta to Separate
   Hold the placental end of the clamped cord and maintain slight tension on the cord. There should be no attempt to pull the placenta out, but just enough tension on the cord so you can feel when the placenta separates and the cord advances.

2. Determine Whether the Placenta Has Separated
   Wait until there are indications that the placenta has separated. This usually occurs within 5 to 10 minutes after the cord is clamped. Indications of placental separation from the uterus include the following:
   • Gush of blood from the vagina
   • Cord advances from the vagina
   • Placenta becomes visible at the introitus

3. Deliver the Placenta
   Delivery of the placenta may occur after a few spontaneous pushes from the woman. If it does not, place a gloved finger in the vagina. If the placenta can clearly be felt or seen, pull gently on the cord and remove the placenta.

 Do not pull on the cord until you can see or feel the placenta in the vagina.

8. What Do You Do if Spontaneous Delivery of the Placenta Does Not Occur Within 30 Minutes?

A. As Long As There Is Little or No Bleeding
   Do nothing. As long as there is no bleeding, there is no reason for concern until more than 30 minutes after delivery of the baby has elapsed. During this time, do not pull on the cord. Do not push on the fundus. Be aware that retained placenta for more than 30 minutes after delivery may be a sign of placenta accreta, a condition where the placenta is abnormally adherent to the uterine muscle. Attempts to manually remove a placenta accreta can result in significant, life-threatening blood loss. If there is minimal bleeding and the placenta has not yet delivered, await the arrival of an obstetric physician before attempting removal.

   Manual removal usually requires anesthesia.

   Preparations for manual removal include the following:
   • Start an intravenous (IV) line if one is not already in place.
   • Call for anesthesia.
   • Move the patient to a room where general anesthesia can be administered and manual removal, or even a laparotomy, can be performed.
   • Consider obtaining blood for possible transfusion.

B. Whenever Profuse Bleeding Is Present or Develops

Call for help. Anesthesia, volume expansion, and surgical and medical support are needed urgently.

If the patient is bleeding heavily, or if profuse bleeding starts, the placenta must be removed. Do not attempt manual removal without anesthesia and surgical support, unless the hemorrhage is so great that you fear the woman will soon bleed to death.

If you believe the woman's life is in danger, proceed immediately with manual removal. Simultaneously begin volume expansion and other measures to respond to maternal blood loss. The placenta must be removed from the uterus because the bleeding cannot be controlled until the placenta has been delivered.

See Unit 2, Obstetric Hemorrhage and Unit 9, Abnormal Labor and Difficult Deliveries, in this book, for additional information about management of obstetric hemorrhage and abnormal third stage of labor.

Self-test

Now answer these questions to test yourself on the information in the last section.

A1. Give at least 2 signs that the baby is coming.

_____

_____

A2. What is the first thing you should do after the head of a baby in vertex presentation is delivered?

_____

_____

A3. What should you do immediately if the shoulders of a vertex presentation do not deliver after 3 to 5 strong pushes?

_____

_____

A4. Give at least 2 indications the placenta has separated.

_____

_____

A5. A woman begins bleeding profusely after delivering a term newborn, but before the placenta is delivered. The only way to control the bleeding is to

_____

Check your answers with the list that follows the Recommended Routines. Correct any incorrect answers and review the appropriate section in the unit.

Preparation for Maternal/Fetal Transport

1. What Is Maternal/Fetal Transport?

Maternal/fetal transport, sometimes called intrauterine transport, occurs when a pregnant woman is referred for delivery at a regional perinatal center. Depending on the woman's condition and available resources, she may be transported by private automobile, local rescue squad, community hospital ambulance and personnel, or specialized maternal transport vehicle and personnel based at the regional center.

2. Why Is Maternal/Fetal Transport Important?

If maternal, fetal, or neonatal intensive care is anticipated, referral to a regional medical center may be desirable for several reasons.

- Women and/or fetuses with certain conditions may require intensive care with highly specialized equipment and personnel and evaluation techniques for extended periods.
- Intrauterine transport is often less stressful for a baby than neonatal transport might be.
- Improved maternal and neonatal outcomes have been demonstrated when high-risk pregnant women give birth in regional medical centers.
- Maternal/fetal transport allows a mother and baby to be close to each other soon after delivery.
- Maternal/fetal and neonatal transport to a higher level of care provides cost-effective use of highly sophisticated, expensive medical equipment and resources for patients who also require high staff-to-patient ratios.

3. What Are the Goals of Preparing a Pregnant Woman or Fetus for Transport?

The primary goal in preparing a pregnant woman and her fetus for transport to a regional center is to stabilize both of them. It is also important to decide which mode of transportation is most appropriate and make provisions for needed therapy en route.

 A woman and/or fetus in unstable condition should not be transported, regardless of how close the regional center is to the referring hospital.

Likewise, the primary goal in preparing a baby for transport is to stabilize the newborn's condition. It is more important to stabilize a baby and wait for a regional center's neonatal transport team to arrive at the birth hospital than to rush an unstable newborn to a regional medical center.

 Stability of a baby's condition is far more important than speed of transport.

Transport of a newborn is covered in detail in Book III: Neonatal Care, Unit 10, Preparation for Neonatal Transport.

4. Which Women Should Be Transported for Delivery at a Regional Perinatal Center?

Although each patient needs to be evaluated on an individual basis, general guidelines can be given for patients who are likely to require maternal/fetal or neonatal intensive care. Conditions for which maternal transfer might be advisable include, but are not limited to, the following:

- Maternal medical problems such as cardiovascular, thyroid, or neurologic problems
- Chronic or pregnancy-specific hypertension
- Rh (or other) sensitization
- Maternal diabetes mellitus
- Third-trimester bleeding
- Premature rupture of membranes at less than 34 weeks' gestation or less than 2,000 g estimated fetal weight
- Multifetal gestation at preterm gestational age and/or 3 or more fetuses at any gestational age
- Intrauterine growth restriction

361

- Post-term pregnancy
- Severe maternal infection such as hepatitis, pyelonephritis, influenza, human immunodeficiency virus, pneumonia, etc
- Maternal kidney disease with deteriorating renal function
- Maternal drug dependency
- Fetal malformation
- Hydramnios
- Oligohydramnios
- Abnormal results from tests of fetal well-being

 Whether maternal/fetal transport is advisable should be decided jointly by the patient's referring physician and the receiving regional center specialist.

Points to discuss prior to transport include the following:

- Is transfer of this woman appropriate at this time, considering the specific circumstances and maternal/fetal condition?
- When is the best time for the transport to begin? (Now? After additional therapy is provided to the woman? Other time frame?)
- What mode of transport is most appropriate for this woman (private car or medical supervision during transfer)?
- Are any specific preparations needed before transfer of this woman? Items to consider include
  - Intravenous fluids, and IV medications (as appropriate)
  - Medication administration
  - Blood transfusion
  - Recommended position for the woman during the transport
  - Fetal assessment

5. Which Pregnant Women Should *Not* Be Transported?

Generally, women in labor should not be transported. Delivery under controlled circumstances at a referring hospital is almost always preferable to delivery en route.

Exceptions may be made on an individual basis with mutual referring hospital and regional center staff agreement. Such exceptions may include women in early labor or women whose preterm labor has been stopped with tocolytic medications for whom there is a short transit time between the referring hospital and the regional center.

As noted earlier, transport should not be undertaken if a woman's condition cannot be stabilized. Transport also should not be undertaken if needed therapy cannot be provided during transfer. The level of care required in the hospital needs to be provided during transport.

 Maternal transport should not be undertaken if there is a significant risk of delivery occurring during transfer or if essential care cannot be provided throughout the transfer process.

6. What Should You Do to Prepare a Pregnant Woman for Transport?

Maternal stability needs to be achieved before transport is begun. This includes

- Stable vital signs
- Cessation of bleeding

- Suppression of seizure activity
- Control of metabolic status
- Control of hypertension

If maternal/fetal transport is undertaken for a woman whose condition might deteriorate during the journey, she should be accompanied by trained personnel with appropriate equipment. Minimal support for maternal transport in these circumstances includes

- Blood pressure monitoring equipment
- Intravenous infusion apparatus, with an IV line in place before transport starts
- Appropriate medications
- Oxygen supply

Although maternal/fetal transport should not be undertaken if delivery during transit is likely to occur, complete neonatal resuscitation equipment should also be available. This should be specific neonatal equipment and separate from any equipment or supplies that might be needed for maternal care during transport.

7. How Do You Make an Obstetric Referral?

Write the hospital name and telephone number you would use to make a prenatal referral, or obtain consultation regarding a high-risk obstetric patient. It may be beneficial to develop a paper or computer referral form, including one for a nurse-to-nurse report, to ensure standardization of communication and process regarding a maternal/fetal or neonatal transport.

Self-test

Now answer these questions to test yourself on the information in the last section.

B1. Give at least 3 reasons why maternal/fetal transport is important.

_____

_____

_____

B2. Name at least 6 conditions where a maternal/fetal transport might be advisable.

_____

_____

_____

_____

_____

_____

B3. A woman in _____ condition should not be transported.

B4. In addition to trained personnel, what equipment should be available during transport for the care of a pregnant woman who requires medical care during the transfer?

_____

_____

_____

_____

_____

Check your answers with the list that follows the Recommended Routines. Correct any incorrect answers and review the appropriate section in the unit.

Imminent Delivery and Preparation for Maternal/Fetal Transport

Recommended Routines

All the routines listed below are based on the principles of perinatal care presented in the unit you have just finished. They are recommended as part of routine perinatal care.

Read each routine carefully and decide whether it is standard operating procedure in your hospital. Check the appropriate blank next to each routine.

Procedure Standard in My Hospital

Needs Discussion by Our Staff

_____ _____ 1. Establish guidelines for a kit for imminent delivery.
- Standard contents
- Designated storage locations (immediately accessible to, or in, each labor room)
- Maintenance of sterility of contents and replacement of kits

_____ _____ 2. Establish a protocol for response to imminent deliveries, including a system for notifying obstetric, pediatric, anesthesia, and/or other personnel, as needed.

_____ _____ 3. Ensure that information about how to make an obstetric referral is available at all times.

_____ _____ 4. Establish guidelines for
- Maternal condition prior to transport
- Equipment and supplies to be available during transport

Self-test Answers

These are the answers to the self-test questions. Please check them with the answers you gave and review the information in the unit wherever necessary.

A1. Any 2 of the following:
- Presenting part is visible in the vagina (almost always the baby's scalp and hair)
- Perineum bulges
- Anus dilates, and the anterior wall of the rectum is visible
- Woman cries out that the baby is coming

A2. Check for a nuchal cord.

A3. *Quickly* do the following:
- Put the head of the bed flat (if not already flat).
- Have the woman grasp behind her knees and pull them to her chest (McRoberts maneuver).

A4. Any 2 of the following:
- Gush of blood from the vagina
- Cord advances from the vagina
- Placenta becomes visible at the introitus

A5. Remove the placenta.

B1. Any 3 of the following:
- Allows highly specialized monitoring and evaluation for women and/or fetuses with uncommon conditions.
- Cost-effective use of medical equipment, personnel, and specialty services.
- Often less stressful for the baby than neonatal transport.
- Allows the mother to be near her baby soon after delivery.
- Recent data have shown improved maternal and neonatal outcomes when high-risk pregnant women give birth in regional medical centers.

B2. Any 6 of the following:
- Medical problems in the woman, such as cardiovascular, thyroid, or neurologic problems
- Chronic or pregnancy-specific hypertension
- Rh or other blood group sensitization
- Maternal diabetes mellitus
- Third-trimester bleeding
- Premature rupture of membranes at less than 34 weeks' gestation or less than 2,000 g estimated weight
- Multifetal gestation at preterm gestational age and/or 3 or more fetuses at any gestational age
- Intrauterine growth restriction
- Post-term pregnancy
- Severe maternal infections, such as hepatitis, pyelonephritis, human immunodeficiency virus, pneumonia, etc
- Maternal kidney disease with deteriorating renal function
- Maternal drug dependency
- Fetal malformation
- Hydramnios
- Oligohydramnios
- Abnormal results from antenatal test(s) of fetal well-being

B3. A woman in unstable condition should not be transported.

B4.
- Blood pressure monitoring equipment
- Intravenous infusion apparatus, with an intravenous line in place before transport starts
- Appropriate medications
- Oxygen supply
- Neonatal resuscitation equipment

Unit 10 Posttest

If you are applying for continuing education credits, a posttest for this unit is available online. Completion of unit posttests and the book evaluation form are required to achieve continuing education credit. For more details, visit www.cmevillage.com.

PCEP

Perinatal Continuing Education Program

Pretest Answer Key
Book II: Maternal and Fetal Care

Unit 1: Hypertension in Pregnancy

1. A
2. True
3. False
4. True
5. True
6. True
7. False
8. False
9. D
10. A
11. D
12. C
13. B
14. Yes No
   - X ___ Urine positive for protein
   - ___ X Weight gain of 1 lb/week
   - X ___ Persistent headache
   - X ___ Right upper abdominal pain
   - X ___ Blurred vision
   - X ___ Uterine contractions
15. Yes No
   - X ___ Use serial ultrasound examinations to assess fetal growth.

- ___ X Check liver transaminases monthly, starting at 28 weeks' gestation.
- X ___ Check creatinine clearance and blood urea nitrogen monthly, starting at 28 weeks' gestation.
- X ___ Use narcotic analgesia liberally during labor.
- X ___ Consult with maternal-fetal medicine specialist if pre-eclampsia develops.
- ___ X Plan for cesarean delivery.

16. Yes No
   - ___ X Provide invasive cardiac output monitoring for 1 to 2 days.
   - X ___ Continue magnesium sulfate infusion for 12 to 48 hours.
   - X ___ Arrange for home blood pressure monitoring for 1 to 2 weeks.
   - ___ X Continue hospitalization and bed rest for 1 to 2 weeks.

Unit 2: Obstetric Hemorrhage

1. True
2. True
3. True
4. True
5. True
6. False
7. False
8. False
9. B
10. D
11. Yes No
   - X ___ Hematocrit
   - ___ X Serum creatinine
   - ___ X Bilirubin
   - X ___ Blood pressure
   - ___ X Blood culture
12. False
13. True
14. True
15. True

369

16. True

17. D

18. D

19. B

20. C

21. A

Unit 3: Perinatal Infections

1. Yes No

  X   ___ Baby with congenital rubella infection

  ___   X Baby with chlamydial conjunctivitis

  ___   X Baby whose mother has untreated gonorrhea at the time of delivery

  X   ___ Baby with suspected herpes infection

  ___   X Congenital cytomegalovirus infection

2. B

3. False

4. True

5. True

6. False

7. True

8. False

9. False

10. True

11. True

12. D

13. C

14. A

15. A

16. True

17. True

18. D

19. B

Unit 4: Various High-Risk Conditions

1. D

2. False

3. True

4. True

5. True

6. False

  X   ___ Systemic lupus erythematosus

  X   ___ Severe maternal hypertension

  X   ___ Multifetal gestation

  ___   X Placenta previa

7. Yes No

  X   ___ Prenatal visit every week during the third trimester

  X   ___ Extra iron and folic acid supplementation

  ___   X Amniocentesis for chromosomal analysis

  X   ___ Serial ultrasound evaluations of fetal growth

8. Yes No

  ___   X Hydramnios

9. False

10. False

11. True

12. True

13. A

14. A

15. C

16. B

17. D

18. B

19. False

20. False

Unit 5: Abnormal Glucose Tolerance

1. False
2. False
3. False
4. False
5. True
6. True
7. False
8. False
9. True
10. True
11. False
12. True
13. B

14. Yes   No
   - _X_   ___ Neonatal hypoglycemia
   - _X_   ___ Birth trauma
   - ___   _X_ Neonatal diabetes mellitus
   - _X_   ___ Neonatal hyperbilirubinemia

15. Yes   No
   - _X_   ___ Pre-pregnancy weight of 200 lb or more
   - ___   _X_ Eastern European heritage
   - _X_   ___ Gestational diabetes mellitus in a previous pregnancy
   - _X_   ___ Maternal age of 35 years or older

16. Yes   No
   - _X_   ___ Begin testing for fetal well-being at approximately 28 weeks.
   - ___   _X_ Consider use of insulin if blood glucose is consistently 80 to 100 mg/dL
   - ___   _X_ Plan to deliver at 36 to 37 weeks' gestation unless tests of fetal well-being indicate a need for earlier delivery.
   - _X_   ___ Estimate fetal weight prior to undertaking vaginal delivery.

Unit 6: Premature Rupture and/or Infection of the Amniotic Membranes

1. Yes   No
   - ___   _X_ Amniotic fluid embolism
   - _X_   ___ Umbilical cord compression
   - _X_   ___ Neonatal sepsis
   - _X_   ___ Abruptio placentae
2. True
3. False
4. False
5. False
6. True

7. Yes   No
   - _X_   ___ Assess cervical dilatation and effacement.
   - _X_   ___ Obtain samples for group B beta-hemolytic streptococcus, *Chlamydia,* and gonorrhea testing.
   - _X_   ___ Collect amniotic fluid from the vaginal pool to test for phosphatidyl glycerol.
   - ___   _X_ Place internal fetal heart rate and uterine contraction monitoring devices.

8. A

9. Yes   No
   - _X_   ___ Start antibiotics.
   - _X_   ___ Use sterile speculum examination to check for prolapsed umbilical cord.
   - _X_   ___ Obtain urine for analysis and culture.
   - _X_   ___ Periodically palpate the uterus.
   - _X_   ___ Give corticosteroids.
   - ___   _X_ Perform digital cervical examination to assess cervical dilatation.

10. False
11. False
12. True

Unit 7: Preterm Labor

1. False
2. False
3. True
4. True
5. True
6. True
7. B
8. D
9. Yes   No

Yes	No	
X	___	Hypertension
X	___	Urinary tract infection
X	___	Cigarette smoking

Yes	No	
___	X	Previous cesarean delivery
X	___	Maternal cocaine use
X	___	Uterine malformation

10. A
11. False
12. True
13. True
14. False
15. False
16. False

Unit 8: Inducing and Augmenting Labor

1. True
2. True
3. True
4. True
5. False
6. B
7. D
8. B
9. C
10. D
11. C
12. True
13. False
14. False

Unit 9: Abnormal Labor Progress and Difficult Deliveries

1. D
2. A
3. True
4. True
5. True
6. True
7. False
8. True
9. False
10. Yes   No

Yes	No	
___	X	Estimated fetal weight of 4,000 g (8 lb, 13 oz) or more
X	___	Maternal anesthesia
X	___	Complete cervical dilation
X	___	Evaluation of fetal size, presentation, and position
___	X	Oxytocin augmentation of labor

11. Yes   No

Yes	No	
___	X	Arrested second stage with normal contraction pattern
X	___	Hypotonic uterine dysfunction during the active phase
___	X	Hypertonic uterine dysfunction during the latent phase
___	X	Maternal fatigue with weak pushing efforts but normal labor pattern

12. B
13. Yes   No

Yes	No	
___	X	Begin broad-spectrum antibiotics.
X	___	Investigate for abruptio placentae.
X	___	Check cervical dilatation every 15 to 30 minutes.

X	___	Prepare for delivery.	20. True
X	___	Anticipate need for neonatal resuscitation.	21. True
___	X	Place the woman in reverse Trendelenburg position.	22. False
___	X	Administer large doses of narcotic analgesia to the laboring woman.	23. True

20. True
21. True
22. False
23. True
24. True
25. False
26. C
27. D
28. D

14. Yes   No
   ___ X Abruptio placentae
   X   ___ Birth trauma
   ___ X Growth-restricted fetus
   X   ___ Prolapsed umbilical cord
15. False
16. False
17. True
18. False
19. True

29. Yes   No
   ___ X Begin oxytocin augmentation.
   ___ X Drain the hydrocephalus with a needle and monitor labor for fetal descent.
   ___ X Advise the parents that hydrocephalus is a fatal malformation.
   X   ___ Perform cesarean delivery.

Unit 10: Imminent Delivery and Preparation for Maternal/Fetal Transport

1. Yes   No
   ___ X Move the woman immediately to the operating room.
   X   ___ Ask the woman to grasp her legs behind the knees and pull them to her chest.
   ___ X Tell the woman to rest and try pushing again in several minutes.
   ___ X Put the head of bed flat.
   X   ___ Press down on the woman's abdomen, just above the symphysis pubis, while gentle downward traction is placed on the baby's head by a second person.
2. A
3. Yes   No
   X   ___ Tell the woman that she will need to push, or stop pushing, as you direct.

   ___ X Ask the woman to assume knee-chest position until her physician arrives.
   X   ___ Call for help, but do not leave the woman.
   X   ___ Assist the woman to deliver where she is.
   ___ X Move the woman immediately to a delivery room.

4. False
5. True
6. False
7. D
8. C
9. False
10. False
11. False

373

Index